Long-Term Prescribing

Long-Term Prescribing

Drug management of chronic disease and other problems

Edited by ERIC WILKES

OBE, MA, FRCP, FRCGP, FRCPsych, DObstRCOG
Professor of Community Care and General Practice
University of Sheffield

faber and faber

First published in 1982
by Faber and Faber Limited
3 Queen Square London WC1
Printed in Great Britain by
Fakenham Press Limited, Fakenham, Norfolk
All rights reserved

© *Faber and Faber Limited 1982*

British Library Cataloguing in Publication Data

Long-term prescribing
  1. Chemotherapy
  I. Wilkes, Eric
  615.5'8   RM262

  ISBN 0–571–11898–4
  ISBN 0–571–11899–2 Pbk

Contents

Contributors

J. N. Agate CBE, MA, MD, FRCP
Consultant in Geriatrics
Ipswich Hospital, Ipswich

P. B. Anderson MA, BM, BCh, MRCP
Consultant Physician and Honorary Clinical Lecturer
in Medicine
University of Sheffield

R. A. L. Brewis MD, FRCP
Consultant Physician, Royal Victoria Infirmary and
Senior Lecturer in Medicine
University of Newcastle upon Tyne

Pamela Buck MB, BS, MRCOG
Lecturer in Obstetrics and Gynaecology
University of Sheffield
Presently Senior Lecturer in Obstetrics and
Gynaecology, University of Manchester

I. D. Cooke MB, BS, DGO, FRCOG
Professor, Department of Obstetrics and Gynaecology
University of Sheffield

Colin B. Brown BSc, MB, MRCP
Consultant Renal Physician
Royal Hallamshire Hospital, Sheffield

Sheila L. B. Duncan MD, FRCOG
Reader, Department of Obstetrics and Gynaecology
University of Sheffield

J. R. Hampton, DM, MA, DPhil, FRCP
Professor of Cardiology
University of Nottingham

C. A. Hardisty MD, MRCP
Consultant Physician
Middlesbrough General Hospital

G. P. Hosking MB, MRCP, DCH
Consultant Paediatric Neurologist and Honorary
Clinical Lecturer in Paediatrics
University of Sheffield

A. Johnson MD, MRCOG
Consultant Obstetrician and Gynaecologist
The Jessop Hospital for Women, Sheffield

D. I. R. Jones MD, MRCGP
General Practitioner, Sheffield *formerly* Senior
Lecturer in General Practice
University of Sheffield

George R. Kinghorn MB, MRCP
Consultant Physician
Sheffield Department of Genito-Urinary Medicine

A. J. Nicholls MB, MRCP
Senior Registrar in Nephrology
Royal Hallamshire Hospital, Sheffield

L. E. Ramsay MB, ChB, MRCP
Consultant Physician and Associate in Medicine
University Department of Therapeutics
Royal Hallamshire Hospital, Sheffield

John Richmond MD, FRCP, FRCP(Ed)
Professor of Medicine
University of Sheffield

R. W. Ross Russell MD, FRCP
Consultant Physician to the Department of Neurology
St Thomas' Hospital, London

Albert Singer DPhil (Oxon), PhD, FRCOG
Consultant Gynaecologist, Royal Northern Hospital
and Whittington Hospital, London
and Honorary Senior Lecturer, University College
Hospital, London

I. B. Sneddon CBE, MD, FRCP
Honorary Consultant Dermatologist
Royal Hallamshire Hospital, Sheffield

Joan Sneddon MD, MRCPsych
Senior Lecturer in Psychiatry and Consultant
Psychiatrist
University of Sheffield

M. P. Taylor FRCGP
General Practitioner and Associate in General Practice
University of Sheffield

M. Thompson MD, FRCP
Consultant Rheumatologist and Lecturer in
Rheumatology
University of Newcastle upon Tyne

D. R. Triger MA, BM, BCh, DPhil, FRCP
Consultant Physician in Gastro-enterology and
Senior Lecturer in Medicine
University of Sheffield

Robert G. Twycross MA, DM, FRCP
Consultant Physician, Sir Michael Sobell House
The Churchill Hospital, Oxford

J. P. H. Wade MD, MRCP
Registrar, Department of Neurology
St Thomas' Hospital, London

J. D. Ward BSc, MD, FRCP
Consultant Physician
Royal Hallamshire Hospital, Sheffield

E. Wilkes OBE, MA, FRCP, FRCGP, FRCPsych,
DObstRCOG
Professor of Community Care and General Practice
University of Sheffield

Introduction

ERIC WILKES OBE, MA, FRCP, FRCGP, FRCPsych, DObstRCOG

One of the many reasons for the introduction of a National Health Service over thirty years ago was the fact that modern medicine was getting too costly a burden for the average citizen to sustain. Therefore, the delivery of medical care had no choice but to become a political act.

At that time we were at the beginning of an unprecedented era of development not only in the cost but also in the effectiveness of modern drugs, and doctors, patients and administrators all had – and indeed still have – a lot to learn.

The more experienced doctors could remember the exaggerated hopes that had inevitably greeted the newer drugs from phenobarbitone to chlorpromazine, cortisone and the tetracyclines. We had to learn that drugs are hardly ever quite as marvellous as at first they seem. Now in the aftermath of disillusion and in a world of 'me-too analogues we know that only ineffective drugs are safe: and since the majority of general practice consultations are to do with conditions that are either self-limiting or incurable, we see now that we took for granted the safety and cheapness of the salicylate or rhubarb mixtures we were prescribing then. The bottle of medicine had for long been the symbol of either cure or, at least, goodwill, the prescription was an integral part of the consultation; and this attitude was extrapolated improperly by doctor and patient to the potentially more helpful and, therefore, more costly and damaging drugs we use and abuse today.

The sociologists' criticism of the doctor as a harassed pusher of dangerous chemicals is presented sometimes with an unattractive petulance that masks the validity of their argument. A major factor that our critics neglect to emphasise is that valid criticisms, from Ivan Illich on, are always to some degree out-of-date. The doctors are conscious of the scores of hospital admissions due not to disease but to treatment: but to a variable degree they are imprisoned by their patients' expectations, and politicians in a democracy are determinedly confusing wants and needs. We have learned, for example, that older people, and especially the bereaved, are apprehensive and lonely just when their physiological sleep-pattern is more intermittent and brief. They wish to hibernate through half the day and complain that they cannot sleep, and every practitioner has had difficulty in weaning sensible and stable patients from the sleeping pills to which they are, they would say, entitled and to which, the doctors would say, they are habituated.

While the system demands of our family doctors not far short of 250-million consultations per year, clearly it is easier and quicker to prescribe than to educate. Marsh's paper (1977) demonstrates the art of the possible; and, at a more anecdotal level, an experienced doctor who took over a traditional single-handed practice reduced in 18 months a repeat prescription routine from 130 each week down to three. There are other welcome signs of change. It may be regrettable that two-thirds of patients still have a prescription accompanying their consultation, but the patients, like the doctors are beginning to query the value or need of drugs. At the same time the vocationally-trained doctor is gradually becoming a more senior and influential figure in the modifying of practice habits and attitudes more fitted to the world of 'Mist Gent Alk'. Indeed, at times, patients are being offered counselling when they present with everyday ills in a way that is inappropriate yet novel.

A typical half-million patients, with about 16 per cent of them over 65 years of age, will have a total bill for general medical services of nearly £7,000,000. The pharmaceutical services for such a population will cost £11,000,000 yearly. This will include the prescribing of over 4 million items in a year at an average cost of £20 for each patient on the doctors' lists.

With so many quite new drugs costing so much of the national wealth, it is necessary to prescribe as efficiently as possible for those long-term disorders so characteristic of an ageing society: and this is the main purpose of this book. It is aimed at the doctors who have been away from medical schools long enough to feel anxious about their impossible struggle to keep up-to-date, but who do not wish to short-change their patients when it comes to the modern treatment of conditions that may imperil the duration or the quality of life.

The book does not pretend to be a complete pharmacology and therapeutics text-book; and, indeed, if new drugs are used as a result of the opinions expressed, they should be used only after a look at such standard references as the *Drug Data Sheets*, the new *National Formulary*, or the invaluable Martindale's *Extra Pharmacopoeia*.

Pregnancy, breast-feeding, and contraception pose problems of major importance in general practice prescribing; and the elderly, depressed, bronchitic hypertensive who comes up with angina seems to be as terrifying a therapeutic jigsaw as the rarer patient on anticoagulants: so chapters on the elderly and drug interaction also seemed advisable.

The main thrust of the book, however, is with the basic management of the main chronic diseases, and we have been fortunate in obtaining contributions from those colleagues who are neither so senior as to be out of touch nor so junior as to be naïve.

The prevention of ischaemic heart disease or hypertension may in theory be within our grasp: but the massive difficulties involved in changing lifestyles make it easy to over-estimate the impact of any educational campaign no matter how costly or sophisticated its technique. It will therefore be necessary for us to keep under review the value and the limitations of the helpful but imperfect drugs at our disposal.

Chronic chest disease will remain a major problem also for decades: and although smoking will gradually be a contemptible addiction of the degenerate old, rather like opium with the Chinese, it is likely to take a few more decades to decline. It is interesting that the oxygen therapy of today – until now a tedious and expensive placebo – is likely, in highly selected cases and over 15 hours per day, to be the major recent advance in this area.

Such a comment should not lead us to underestimate the value of our modern drugs in asthma control. If we use them to full effect, and with the involvement of the well-briefed patient, the admission to hospital of patients in or near a condition of status asthmaticus should be so exceptional and rare as to stimulate a careful review as to how such mis-management has been allowed to take place.

However slow we may be to exploit to the full the considerable resources at hand for dealing with asthma, it is fair to say that our anticonvulsant therapy should have been more brutally remodelled over the last five years, but remains antique and unsatisfactory. Phenobarbitone and phenytoin are still probably over-prescribed, instead of being restricted mainly to the elderly well-controlled epileptic. Carbamazepine and sodium valproate are genuinely important advances and most practices would face an audit of their epileptic management with justifiable apprehension.

In chronic disease processes of the gut and the kidney the expansion of our knowledge has not yet been accompanied by any great improvement of simple treatments: but a realistic appraisal of what is likely to be of help is now possible and merits again a detailed review. The changing face of gastro-intestinal disease may owe more to alcohol-related consequences than to dramatic innovations, but endoscopy has at last allowed us on a massive scale to monitor the effects of our treatment, and permits the worth of new drugs like cimetidine fairly quickly to be placed somewhere between world-beater and costly menace. The nephrologist is even newer to us than the endoscopist and his knowledge is therefore not so easily exploited. The diagnosis of renal disease depends more than ever now on renal biopsy and detailed histology. We must try and get important renal pathology referred sooner, but such a laudable intention will not make the insidious clinical onset any easier to diagnose.

The introduction of so many new non-steroid anti-inflammatory analgesics, authoritatively reviewed in the chapter on rheumatic diseases, may give some hope and comfort to many of our patients; but in an unknown but increasing proportion it may be leading them to an analgesic nephropathy as well. Such a situation typifies the therapeutic tight-rope we need to walk, with gross over-treatment on one side and inexcusable neglect on the other. Perhaps in these circumstances the good physician can only be defined as one who keeps making different, as opposed to the same, mistakes.

The multiplicity of psychotropic drugs developed over the last 10 or 15 years makes this sort of dilemma inescapable. We have more than trebled our prescribing of anti-depressives, but the 'me-too' drugs claiming fewer side-effects and more rapid onset of action here, have produced on the whole an unimpressive performance: and despite some newer valuable drugs as mianserin (which can be used with most hypotensive drugs except clonidine) or flupenthixol, the reader may get reassurance that the older-established drugs have not been rendered as out-dated as the marketing literature might suggest.

The management of diabetes or of thyroid disorders also has not radically changed. The use of insulin in a syringe-driver may make the regulation of blood sugar to more physiological levels at last possible, but at this stage we are perhaps more bemused by the different insulins rather than possible advances in technology; and the more effective education of patient, family, nurse and general practitioner seems likely to produce better care through nothing more dramatic than the conscientious implementation of established regimens and an improvement in follow-up arrangements.

New hormonal weapons, by contrast, have greatly modified the management of gynaecological problems: and since we have never had so many post-menopausal women as today we clearly need a cautious survey of the indications and complications of hormone replacement therapy.

A similarly reasoned look at cytotoxic therapy should also be of interest to all practitioners: for just as we have learnt a good deal of late about the needs of the dying patient, so we have also seen that an overdose of indiscriminate enthusiasm in a medical oncologist can be as damaging and unhelpful to the patient as an overdose of cytotoxic drugs. It is just this sort of overview, not only of the needs and resources of the patient, but also of the specialist skills of his colleagues, that need to be integrated and programmed by the general practitioner. We must be increasingly and authoritatively involved in the fascinating challenge of long-term drug management. It is hoped that this book – although at times selective, dogmatic, even idiosyncratic – will be a reliable and helpful companion along the way.

REFERENCE

Marsh, G. M. (1977). Curing minor illness in general practice. *British Medical Journal*, **2**, 1267–9.

Chapter 1 Ischaemic heart disease

J. R. HAMPTON DM, MA, DPhil, FRCP

Ischaemic heart disease (IHD) is one of the major causes of death in Western society, but it is not – or should not be – a major cause of disability. Atheroma of the coronary arteries becomes almost universal with increasing age, yet many patients are asymptomatic. When IHD causes death, death is often sudden or occurs after a brief illness, and patients who survive a heart attack are more often than not completely free of symptoms. In this chapter I shall use the term *ischaemic heart disease* to include any cardiac problem that results from atheroma of the coronary arteries; *coronary heart disease* (CHD) is an American term with the same meaning. I shall use the old-fashioned word *heart attack* to include sudden cardiac events, most of which are due to blockage of a coronary artery by thrombus; I shall, however, avoid *coronary thrombosis* for some patients die suddenly and no thrombosis can be demonstrated, and I shall also avoid *myocardial infarction* for this is a pathological term that can only properly be applied after an autopsy.

Drug therapy in IHD has to be considered from two points of view: the role drugs have to play in prophylaxis, and their role in the treatment of symptoms. We can think of IHD in three clinical phases, before the heart attack, the heart attack itself, and following recovery from the heart attack. Obviously in individual patients the long-term illness may not follow such a sequence – for example, a patient with angina may never have a heart attack, and heart failure does not only occur after a heart attack – but the drug therapy of such problems is the same at any stage.

BEFORE THE HEART ATTACK

1. Prevention

Attempts to prevent an individual developing the symptoms of IHD are sometimes called *primary prevention*; *secondary prevention* is a term used to describe measures to prevent a second attack. Primary preventive efforts therefore involve healthy people, and involve all the problems of persuading people to see themselves as potential patients.

Several things have been identified as 'risk factors' for IHD in healthy subjects. This means that their presence is associated with an increased risk of developing symptoms (either angina or a heart attack) but it does not necessarily follow that these factors *cause* the disease. It may well be that some or all of them are merely 'markers' for some other characteristic that is the real culprit; a risk factor can only be accepted as causal if its removal can be shown to lead to the elimination of the excess risk with which it is associated.

SMOKING
The risk of having a heart attack is directly related to the number of cigarettes smoked. Stopping smoking reduces the risk, and smokers who have had one heart attack have less chance of a second if they stop smoking. Smoking can therefore be accepted as a *causal* risk factor, just as it is a cause of lung cancer. Since smoking causes both ischaemic heart disease and lung cancer, persuading his patients to stop smoking is probably the greatest service a doctor can do for them.

HYPERTENSION
The higher the blood pressure, the greater the risk of a heart attack. However, it is not yet clear whether control of blood pressure eliminates the excess risk. There is a possibility, not yet proven, that blood pressure control with diuretics does not reduce the mortality for heart attacks while control with beta-blockers does. But the most important thing about blood pressure is its relationship to stroke, and here it is undoubtedly a causal risk factor. High blood pressure must be detected and treated to reduce the risk of stroke, and any useful effect this has on mortality from heart attacks can be looked on as an additional bonus.

CHOLESTEROL
A high blood cholesterol level is a risk factor for IHD, and arguments have raged for 20 or more years whether hypercholesterolaemia of itself causes a heart attack. There is a general belief now that the blood cholesterol level is not of major importance: certainly the majority of heart attacks occur in patients with cholesterol levels

that are within the normal range. It has been shown that if clofibrate (Atromid) is given for a prolonged period to subjects whose cholesterol level is in the upper third of the normal range, their chances of having a heart attack are reduced. This might be interpreted as proving that hypercholesterolaemia is a causal risk factor, but clofibrate has effects other than on lipids and it is not impossible that one of these effects is the important one. However, the argument is academic, for in the treated patients there was an excess of gastro-intestinal cancers and of gallstones. For this reason treatment with clofibrate was not associated with any reduction of overall mortality, and the drug clearly has no place in the treatment of subjects with modestly elevated blood cholesterol levels. Whether it should be used to treat those few patients who have very high cholesterol levels indeed is not known, and the place of other lipid lowering agents (mainly resins which are very unpalatable) is not clear either.

OBESITY

Obesity is a risk factor for IHD, but it has never been shown to have a causal relationship. It does, however, cause a lot of non-cardiac problems which entirely justify fat people trying to lose weight.

EXERCISE

Lack of physical exercise is certainly a risk factor for IHD. The best evidence for this relates to groups of workers with very heavy jobs (lumberjacks and dock workers) but a survey of the spare time activities of civil servants has also shown that those who spend their weekend in some physical pursuit have a lower risk of IHD than their more slothful colleagues. Unfortunately, of course, it does not necessarily follow that if an inactive man suddenly takes up regular exercise he will increase his expectation of life, for it may be that people who like to take exercise are different in some other important way from those who do not.

Much of the present enthusiasm for exercise seems to stem from confusion about the relationship between physical fitness and health. Physical fitness is a physiological state that can apply equally to healthy and ill subjects. Physical fitness is relative, not absolute; it implies that more exertion can be undertaken for less cardiac work. Thus a fit subject can carry out a given task with a slower heart rate and a lower blood pressure than an unfit one, and if a patient's activities are limited by heart disease then he will be able to undertake more physical exertion if he trains and becomes fit. The mechanism of physical fitness is not completely understood, but it is a property of skeletal rather than cardiac muscle. It seems that regular exercise of the skeletal muscle causes biochemical changes that lead to the muscle cells becoming more efficient at extracting oxygen from the blood, so that for a given blood supply (that is, for a given amount of cardiac work) a 'trained' muscle can do more work than an 'untrained' one.

There is no question that physical fitness brings a state of mental and general well-being, and for this reason alone physical training can be recommended. Encouragements to exercise such as 'Run for your life' must, however, be taken with a pinch of salt.

2. Angina

NITRATES

Glyceryl trinitrate (trinitrin) remains the mainstay of the treatment of angina. Sublingually in a dose of 0.4mg pain is rapidly relieved, and, indeed, if pain is not relieved within two or three minutes the diagnosis of angina must be questioned. Patients should be encouraged to use as many tablets each day as necessary, and to take one before embarking on any activity that might be expected to cause pain. Trinitrin paste rubbed on the chest is highly effective in preventing nocturnal angina, though is less useful by day.

The various long-acting nitrate preparations are relatively inefficient unless used in high doses.

BETA-BLOCKERS

Any patient who needs more than an occasional trinitrin tablet should be treated prophylactically with a beta-blocker. There are about 15 of these drugs on the British market and all are effective; all cause side-effects such as a general feeling of lethargy (which usually passes off in a week or two) and cold hands and feet. All should be considered potential cardiac depressants and should be used with care in the presence of heart failure. The one with the longest track record, propranolol (Inderal), is more likely than the others to cause bronchospasm, but all can do this.

Propranolol is the cheapest and has the advantage of easy titration of dose against symptoms. The starting dose is 40mg t.d.s., and this can be increased slowly to 160mg t.d.s. This drug has the disadvantage of a short half-life; of the beta-blockers that only need to be taken once daily atenolol (Tenormin) is probably the most effective hypotensive and therefore possibly the best for angina as well. The starting dose of atenolol is 50mg daily but the dose response curve is flat, and there is probably little point in exceeding 200mg daily.

NIFEDIPINE (Adalat)

This drug blocks the influx of calcium into heart muscle cells. In some people it has a dramatic effect on angina, but in others it is disappointing. Possibly it works best when angina results from coronary artery spasm rather than from a fixed obstruction like atheroma. It is worth trying (10 or 20mg t.d.s.) but there is no point in persisting unless it is obviously beneficial.

DIURETICS

Nocturnal angina – and to a less extent that occurring during the day – may be due to heart failure. Patients with night pain should be given a diuretic; sometimes a short-acting drug like bumetanide (1mg at 6.00 p.m.) may be helpful.

THE PLACE OF SURGERY

Narrow segments of coronary arteries can be by-passed by the insertion of pieces of saphenous vein between the aorta and the distal part of the coronary artery. One, two, or three such by-passes can be inserted and the operative risk should be less than five per cent. At least 80 per cent of patients so treated can expect complete relief of pain, and the operation should be recommended without hesitation to any patient who is otherwise well, who is not in heart failure, and whose angina is not controlled after an intensive trial of medical treatment. Just what constitutes adequate control of pain is clearly an individual matter, and will depend on the patient's lifestyle and expectations. While excellent for symptoms, it is not clear that coronary vein by-pass grafting prolongs life. It probably does when either the main left coronary artery is stenosed, or when all three main arteries (right, left anterior descending, and left circumflex) are stenosed and can be grafted. Patients with disease of only one or two vessels will probably not benefit in terms of longevity. Unfortunately, there is no way of selecting those patients with 'main left' or 'three vessel' disease, except by coronary angiography and it is not a practical proposition to attempt this procedure on all patients with symptoms of IHD. For the moment, coronary angiography is best reserved for young patients and for those with angina that is not responding to medical treatment.

THE ACUTE HEART ATTACK

Half the patients who have a heart attack die from it, and half the deaths that occur do so within two hours of the onset of symptoms. Anyone alive at the end of the first day has a good chance of survival. Death results either from a dysrhythmia (ventricular fibrillation or asystole) or from the failure of the heart to act as a pump because too much muscle has been destroyed. Dysrhythmias are treatable, and any patient seen within the first two hours should be admitted to a hospital where a defibrillator is available and where there are staff who know how to use it. Patients who are seen by their general practitioner at home who have had their symptoms longer than four hours (and people who call general practitioners rather than dialling 999 for an emergency ambulance have often had symptoms for at least this period) can be safely kept at home provided they do not have a dysrhythmia that clearly needs hospital treatment.

Pain relief

Pain is the patient's main problem and no general practitioner should contemplate home management unless he can visit often enough to ensure adequate analgesia. Powerful agents are required in the first 24 hours and diamorphine (heroin) 5mg intravenously (IV) is probably still the drug of choice because of its euphoric effect. It does, however, have the administrative disadvantage of being a controlled drug, and for this reason alone the more expensive buprenorphine (Temgesic) 0.3mg IM or IV is perhaps the ideal drug for domiciliary use.

Dysrhythmias

WHEN TO TREAT

It used to be thought that dysrhythmias gave a warning of impending cardiac arrest due to ventricular fibrillation or asystole. This is now known not to be the case, and the day of treating asymptomatic ventricular extrasystoles is over. A dysrhythmia must, of course, be treated if it is impairing the function of the heart; this will usually show itself as heart failure or angina. A dysrhythmia should also be treated if it seems likely that haemodynamic embarrassment will occur sooner or later: the supraventricular tachycardias, for example, may cause no problems initially but may lead to heart failure or death after an hour or two.

There is no convincing evidence that any drug can usefully be given prophylactically for dysrhythmias in patients with acute heart attacks.

SINUS RHYTHM

Sinus tachycardia is a sign of pain, anxiety, or heart failure: it should not be treated as a dysrhythmia. Sinus bradycardia (rate less than 40 per minute) is unimportant provided the patient has no symptoms and there are no associated dysrhythmias. Sometimes it is a sign of vagal over-activity, and may then be associated with pallor and hypotension; it should then be treated with atropine 0.6mg IV.

CONDUCTION DISORDERS

First degree, second degree and bundle branch blocks do not need treatment. Complete (third degree) block needs treating if the ventricular rate is less than 50 per minute. Although an infusion of isoprenaline may buy time, this dysrhythmia is best managed with the insertion of a temporary transvenous pacemaker.

SUPRAVENTRICULAR DYSRHYTHMIAS

Supraventricular ectopics never need treating. The most common dysrhythmia that may need treatment is atrial fibrillation, and here digoxin is the drug of choice. The aim is merely to control the ventricular rate: digoxin has little part to play in the management of heart failure. Initial treatment can be given intravenously if the ventricular rate is above 150 per minute and the patient is ill, but IV digoxin must be used with care, and the dose should never exceed 0.5mg. Orally the initial dose is 0.5mg followed by 0.25mg two hours later. The 'digitalising' dose depends on the patient's renal function (the older the patient the worse this is likely to be) and weight. The maintenance dose of digoxin is that which keeps the ventricular rate below 100 per minute, without causing anorexia or nausea. A healthy middle-aged man might need 0.25mg daily or even 0.25mg b.d., but a little old lady might only need 0.0625mg daily.

Atrial flutter, atrial tachycardia and nodal (junctional) tachycardia can be treated with digoxin but an IV beta-blocker or IV disopyramide works more rapidly. The best IV beta-blocker is still practolol (dose 5 mg, repeated at ten-minute intervals up to 20mg). Disopyramide (Norpace; Rhythmodan) may induce heart failure, and 50mg IV should be given over ten minutes.

Supraventricular bradycardias – and in the acute heart attack situation this usually means nodal escape rhythms – are best treated with atropine.

VENTRICULAR DYSRHYTHMIAS

Ventricular extrasystoles do not need treating unless they are occurring so frequently that there is reason to believe that they are making the heart inefficient. Ventricular tachycardia is best treated with lignocaine 100mg IV (repeated after five minutes if necessary) and recurrent attacks can be controlled by an intravenous infusion of lignocaine at 2–3mg per minute. Second-line drugs for ventricular tachycardia are the beta-blockers, disopyramide, and mexiletine.

CARDIOVERSION

The correction of a dysrhythmia by direct current shock is clearly a hospital (or sometimes a special ambulance) procedure. It is the only way to correct ventricular fibrillation, and electrical treatment should be used in preference in any patient with a tachydys-rhythmia who has pulmonary oedema. It is a good general principle that all antidysrhythmic drugs with the exception of digitalis are cardiac depressants, so the sicker a patient the sooner one should turn away from drugs and towards cardioversion.

Heart failure

When a heart attack causes severe pump failure a clinical syndrome may be seen that some people call *cardiogenic shock*. Unfortunately people use this term differently, and on the whole those who claim that effective treatment exists are those with loose definitions. The fully-developed picture of breathlessness, a cold clammy skin, an unrecordable blood pressure, clouding of consciousness and failure of urine production is nearly always fatal. On the other hand, patients in the early stages of a heart attack often exhibit one or two of these features, and respond dramatically to pain relief and reassurance. There is no really useful treatment for severe pump failure, and the old view that such patients may be 'too sick to travel to hospital' is probably the correct one.

Acute pulmonary oedema, demonstrated by breathlessness, peripheral vasoconstriction (and therefore sometimes a high blood pressure) and pulmonary crepitations should be treated with oxygen, diamorphine, intravenous aminophylline (250–500mg given slowly) and intravenous diuretics (frusemide 20–40mg). Many patients with heart attacks are given diuretics unnecessarily on the basis of lung crepitations alone, and this is undesirable as diuretics can occasionally cause profound hypotension.

Once the acute pulmonary oedema has been treated, maintenance therapy depends on the size of the problem. Digoxin is not much use for heart failure compared with diuretics, and it is easier to think of it now as an antidysrhythmic compound. Mild heart failure can be managed with a thiazide, and the simplest and cheapest is bendrofluazide 5–10mg daily. Most people do not need potassium supplements, although it must be remembered that old people are particularly prone to hypokalaemia. If a thiazide is insufficient, a combination tablet containing a thiazide and a distal-loop potassium retaining diuretic is the next thing to try (Moduretic; Dyazide; Aldactide). If breathlessness, oedema, and a raised jugular venous pressure persist despite one of these preparations it is necessary to change to frusemide (Lasix) beginning at 40–80mg daily and increasing slowly; either potassium supplements or a potassium-retaining diuretic (such as amiloride 5 or 10mg daily) must be added.

There is at present considerable interest in the manipulation of either venous return ('pre-load reduction') or of the systemic resistance ('after-load reduction'), or more simply, blood pressure reduction. There is no doubt that judicious use of venous or arterial dilating drugs can cause a considerable haemodynamic improvement in patients with heart failure, with short-term clinical benefits. Whether such therapy has any place in long-term treatment remains to be seen.

AFTER THE HEART ATTACK

Recovery from a heart attack begins very rapidly. Most patients are pain free within 24 to 48 hours, and there is no reason why they should be kept in bed longer than this. They can be allowed to walk around the bedroom on the third day, and by the end of a week should be mobile around the ward or the house. Patients without complications can be discharged from hospital after a week, and their activity should then be progressively increased. After a further month most patients should be able to walk a mile without trouble, should be performing all normal activities, and all except (perhaps) those with very heavy jobs should be ready for work.

The outlook for a patient who recovers from a heart attack depends mainly on his or her age, and on the amount of heart muscle that has been damaged. Patients who during the initial attack develop evidence of heart failure fare considerably worse than those whose course is uncomplicated. It is perhaps for these reasons that pre-existing risk factors have little influence on long-term outcome. There is no benefit from cholesterol manipulation after a heart attack, and while control of hypertension and obesity and encouraging exercise are all important on other grounds, they probably do not affect the chances of a second attack. Stopping smoking, however, is undoubtedly beneficial.

Attempts to prevent second heart attacks therefore mainly involve the administration of drugs, and two main categories of drug seem logical to try. It seems reasonable to attempt to prevent thrombosis of a coronary artery, and to prevent the dysrhythmias that are responsible for the many early deaths from heart attacks.

Antithrombotic drugs

ANTICOAGULANTS

Anticoagulants are drugs that affect clotting. The ones commonly used are heparin (which has to be given intravenously) and warfarin. These drugs do not affect the formation of thrombi, which are made up of aggregates of platelets, so they would not necessarily be expected to be useful in a thrombotic disease like a heart attack, as opposed to a clotting disease like deep vein thrombosis and pulmonary embolism. Many studies of the use of anticoagulants after heart attacks were carried out in the 1950s and 1960s, and on the whole ended in disillusionment. However, the results were probably as good as those obtained with other compounds more recently, and the anticoagulants almost certainly do confer a long-term benefit on survivors of myocardial infarction. The benefit seems greatest in young men (under 55 years) and particularly in those who have had more than one heart attack. There is no early reduction in mortality, and treatment can be commenced any time in the first few weeks; once started it should be continued for two or three years.

ANTI-PLATELET AGENTS

Of the anti-platelet (and therefore, one hopes, antithrombotic) compounds, *aspirin* has received most attention. Several trials have shown a reduction in mortality among treated patients but none have reached the conventional level of statistical significance. The largest study of aspirin (AMIS – Aspirin Myocardial Infarction Study) showed no benefit from treatment at all, and probably aspirin is valueless. Another anti-platelet compound, *dipyridamole* (Persantin) is under investigation, and in combination with aspirin it has been found to reduce mortality if treatment is begun within a few months of the heart attack (PARIS – Persantin Aspirin, Reinfarction Study). The value of dipyridamole is, however, still far from clear.

Sulphinpyrazone (Anturan), a drug developed many years ago as a uricosuric for the treatment of gout, has anti-platelet properties, and there are theoretical reasons for supposing it might have a clinically useful antithrombotic effect. A large North American study (ART – Anturan Reinfarction Trial) produced the unexpected result that sulphinpyrazone treatment begun one month after a heart attack reduced mortality in the next six months, not by preventing re-infarction (which might be supposed to result from coronary artery thrombosis) but by reducing the incidence of sudden death. Such an unexpected answer must always be regarded with some suspicion, and several aspects of the trial are open to criticism. Nevertheless, if this effect of sulphinpyrazone is real, then it is both interesting from the point of view of mechanisms of death and important clinically. Further studies with sulphinpyrazone are awaited.

The basic problem with all anti-platelet agents is that

it is far from clear just what properties a drug needs to have if it is to be clinically useful. Once a drug has been found to have a definite clinical effect we shall learn a lot about thrombosis from the drug's mode of action, and it should then be possible to produce new and more effective compounds.

ANTI-DYSRHYTHMIC DRUGS

Beta-blockers may possibly be useful for the secondary prevention of heart attacks. Although of no prophylactic use in the acute stages, two studies (involving alprenolol, and the now-withdrawn compound, practolol) have suggested that if treatment is begun after a month mortality is reduced over the following year. The benefit is not great and indeed may not be real; at present the routine use of beta-blockers for this purpose cannot be recommended.

CONCLUSIONS

There are no drugs that can or should be administered to healthy asymptomatic people to prevent ischaemic heart disease. While high blood pressure should certainly be treated, more benefit can be anticipated from the prevention of strokes than of heart attacks. No drugs are available that can be given prophylactically to reduce the likelihood of death during an acute heart attack, and the benefit from long-term treatment of survivors of heart attacks is at best marginal. Symptomatic treatment of patients with ischaemic heart disease is, however, highly effective.

Chapter 2 Hypertension

LAWRENCE E. RAMSAY MB, ChB, MRCP

INTRODUCTION

It is beyond argument that the management of patients with high blood pressure has improved remarkably in the last 40 years, and a look at changes over the last decade suggests that the improvement is continuing. We now know reasonably clearly who needs treatment and who does not, and we can quantify, at least on average, the benefits of treatment as regards reduction of cardiovascular morbidity and mortality. There is a broad measure of agreement on those methods which are effective in lowering the blood pressure, and on the choice of drugs. The antihypertensive drugs available now are much simpler to prescribe, and, more important, much less of a burden to patients, than were their predecessors. Against this background it is perhaps understandable that some doctors consider treatment easy and regard the management of hypertension as a completed success story. They err in taking far too narrow a view of the aims of medical care. The true situation has been shown by population surveys from several developed countries, including Britain. The findings have been remarkably consistent, and can be summarised as a 'rule of halves'. Half of all hypertensive subjects are undetected; half of those known to be hypertensive are not on treatment; and half of those on treatment have unsatisfactory blood pressure control. The upshot is that seven of every eight people with hypertension are getting no protection, or suboptimal protection, against the risk of premature vascular disease.

Viewed in this way it is clear that effective management of hypertension must have three major components:

1. Identification of all those in the population who will benefit from treatment.
2. Impeccable management of individual patients.
3. Persuading patients who feel well to stay under long-term medical care.

The major part of this chapter is concerned with the management of the individual patient, simply because that is where the bulk of present knowledge lies.

Nevertheless, it must not be forgotten that if all doctors applied the very highest standard of care to every hypertensive patient presenting in the course of ordinary practice, only 25 per cent of those who would benefit from treatment will actually receive it. The development of methods for comprehensive identification of those who need treatment, and for keeping patients under effective care, is in its infancy.

There is, nevertheless, considerable scope for improvement in the management of those hypertensive patients who have been identified. The 'rule of halves' tells us that half of those on treatment remain hypertensive, and several surveys in general practice, general medical clinics, and hypertension clinics have confirmed that control of blood pressure is often less than perfect. In my view one important cause of unsuccessful treatment is unnecessary over-elaboration of the whole process. Time and energy are diverted to investigation, constructing 'risk profiles', giving advice which has no sound basis, or an overcautious treatment regimen, at the expense of the main object of the exercise, which is, of course, to lower blood pressure. That objective is best attained by simple evaluation, simple advice, simple treatment, and simple follow-up.

WHY SCREEN?

Approximately 10 per cent of the adult population of Britain below 70 years of age have diastolic blood pressures averaging 100mmHg or higher (phase 5, disappearance). There is evidence (discussed later) that effective treatment of this group would substantially reduce the incidence of death and disability from vascular disease, particularly strokes, in the population. Current methods of detection identify only a quarter of those who stand to benefit from treatment. At present hypertension is diagnosed in patients who present with symptoms traditionally linked with hypertension (headache, dizziness, palpitations, epistaxis, etc) although these symptoms are now known to be coincidental; in patients who present with complications of hypertension, which could have been prevented; and in those screened for specific purposes, for example, insurance, employment, or pre-operative evaluation.

The pattern of treatment which emerges from this system of case finding is irrational. Among treated patients women outnumber men considerably, although the prevalence of hypertension in the population is similar in the sexes. Elderly patients form a large proportion of those treated, although there is at present no evidence that they actually benefit from treatment. Since hypertension, even of severe degree, usually remains asymptomatic until complications occur, there is little prospect that the rate of ascertainment can improve within the present framework. Given that hypertension is common, asymptomatic and largely undiagnosed, and that its complications are common, important and largely preventable, the case for some form of screening seems indisputable.

HOW TO SCREEN

Ideally we need to know the blood pressure of every adult less than 70 years old in the population and, if the pressure is normal, the measurement needs to be repeated every five years. Those with a reading of 150/90mmHg or higher need further evaluation, and some will need treatment. This is obviously a mammoth task, but at least there are some pointers as to how it should be tackled. It seems clear that screening is best undertaken by those in a position to continue the further evaluation and management. When special teams are imported into the community the follow-up and treatment rates have generally proved disappointing. In Britain the existing system of general practice is in some ways ideal for the task. Each member of the population relates to a single doctor or practice; practice lists are reasonably stable and definable; and a large proportion of the population comes into contact with the practice within a relatively short period of time. Thus a general practitioner who measured the blood pressure of every person who crossed his threshold (for any reason) would screen about 70 per cent of those at risk in one year, and 90 per cent within five years. In theory, then, he could screen 90 per cent of his list on a casual basis, and complete the task by a deliberate effort to reach the remaining 10 per cent. In fact, this needs considerable organisation within the practice, including delegation of screening measurements to ancillary staff who need to be trained, documentation, a system for follow-up, and of course, provision for the extra work of managing those found to be hypertensive. Detailed discussion of these aspects is available in the excellent text by Tudor Hart (1980).

DIAGNOSING HYPERTENSION

As blood pressure is a continuously distributed variable in the population it is fashionable to point out that hypertensive patients cannot be separated clearly from normotensive people, but the practising doctor must do just that. He needs to classify each person arbitrarily into one of three categories: hypertension needing treatment (broadly, diastolic averaging 100mmHg or higher); hypertension needing observation (diastolic averaging 90–99mmHg); and normotension. Blood pressure shows large variations within individual subjects over time, and the crucial question is how many readings are needed to classify the person satisfactorily. Before discussing this it is worth mentioning that all measurements should be taken by a careful observer, with an accurate and well-maintained instrument, using a cuff of appropriate size on a supported and unconstricted arm. It is best to measure diastolic pressure at the disappearance of sounds (phase 5) for purely practical reasons. First, disappearance is more reproducible than the point of muffling (phase 4), and, secondly, the literature on the epidemiology and therapy of hypertension has used phase 5 values increasingly. Those who use phase 4 readings have to adjust their diastolic values by subtracting approximately 8mmHg, to obtain equivalent phase 5 readings.

A single casual blood pressure measurement has prognostic value for subsequent vascular disease, and this has misled some doctors into believing that a single high reading deserves treatment. While a single reading does indeed have some prognostic value, the accuracy of prognosis is much better if the mean of several measurements is used. Approximately one-third of those classified as hypertensive by a single reading will, in fact, prove to be normotensive as judged by the mean of several readings (Armitage et al, 1966). Repeated measurements at *separate visits* have more power in classifying patients correctly than repeated readings during one visit (Armitage et al, 1966). In general, the average of three single readings taken on separate visits gives satisfactory classification. Additional measurements should be obtained when the readings show unusual variability, when a downward trend is evident, and when the mean value falls close to the decision threshold (e.g. 100mmHg diastolic). Additional readings are also advisable when the systolic pressure may influence the therapeutic decision, as the variability of systolic pressure is larger than that of the diastolic. The doctor who feels that readings at three or more visits are rather tiresome ought to consider the alternative – a lifetime of visits for supervision of treatment which is possibly unnecessary.

FURTHER EVALUATION

History and examination

When the initial blood pressure reading is only mildly elevated it is wise to postpone full evaluation until hypertension has been confirmed by repeated measurements, otherwise considerable effort will be wasted on the third of patients who are eventually classified as normotensive. The history and physical examination should be directed particularly towards the following points.

COMPLICATIONS OF HYPERTENSION

These should be sought carefully, as they dispel any doubt about the need to lower the blood pressure. The history should seek symptoms suggesting cerebrovascular disease, left ventricular failure, renal impairment, previous myocardial infarction, angina, intermittent claudication or visual failure. The important points in examination are the state of the heart (displaced, heaving apex beat; fourth heart sound), the lung bases (crepitations which do not clear on coughing), and the optic fundi. It seems odd that ophthalmologists examine the fundi in a darkened room with the pupils widely dilated, whereas physicians and general practitioners often seem content to glimpse the fundi through pinpoint pupils in a brightly lit room. The point of major importance in the fundi is the recognition of haemorrhages, cotton-wool exudates and papilloedema, as the presence of any of these greatly increases the urgency of the situation. Hard exudates by themselves have less prognostic significance, and I doubt whether identification of vessel changes alone (e.g. arterio-venous nipping) is of value except, perhaps, in patients under the age of forty.

UNDERLYING CAUSES OF HYPERTENSION

The diagnosis of secondary hypertension depends more heavily on clinical acumen now than it did when more extensive routine investigation was the rule. Drug ingestion is by far the most common cause of curable hypertension. In order of importance, oestrogens, non-steroidal anti-inflammatory drugs (e.g. phenylbutazone, indomethacin), steroids, carbenoxolone, and analgesic abuse are recognised offenders. A documented recent onset of moderate or severe hypertension, or an abrupt worsening of mild hypertension, is a strong pointer to an underlying cause and the history of previous measurements should be reviewed. Symptoms of past or present renal disease should be sought by direct enquiry, as should features suggesting phaeochromocytoma (the five Ps: paroxysms of pallor,

palpitation, perspiration or pain in chest or head). In the examination, diagnoses of Cushing's syndrome (general appearance) or coarctation (femoral pulses) depend almost entirely on the physical findings. The comfortable cushion of a routine IVP has been removed in recent years, and palpation of the abdomen for polycystic kidneys, hydronephrosis or renal tumour should perhaps be more careful than it needed to be previously. A continuous or systolic-diastolic bruit in the abdomen suggests renovascular hypertension, but short systolic bruits are common and have little diagnostic significance.

FACTORS INFLUENCING CHOICE OF TREATMENT

The importance of obesity, salt intake, alcohol use and smoking habits is discussed later. The patient's occupation should be noted. The most important point in the treatment history is the careful recording of previous adverse reactions. Patients are caused discomfort and even serious illness depressingly often through what is called, politely, 'accidental re-challenge'. Finally, co-existent medical problems may have an important influence on the choice of drugs, e.g. asthma contra-indicating beta (β)-blockers, or previous depression contra-indicating methyldopa. The real difficulty is how to keep these relevant facts to the forefront of one's mind during many years of management. A simple problem list, which includes all previous drug failures, should be scrutinised as a matter of routine whenever treatment is altered. It is unsafe to treat chronic conditions such as hypertension without this safeguard.

Routine investigation

A reduction in the amount of routine investigation is an important simplification of management which has evolved in recent years, and it has been said that the doctor who does no investigations and treats the hypertension will rarely do harm. While hypertension is very common, curable causes other than drugs are very rare. For example, Berglund et al (1976) unearthed only two cases of 'curable' hypertension by investigating 689 hypertensive patients detected in a population survey, and neither patient was in fact cured by surgery. Extensive routine investigation of every hypertensive patient is therefore impractical and unrewarding, although it is worth repeating that a selective policy of investigation puts greater demand on clinical acumen. A blood urea, plasma potassium, and urine testing for protein and blood form an acceptable minimum of investigation. The need for a routine chest x-ray and cardiogram has been questioned recently, and they are not essential in every patient. However, they should be done in borderline cases before deciding not to treat, as the presence of left ventricular hypertrophy on the ECG, or cardiomegaly on the chest x-ray, would swing the decision firmly towards treatment. It should be remembered that black people often have 'abnormal' cardiograms by conventional criteria, and their ECGs need cautious interpretation.

Special investigations

GENERAL INDICATIONS
Renal hypertension, phaeochromocytoma and primary aldosteronism (Conn's syndrome) should be considered in certain high yield groups, namely:

1. Accelerated hypertension (haemorrhages and exudates ± papilloedema).
2. Recent onset, or abrupt worsening, of hypertension.
3. Resistant hypertension (to a good regimen of three drugs).
4. Moderate or severe hypertension when aged less than 30 years.
5. Suggestive features in the history, examination or simple investigations.

INTRAVENOUS PYELOGRAM
Even in hospital practice the yield from routine IVPs is unacceptably low (Atkinson and Kellett, 1974), and it should be performed only when there is a clue in the clinical evaluation, when blood urea or urinalysis is abnormal, and in the circumstances listed above. A rapid-sequence IVP should be requested specifically as this will show some abnormality in 80 per cent of patients with renovascular hypertension. However, a normal IVP does not exclude this diagnosis.

PHAEOCHROMOCYTOMA
This need not be excluded routinely. The indications for a screening test are paroxysmal symptoms; unusually labile hypertension; a paradoxical response to treatment; unexplained weight loss; hypertension in pregnancy (because phaeochromocytoma is often fatal during pregnancy); and the general indications mentioned above. A single 24-hour urine test using appropriate methods is sufficient to exclude the diagnosis provided the patient is hypertensive during the collection (Engelman, 1977). When investigating intermittent hypertension with paroxysmal symptoms the patient should start the urine collection during an attack. Interference by drugs and the need for dietary restriction lead to a variation in laboratory policies, so these should be checked beforehand.

PRIMARY ALDOSTERONISM
This should be considered when there is severe muscle weakness, tetany, polyuria and polydipsia; hypokalaemia unrelated to diuretic treatment; and severe hypokalaemia (< 2.7mmol/litre) during diuretic treatment. Further investigation needs hospital referral, and is not easy even in the hospital setting.

WHO NEEDS TREATMENT?

Controlled trials
Treatment is clearly indicated when complications are present, but for the majority of patients who have no complication the decision is more difficult. Following publication of the Veterans Administration Study (1970) there was a fair measure of agreement that patients with diastolic blood pressures averaging 105mmHg or higher should have treatment. The management of those with milder hypertension (diastolic averaging 90–104mmHg) has been problematical, because they are known to be distinctly at risk from vascular complications, yet benefit from blood pressure reduction had not been shown. Results from two major studies examining this problem have been published recently.

THE HYPERTENSION DETECTION AND FOLLOW-UP PROGRAM (1979a, b)
This reported a study comparing the effect of a therapeutic programme which included systematic antihypertensive treatment with that of ordinary medical care over a period of five years. Patients with entry diastolic pressures between 90–104mmHg, whose management included systematic antihypertensive treatment, showed a significant 20 per cent reduction in mortality. The results seem to have been accepted (and acclaimed) as the final answer to the question in the United States, but sadly the study had many unusual features which cast considerable doubt on its relevance to ordinary practice in Britain. The management of the two patient groups differed in important respects other than antihypertensive treatment, and it is not at all clear how much of the reduction in mortality can be attributed to lowering of blood pressure. The reduction in non-cardiovascular deaths was almost as large as that in cardiovascular deaths. Further, the benefits of the special treatment programme were largest in black patients, and in fact white women showed no benefit whatever from special treatment.

THE AUSTRALIAN TRIAL ON MILD HYPERTENSION (1979, 1980)

This was a more conventional placebo-controlled study of antihypertensive treatment in patients with diastolic pressures averaging 95–109mmHg. Patients treated with antihypertensive drugs showed a significant reduction in total mortality, largely through a two-thirds reduction in cardiovascular deaths. The main impact of treatment was on cerebrovascular events, and, in keeping with previous controlled trials, there was no significant effect on the incidence of ischaemic heart disease. The advantages of treatment were most clear cut in older patients (50 to 69 years) and in men. It is important to note that patients with initial diastolic pressures of 95–99mmHg showed no significant reduction in fatal or non-fatal vascular complications, and that this group actually had a non-significant *increase* in the incidence of myocardial infarction.

These studies do not provide the final answers, and leave considerable scope for differences of opinion: but they provide reasonable evidence that patients less than 70 years old with diastolic pressures averaging 100mmHg or higher will benefit from reduction of blood pressure. Below this level (diastolic 90–99mmHg) it remains to be shown that there is any benefit from treatment. It is my practice to keep patients with diastolics averaging 90–99mmHg under supervision, and to recommend only those methods of treatment which do not involve drugs.

Systolic blood pressure has at least as much prognostic value for vascular complications as the diastolic pressure, and the blood pressure of those with systolic pressures averaging 170mmHg or higher should probably be lowered, even if the diastolic is below 100mmHg. The proviso that systolic pressure is more variable than diastolic pressure, and needs more readings to classify the patient safely, has already been mentioned. The policy for treating patients aged 70 years or more is discussed later.

The 'risk factor' approach

It is commonly suggested that the level at which hypertension is treated should be varied according to the presence or absence of certain risk factors. I believe that this concept is *not* soundly based, and will consider the various risk factors in turn.

SEX

For a given level of blood pressure women have a better prognosis than men, and some suggest that the level for intervention should be 5–10mmHg higher in women, or should be lower in men. In fact the excess mortality in males is due to ischaemic heart disease, and at a given blood pressure level the prognosis as regards stroke is similar in men and women. Since the major impact of antihypertensive treatment is on stroke, and we have as yet no definite evidence that coronary heart disease can be prevented, the logic of treating the sexes differently is doubtful.

AGE

Many recommend that young patients should be treated at lower levels of blood pressure than the middle-aged. The Australian Trial showed benefit most clearly in older patients, and this has been noted also in previous controlled trials. The risks of 30 to 40 years of treatment with diuretics or β-blockers are entirely unknown, and I would hold to an average diastolic of 100mmHg or higher regardless of age.

CIGARETTE SMOKING

This is an important and remediable risk for vascular disease, and it undoubtedly magnifies the risks of hypertension. The appropriate treatment is advice and encouragement to quit smoking, not more aggressive treatment of hypertension.

PLASMA LIPIDS

Plasma total cholesterol, and particularly the ratio total cholesterol: high density lipoprotein, are predictors of vascular disease, and it is often suggested that they should be measured routinely in hypertensive patients. This might have some merit if the results were used simply to identify high-risk patients. However, it is entirely unclear how the results should modify the treatment of hypertension. If lipids are thought to be *really* important, we should probably be *less* willing to treat mild hypertension when they are abnormal, as there is no doubt that thiazides and β-blockers both affect the lipid 'profile' adversely (Anon, 1980). Some suggest that abnormal lipids should be treated by dietary modification or even by drugs, but there is no evidence that this is beneficial, and it may be harmful (Committee of Principal Investigators, 1980).

My objections to the risk factor approach are threefold. First, it has no support from the controlled trials which are available. Secondly, it elaborates treatment unnecessarily at a time when the majority of hypertensive people in the population are not getting the simple effective treatment they need. Thirdly, with respect to 'treatment' of plasma lipoproteins, the hypertensive patient will be advised to make several substantial changes to his way of life. He may be advised to take tablets regularly, reduce his weight, eat less salt, stop smoking and cut his alcohol consumption. These measures all have some rational basis, but in the best hands compliance varies from about 10 per cent (for stopping smoking) to about 70 per cent (for regular tablet-taking). It seems unwise and unkind to dilute this sound advice, which is poorly accepted, with further measures which have no proven benefit. I can see no case for routine measurement of plasma lipoproteins in hypertensive patients.

TREATMENT WITHOUT DRUGS

Weight reduction and moderate salt restriction are effective in lowering blood pressure, and deserve detailed and more enthusiastic consideration for several reasons. They are inexpensive and non-toxic, and can therefore be recommended readily to those with diastolic pressures averaging 90–99mmHg, in whom benefits of drug treatment are unproven. In addition a proportion of patients with higher diastolic pressures will become normotensive with these measures alone. They are welcomed by at least some hypertensive patients, who wish to know what they can do to help themselves. Finally, these methods of treatment are not widely advocated, perhaps because they are more time consuming than prescribing tablets, but probably because the enormous commercial promotion in the field of hypertension has all been towards the use of drugs.

Weight reduction
Blood pressure falls on average by 2.5/1.5mmHg for each kilogram of weight lost (Ramsay et al, 1978). In an impeccably controlled study Reisin et al (1978) reported mean falls in blood pressure of 19/18mmHg in untreated hypertensive patients, and 30/20mmHg in those taking antihypertensive drugs, for an average weight loss of 9kg (1.5 stone). These responses compare favourably with those to any antihypertensive drug in common use. The average weight of consecutive patients referred to one hospital blood pressure clinic was 10.1kg above the ideal for sex and height (unpublished data), so that most hypertensive patients would benefit from weight reduction. The main argument against the value of weight reduction has been the difficulty in obtaining compliance, as only one-third of patients respond to the appropriate advice with substantial weight loss. This argument is invalid on two counts. First, poor compliance is also an important problem with drug treatment (Sackett et al, 1975; Marshall and Barritt, 1977), but it has never been suggested that drug treatment should be abandoned for this reason. It remains to be shown that patients comply better with tablet taking than they do with weight reduction, *given equal enthusiasm by the prescriber.*

Secondly, it is wrong to deny valuable advice to the one-third of patients who will benefit because the remaining two-thirds will not, or cannot, comply.

Salt restriction
The effect of a palatable reduction of salt intake on blood pressure is more modest. Morgan et al (1978) showed that moderate restriction reduced the diastolic pressure by an average of 9mmHg in mild hypertension. The full effect took several months to develop, and was obtained *despite* incomplete patient compliance. A response of this magnitude requires avoidance of added salt at table and exclusion of heavily salted foods from the diet. It seems reasonable to advise all hypertensive patients to give up added salt at table. Exclusion of heavily salted foods should be considered in borderline cases, in those resistant to treatment, and in patients who want to try anything rather than take tablets.

Alcohol
Hypertension and regular alcohol consumption are both common in the population, but there is now overwhelming evidence that they occur together more often than can be explained by chance (Ramsay, 1979). The association is not dependent on possible confounding factors such as age, obesity, salt intake or social class. It is important to appreciate that the association is not with alcohol abuse in the accepted sense. The statistical 'risk' of hypertension starts at an average intake of only three drinks per day. The practical consequence is that hypertension is between two and three times more common in those who drink alcohol regularly. More than one-third of hypertensive men consume on average four or more drinks daily. It is increasingly probable that regular alcohol consumption actually *causes* hypertension in some way, but proof of cause and effect has still to be obtained. In our present state of knowledge it is reasonable to impart these facts to hypertensive patients who drink regularly, and to suggest that an intake averaging less than three drinks per day would be safer (one drink is a single measure of spirits, or half a pint of beer).

Cigarette smoking
Smoking one or two cigarettes elevates blood pressure by about 12/7mmHg for 15 minutes or so, but smoking is not associated with sustained elevation of the blood pressure. In fact the blood pressure of smokers is slightly lower than that of non-smokers, and it actually rises slightly in people who quit the habit. These changes are not simply a function of body-weight. Thus smoking is not a cause of hypertension, and

stopping will not help the blood pressure. The importance of smoking is its additive effect on the risk of vascular disease when it is combined with hypertension. There is sound evidence that stopping cigarettes improves the prognosis even when established ischaemic heart disease or peripheral vascular disease are present, so it is never too late to stop. Accelerated (malignant) hypertension and atherosclerotic renal artery stenosis are strongly associated with smoking.

The psyche

Sedatives have no antihypertensive action at tolerable doses, and should be used only for co-existent psychiatric problems, not to lower the blood pressure. More elaborate treatments of the psyche such as biofeedback can lower the blood pressure, but at present they have little place in ordinary management (Steptoe, 1977). Advice to 'take things easy' or to 'avoid stress' is both unrealistic and meddlesome. The aim of treatment should be to control the blood pressure and let the patient get on with his ordinary life.

Work and exercise

In general patients may continue safely to take exercise which is appropriate to their age and general state of fitness. Isometric exercise (e.g. hand clenching) causes marked elevation of the blood pressure, and extreme forms such as weightlifting are best avoided. For the same reason those whose occupation involves heavy lifting should be kept off work temporarily, or should be found lighter duties, until the blood pressure has been satisfactorily controlled. Uncomplicated hypertension rarely alters a patient's fitness to continue in his occupation. Even those who work at heights or with dangerous machinery can usually carry on safely while taking modern drugs, although it is sometimes necessary to interrupt work for a few days when introducing a new drug to ensure that there is no unexpected adverse effect. Uncomplicated patients under satisfactory control with a simple regimen are considered fit to continue holding Heavy Goods Vehicle or Public Service Vehicle licences. Detailed recommendations on fitness to drive either socially or professionally can be found in the useful booklet *Medical aspects of fitness to drive*, circulated in 1978 to all doctors in the National Health Service.

DRUG TREATMENT

General principles

It is worth re-stating that the treatment of uncomplicated mild or moderate hypertension (diastolic$<$120mmHg) is never a matter of urgency, and that drug treatment should not be started until the mandatory three readings at separate visits have been obtained. Even at higher levels, or when the presence of complications makes it obvious that treatment will be needed, some attempt should be made to get replicate readings before introducing drugs. A conscious effort should be made to keep the drug regimen simple, as this improves compliance. Table 1 shows two examples of 'triple therapy' of equal efficacy, one using six tablets in two daily doses and the other needing 21 tablets in three daily doses. This may seem extreme, but similar examples are, unhappily, not rare. *All* the drugs in common use can be given twice daily, morning and evening, and doses prescribed at other times tend to be taken irregularly, or not at all. With appropriate choice of drugs and tablet strengths a full regimen of three drugs needs only six tablets in the day. Polypharmacy is both necessary and rational in the treatment of hypertension, necessary because even in mild hypertension only half the patients are controlled by a single drug (Veterans Administration Study Group, 1977), and rational because the use of smaller doses of individual drugs in combination reduces the incidence and severity of side-effects.

Drugs are added step-wise until control is achieved, and a treatment 'ladder' with my personal choice of

Table 1 Two examples of 'triple therapy' of equivalent antihypertensive efficacy

Drug	Dose	Tabs/Day	Drug	Dose	Tabs/Day
atenolol	100mg, mane	1	oxprenolol	80mg, 3 t.d.s.	9
bendrofluazide	5mg, mane	1	bendrofluazide	5mg, 1 b.d.	2
hydralazine	50mg, 2 b.d.	4	slow K	600mg, 2 b.d.	4
			hydralazine	25mg, 2 t.d.s.	6
TOTAL TABLETS/DAY		6			21

Table 2 Treatment ladder for the management of hypertension

	Drug and dose	Alternatives
STEP 1:	weight reduction salt restriction reduce alcohol	—
STEP 2:	atenolol 100mg daily *or* bendrofluazide 5mg daily	any other β-blocker, but dose titration may be needed
STEP 3:	atenolol 100mg daily *plus* bendrofluazide 5mg daily	combined diuretic plus β-blocker tablet : dose titration may be needed
STEP 4:	*add* hydralazine 25mg b.d. ↓ 50mg b.d. ↓ 100mg b.d.	methyldopa 125mg b.d.→1g b.d. *or* prazosin 0.5mg b.d.→10mg b.d.
STEP 5:	*add* frusemide 40mg daily *or* spironolactone 100mg daily	*exclude*: non-compliance drug interaction secondary HBP
STEP 6:	*non-urgent*: try other step 4 drugs *urgent*: add minoxidil (men) *or* guanethidine (women)	labetalol

drugs is shown in Table 2. Those working in hospital clinics are often struggling among the steps at the bottom of the table, whereas in general practice only 20 to 30 per cent of patients will go beyond step 3. Many doctors are rather timid about increasing the dose of antihypertensive drugs. In general, responses are related to the logarithm of the dose, so that logarithmic increments, i.e. sequential doubling of the dose, are logical. For example an increase in methyldopa dosage from 1g daily to 2g daily is no different, in pharmacological terms, to an increase from 250mg daily to 500mg daily. Unduly small increments delay control of the blood pressure and tend to dishearten the patient. The aim of treatment is a diastolic pressure maintained at below 90mmHg when lying or standing. The systolic pressure generally looks after itself when the diastolic is lowered, but it is occasionally necessary to increase treatment to lower the systolic below 160mmHg, despite satisfactory diastolic control. In more severe hypertension one must sometimes settle for less perfect control. This need not cause undue despondency, as there is evidence that control to diastolic pressures of 90–104mmHg affords considerable protection against complications in severe hypertension (Taguchi and Freis, 1974).

ACUTE MANAGEMENT OF HYPERTENSION

This is rarely a matter of genuine urgency but when it does happen the following routine is recommended:

A. *Urgent reduction of blood pressure* (needed only occasionally)

Indications:
1. Hypertensive encephalopathy
2. Fulminant hypertensive LVF unresponsive to conventional treatment
3. Eclampsia or impending eclampsia
4. Catecholamine 'crises'*, phaeochromocytoma, clonidine withdrawal, MAOI interactions.

Note *Phentolamine 5mg intravenously for catecholamine crises.

Treatment:
1. Keep patient lying flat for first 24 hours of treatment
2. Labetalol 50mg intravenously over 1 minute. Repeat at 5-minute intervals to a total of 200mg if necessary
3. Frusemide 80mg intravenously if response inadequate. Watch K+

4. Diazoxide 150mg intravenously rapidly. Repeat at 5-minute intervals to a total of 600mg if necessary. Watch blood sugar
5. Nitroprusside infusion – **this needs intensive supervision** and should only be undertaken where such facilities are available.

B. *Rapid reduction of blood pressure*

Indications:

Accelerated (malignant) hypertension, and other situations less urgent than those above.

Aim:

Reduce diastolic blood pressure to 100–110mmHg gradually over 24 hours.

Treatment:

1. Keep patient lying flat for first 24 hours of treatment
2. Oral labetalol: given six-hourly according to sliding-scale:

diastolic BP	dosage of labetalol
> 140mmHg	400mg
131–140mmHg	300mg
121–130mmHg	200mg
111–120mmHg	100mg
< 111mmHg	NIL

3. Oral frusemide 80mg if no response 2 hours after first dose of labetalol. Watch K+
4. Introduce and titrate up usual oral antihypertensive treatment until labetalol 'phased out'.

ROUTINE MANAGEMENT OF HYPERTENSION

First drug: diuretic or β-blocker?

One need not lose much sleep over this question. In a minority of patients the choice is clear, but for the large majority we do not have a correct answer. As many as 70 per cent of patients will end up taking both types of drug in any case. A diuretic is clearly the choice for patients over 60 years of age, and for black patients, as both groups respond relatively well to diuretics and relatively poorly to β-blockers. A diuretic is also needed for those with contra-indications to β-blockade, such as asthma, heart failure and second or third degree heart block. Patients engaged in heavy manual work are also best treated with a diuretic, as β-blockers tend to cause muscle fatigue. β-blockers are the logical choice in patients with co-existent angina, gout or maturity-onset diabetes.

The majority of patients under the age of 60 years have no clear pointer to either diuretic or β-blocker.

The main argument for preferring a diuretic in these patients is the low cost of treatment. Two arguments have been advanced in favour of β-blockers. First, there is a slightly higher chance of controlling mild or moderate hypertension with a single drug; 50 per cent for a β-blocker against 30 per cent for a diuretic. The second argument is that β-blockers *may* reduce the incidence of ischaemic heart disease. The failure of antihypertensive treatment to protect against coronary heart disease in controlled trials has already been mentioned. There is one study suggesting that β-blockade may reduce the incidence of ischaemic heart disease in hypertensive patients (Berglund et al, 1978), but the evidence is far from conclusive. At present I start treatment with a β-blocker in younger patients, hoping to prevent ischaemic heart disease, but with considerable misgivings about the cost of treatment.

β-Adrenergic blockers

All β-adrenergic blockers are effective antihypertensive drugs regardless of their ancillary properties (Davidson et al, 1976). Practolol, one of the earlier β-blockers, caused serious toxicity in the form of an oculomucocutaneous syndrome and sclerosing peritonitis, and for some time afterwards those β-blockers which had been longest in clinical use, propranolol and oxprenolol, were preferred. Since the practolol episode the β-blockers have been under the most intense scrutiny for adverse effects, and serious problems have not yet emerged. The prescribing doctor now has a large number of β-blockers at his disposal, and he has been the target of considerable promotional efforts based variously on the ancillary properties, the ease of use, and the relative cost of these drugs.

Propranolol has had the longest and widest clinical use, and is the standard β-blocker against which others are compared. It has no partial agonist activity and is non-selective in its action. Therefore it blocks both β_1-receptors (e.g. in the heart) and β_2-receptors (e.g. in the bronchi). After absorption from the gastro-intestinal tract it is extensively metabolised during the first pass through the liver, and there is considerable variation between patients in the amount of drug in the plasma and, presumably, at the receptor sites. This variability may explain one major problem when treating hypertension with propranolol, that is the uncertainty as to its effective ceiling dose. At present most doctors seem to go no higher than 640mg daily, but even this needs several dose titration steps if the initial dose is 40mg twice daily. Other non-selective β-blockers without partial agonist activity, such as sotalol, timolol and nadolol, are used less widely.

PARTIAL AGONIST ACTIVITY

Oxprenolol, pindolol and acebutolol have a weak stimulant action on β-receptors, evident only when the background sympathetic activity is low, while acting as β-blockers when sympathetic activity is higher. This property, termed partial agonist activity or intrinsic sympathomimetic activity, confers one discernible clinical advantage, namely a smaller reduction in the resting heart rate. One of these drugs should therefore be considered when bradycardia is present before treatment, or when treatment with β-blockers with no partial agonist activity is complicated by symptomatic bradycardia. These drugs may be less likely than propranolol to cause cold extremities (Marshall et al, 1976), but suggestions that they are relatively safe in patients with asthma or cardiac failure are not soundly based, and would be dangerous to act on.

CARDIOSELECTIVITY

Selective drugs block β_1-adrenergic receptors with *relative* sparing of the β_2-receptors in the bronchi and peripheral vasculature. Atenolol and metoprolol are cardioselective. Neither is completely selective, and selectivity tends to be lost at higher doses. Atenolol or metoprolol should be prescribed when it is essential to use a β-blocker in a patient with reversible airways obstruction, but they should be started only under the closest supervision, and full doses of a β_2-stimulant drug (e.g. salbutamol) should be given simultaneously. There is some evidence that selective β-blockers are less likely than the non-selective drugs to cause cold extremities, tired legs, CNS effects (dreams, depression), or a fall in glomerular filtration rate, and they cause a slightly larger fall in diastolic blood pressure, by about 5mmHg. In theory a selective drug would be preferable in insulin-dependent diabetics, but in practice it is probably safe to use any of the β-blockers in this situation.

PHARMACOKINETIC PROPERTIES

The β-blockers vary widely as regards their plasma half-lives, but the duration of the hypotensive effect during chronic treatment relates poorly to the half-life, or to the duration of β-blockade after single doses. All the β-blockers available can be prescribed satisfactorily in two daily doses, and it is probable that all would be effective if taken as a single daily dose. Slow-release formulations of several β-blockers have appeared recently. These products lower the blood pressure satisfactorily but it is doubtful whether they are really necessary. It is a good commercial policy to introduce a new formulation, with a fresh patent, before expiry of the patent on the parent drug. Therefore doctors should demand stringent proof that any new formulation has a clear advantage before changing their prescribing habits.

DOSE-RESPONSE RELATIONSHIP

It was mentioned above that the effective dose range of propranolol remains uncertain, and this is so for most of the β-blockers. Atenolol seems exceptional, as there is sound evidence that the initial dose of 100mg daily is also the ceiling dose as regards antihypertensive effect, perhaps because the variation in plasma concentration of the drug between patients is very small. The flat dose-response relationship makes atenolol a very simple drug to use in ordinary practice.

THE CHOICE OF β-BLOCKER

This is a difficult problem without a straightforward answer. The factors to consider are the relative safety (extent of clinical use), cost (but note the difficulty of determining equivalent doses), and ease of use (need for dose titration), and the possible merits of ancillary properties such as partial agonist activity or selectivity. There are obviously endless permutations and many uncertainties, and it is no surprise that a consensus has not emerged. Remarkably few writers have been willing to commit themselves to a choice, although they presumably make one in everyday practice. I use atenolol because it is so simple to use, and because I believe on balance that cardioselectivity does have some overall advantage, but I am unhappy about its cost.

CONTRA-INDICATIONS TO β-BLOCKADE

Asthma and cardiac failure of any degree are strong contra-indications to β-blockade. In exceptional circumstances it sometimes proves necessary to use a β-blocker in patients with these conditions, but this should generally be done in hospital. A prolonged P-R interval is not a contra-indication to β-blockade, but higher degrees of heart block are. The effect of β-blockers in patients with irreversible airways obstruction (e.g. chronic bronchitis, industrial lung disease) is not entirely clear. Those with simple chronic bronchitis, defined as chronic sputum production without any reduction in peak flow rate (PFR) or FEV_1/FVC, can be treated safely. If there is mild airways obstruction which is not reversible, as shown by an improvement in pulmonary function tests of less than 20 per cent in response to inhaled salbutamol, a selective β-blocker such as atenolol or metoprolol can be used, but respiratory function should be monitored by serial PFR readings. When airways obstruction is reversed significantly by salbutamol (asthmatic bronchitis), or if it is severe, β-blockers should be avoided.

Intermittent claudication is widely, but wrongly, thought to be a contra-indication to β-blockade. The point is important, because many claudicants also have angina and may be denied treatment they need badly for no good reason. There have been reports of β-blockers causing or worsening intermittent claudication, and they occasionally precipitate superficial skin necrosis in patients with peripheral vascular disease. However, when the effect of β-blockers has been examined in formal studies in patients with claudication, they could not be distinguished from placebo treatment. It is probably better to use a selective β-blocker, and one should keep a close eye on the walking distance, and on the skin of the feet, after starting treatment. I have seen no adverse effect after treating many patients in this way.

Diuretics

In sharp contrast to the situation concerning β-blockers, the choice of diuretic for the treatment of hypertension is perfectly clear. A small dose of the cheapest thiazide diuretic, which, in Britain, is bendrofluazide should be given as a single daily dose, and the tablet should not contain potassium chloride. Those who use anything else are wasting money, but unfortunately prescribing statistics confirm that rational prescribers are in the minority.

THE THIAZIDES

These are simple to use, well tolerated, and will normalise the blood pressure in about 30 per cent of patients with mild or moderate hypertension. None of the thiazides has proved superior in *any* respect to the least expensive, bendrofluazide, which costs less than one pence per day to prescribe. The thiazides have a flat dose-response curve in mild or moderate hypertension, and the prescription of large doses, or divided daily doses, worsens the biochemical disturbances such as hypokalaemia without any benefit as regards further blood pressure reduction.

OTHER MEDIUM POTENCY DIURETICS

These appear on the market with clockwork regularity, enjoy a brief spell of success, then lapse into obscurity. None of them has proved superior to bendrofluazide in any respect. The most recent offerings are indapamide (Natrilix) and xipamide (Diurexan). Indapamide has the pharmacological properties of a medium-potency diuretic, and has proved indistinguishable from the thiazide diuretics in published studies. The cost is twenty times that of bendrofluazide. Remarkably, it has been promoted as an antihypertensive drug and *not*

as a diuretic, and I have seen the ridiculous situation of patients being treated with two diuretics, for example Natrilix plus Navidrex K. It is not clear whether the fault lies with the manufacturer, with the licensing authority, with the ABPI (which monitors promotional methods), or with the prescribing doctor, but it is clear that the patient's interests are not being protected. Xipamide (Diurexan) has a diuretic potency slightly higher than that of the thiazides, and theoretically it could have greater antihypertensive activity (and greater toxicity). However, there are no published studies which show the drug to be superior to the thiazides, and there must be little incentive for the manufacturer to mount the appropriate trials when an easy market can be found without them. The cost of xipamide is ten times that of bendrofluazide.

LOOP DIURETICS

Frusemide (Lasix), bumetanide (Burinex) and ethacrynic acid (Edecrin) have a higher diuretic potency than the thiazides, but they have proved significantly *inferior* to the thiazides in antihypertensive effect, presumably because of their short duration of action. They are relatively expensive, and their dramatic diuretic action is socially disruptive and occasionally precipitates retention of urine in elderly males. The loop diuretics have no place in the management of uncomplicated hypertension, but they do have a useful role when there is co-existent cardiac or renal failure, and in resistant hypertension, as discussed later.

POTASSIUM-SPARING DRUGS

Spironolactone, amiloride and triamterene all act on the distal renal tubule, promoting mild natriuresis and conserving potassium. Their use as potassium-sparing agents is discussed later. Spironolactone has an antihypertensive action equivalent to that of the thiazides when given as a 100mg single daily dose. It is expensive, and commonly causes side-effects, particularly gastro-intestinal disturbance, but it has a valuable role in three uncommon situations: as an alternative to the thiazides when the latter drugs are contra-indicated, for example by allergy, severe gout or glucose intolerance; in resistant hypertension, as discussed later; and in the medical management of primary aldosteronism and other rare states of mineralo-corticoid excess. Amiloride and triamterene have some antihypertensive action, but this seems weaker than that of the thiazides or spironolactone when they are used at the recommended dosage. The adverse effect most to be feared from all three potassium-sparing drugs is hyperkalaemia, which may be fatal, and they must not be used (even in combination tablets) unless renal function is *known* to be normal. They should not be prescribed in conjunction with potassium supplements.

POTASSIUM PROBLEMS

The thiazide diuretics always cause some reduction in the plasma potassium, but it is uncommon for the level to fall below 3.0mmol/litre with conventional doses (e.g. bendrofluazide 2.5–5mg daily). In recent years it has become clear that the fall in plasma potassium does *not* reflect potassium depletion as there is no reduction in total body potassium, even when this is measured by very sensitive methods. In the uncomplicated patient with hypertension treated with a thiazide we are therefore faced with a problem of mild hypokalaemia, but not with potassium depletion. It is not known with certainty whether mild hypokalaemia (plasma potassium 3.0–3.5mmol/litre) is harmless or harmful. However, there is no good evidence that this degree of hypokalaemia causes symptoms, or predisposes to serious side-effects such as cardiac arrhythmias. On the other hand there is considerable evidence that the routine use of potassium supplements or potassium-sparing drugs causes some morbidity, and even mortality. Review articles during the last decade have concluded fairly unanimously that the risks of routine potassium supplementation, small though they may be, exceed the benefits. This conclusion has to a large extent been ignored in ordinary practice, and it seems worth repeating that *patients with uncomplicated hypertension treated with a thiazide diuretic do not need routine potassium supplements.*

It is worth considering briefly the logic of current prescribing practice. Many patients are treated with a combined thiazide and potassium chloride preparation, e.g. Neonaclex K or Navidrex K. The dose of potassium chloride given is 8 or 16mmol daily, depending on whether one or two combined tablets are prescribed. The effect of 16mmol potassium chloride daily is very small, amounting to a rise in plasma potassium of less than 0.2mmol/litre (Ramsay et al, 1980). If the prescribing doctor believes that potassium is *really* important he needs to give much more, perhaps 64mmol (eight Slow K tablets) daily. If he does *not* believe that potassium is important, he should not use it at all. The small doses of potassium which are widely prescribed at the present time can only be regarded as placebo treatment for the doctor.

The specific indications for treatment or prevention of hypokalaemia are as follows:

1. Plasma potassium lower than 3.0mmol/litre.
2. Digoxin treatment, or treatment with other drugs which predispose to arrhythmias (tricyclic antidepressants, phenothiazines, quinidine-like drugs).
3. Patients over 70 years of age, and those with a very poor diet.
4. Chronic liver disease.

In practice it is only necessary to measure the plasma potassium concentration once, about a month after starting treatment, as hypokalaemia then remains constant and does not progress. If the level is below 3.0mmol/litre, which will be the case in less than five per cent of uncomplicated patients, hypokalaemia should be treated. The choice of treatment lies between a large dose of potassium chloride (e.g. eight Slow K tablets daily), which is entirely inconsistent with the principles of simple treatment, or a single daily dose of a potassium-sparing drug (e.g. spironolactone 50–100mg), which is clearly preferable from the point of view of the patient's convenience. The combined tablets Aldactide (containing thiazide+spironolactone), Moduretic (thiazide+amiloride) and Dyazide (thiazide+triamterene) seem reasonably satisfactory *for those few patients who really need prevention or treatment of hypokalaemia.*

OTHER BIOCHEMICAL ABNORMALITIES

The thiazide diuretics cause elevation of serum uric acid, blood urea and cholesterol, and also plasma renin activity, and they tend to cause glucose intolerance. None of these need special monitoring. From time to time it has been suggested that one or other of these abnormalities may impair the prognosis of hypertensive patients, but it must not be forgotten that the controlled trials which have shown the benefits of antihypertensive treatment *all* used thiazides as a cornerstone of treatment. It seems clear that the benefits of diuretic treatment are likely to outweigh any theoretical risks.

The second drug: diuretic plus β-blocker

The fact that 50 to 70 per cent of even mildly hypertensive patients need treatment with two drugs has been mentioned already, and the figure is higher in those with moderate or severe hypertension. Thiazides and β-blockers have an additive effect as regards lowering the blood pressure, but it is of interest that the β-blockers attenuate diuretic-induced hypokalaemia significantly. The average rise in plasma potassium with β-blockade is 0.2–0.3mmol/litre. Recently, several combined tablets containing both diuretic and β-blocker have become available. These combinations should not be used as first drugs in the treatment of hypertension but they seem to be an acceptable choice at this second stage of treatment. They have the merit of convenience for the patient and also reduce the burden of prescription charges. The dose of diuretic is *very* small in some of the combined tablets, and I believe it is best to revert to the separate drugs, and use a slightly larger dose of diuretic, if the response to the combined tablet proves inadequate.

The third drug

WHICH THIRD DRUG?

Problems for both the patient and for the doctor really begin when the blood pressure is not adequately controlled by treatment with a diuretic plus β-blocker. Several candidates are available for use as the third drug, but none of them is entirely satisfactory, and controlled comparative studies to guide the doctor in his choice are not available. In a few patients the choice is dictated by contra-indications. For example, hydralazine is best avoided in patients with severe angina, or methyldopa in patients with a history of depression. However, in most patients the choice is determined by the current fashion or by the doctor's familiarity with individual drugs. The drugs used most widely at the present time are, in order, hydralazine, methyldopa and prazosin (Ramsay, 1980), while clonidine, reserpine and labetalol also deserve brief discussion.

Hydralazine lowers blood pressure by a direct vasodilator action on peripheral arterioles. When first introduced it was used alone and at high doses, and it often caused intolerable side-effects such as headache, flushing, severe tachycardia, or angina. There was also an unacceptably high risk of an illness resembling systemic lupus erythematosus (SLE), and for these reasons the drug was largely abandoned in Britain. The subjective symptoms (headache, flushing, tachycardia) are caused by reflex sympathetic stimulation, and interest in hydralazine was re-awakened when it emerged that this could be prevented by simultaneous treatment with a β-blocker. To reduce the risk of developing SLE the dose is generally limited to 200mg daily. At present hydralazine is widely used in conjunction with a β-blocker, starting with 25mg b.d. and increasing the dose as required to a maximum of 100mg b.d. The centrally-acting sympatholytic drugs, methyldopa, clonidine and reserpine also block the reflex sympathetic effects of hydralazine, but less effectively than do the β-blockers, and hydralazine should rarely be used without concomitant β-blockade.

Use of hydralazine in this way has two main problems. Firstly, its potency as an antihypertensive drug is rather modest, and it often fails to control more severe degrees of hypertension. The second problem is continuing concern about the possibility of drug-induced

SLE. It has become clear that the risk is not negligible with low doses and the figure of three per cent reported recently (Bing et al, 1980) accords with my own experience. The SLE syndrome is characterised by vague ill-health, weight loss, arthropathy, skin rashes and, less commonly, pleurisy or pericarditis. The kidneys and brain are spared. The illness is completely reversible when hydralazine is stopped, but it is nevertheless a severe adverse reaction, and the diagnosis is often delayed because of its insidious onset. The problem facing the doctor who prescribes hydralazine is how to predict which patients will develop drug-induced SLE, or how best to monitor patients so that an early diagnosis is made. As regards prediction, hydralazine-induced SLE tends to develop in women, in patients who are slow acetylators of hydralazine and in those with HLA-DR4 antigen (Batchelor et al, 1980). Using these variables it is probable that a small group of patients at very high risk could be identified, leaving the large majority of patients at negligible risk from SLE. This approach is promising, but quite impractical at present, and in fact it is not routine practice to measure even the acetylator status when prescribing hydralazine. As regards monitoring patients on hydralazine, some have suggested routine measurements of antinuclear factor (ANF) in the blood, for example at six-month intervals, as the development of SLE is preceded by the appearance of ANF. However, the majority of patients developing positive ANF titres will not progress to the SLE syndrome, so that this method is too sensitive, and not specific enough. At present the best answer to this worrying problem seems to be close clinical supervision, with a high index of suspicion towards any unusual illness in a patient taking hydralazine. There is perhaps a case for issuing patients with a card or leaflet, warning about the rare possibility of hydralazine-induced joint pains, skin rash, etc, which could be shown to any doctor they consult while taking the drug.

Methyldopa has been displaced as a drug of first choice because it caused subjective side-effects much more often than either the diuretics or β-blockers. In my clinic 60 per cent of patients reported side-effects, most commonly drowsiness and physical tiredness, and 25 per cent of patients had to discontinue methyldopa within six months of starting it. Despite this it still has an important role as a third drug; in patients who cannot take a β-blocker; and as the drug of choice in pregnancy hypertension. When used as a third drug, added to diuretic and β-blocker, I suspect that its antihypertensive potency is greater than that of hydralazine. The frequency of failure due to side-effects can be reduced by starting at a very low dose, 125mg b.d., and it is not usually worth increasing the dose beyond 1000mg b.d. Like hydralazine it has uncommon but serious adverse reactions during long-term use, including depression, acute and chronic liver reactions, haemolytic anaemia, chronic eczema and parkinsonism.

Prazosin is a post-synaptic α-adrenergic blocker which for practical purposes acts as a vasodilator. It causes less reflex tachycardia than hydralazine, and can therefore be used without a β-blocker, and is said to be better tolerated than methyldopa, although the published evidence does not support this entirely. It received bad publicity when first introduced due to an uncommon but alarming syncopal reaction following the first dose. This first dose effect can be avoided by starting at a low dose, 0.5mg b.d., and by advising that the first 0.5mg dose is taken after retiring for the night. The maximum dose recommended is 10mg b.d. and considerable dose titration is therefore needed in some patients. As far as is known prazosin has no serious adverse effects on long-term use, but experience with this drug is much less than that for hydralazine or methyldopa. On paper prazosin ought to be superior to either hydralazine or methyldopa, but I have not found this to be so in practice. Its antihypertensive potency seems to be rather limited, like that of hydralazine, and it quite often causes subjective side-effects, particularly dizziness. Sound studies comparing hydralazine, methyldopa and prazosin are badly needed.

Clonidine is a centrally-acting drug with a spectrum and frequency of side-effects similar to those of methyldopa. In addition sudden interruption of treatment can cause a dangerous hypertensive reaction accompanied by symptoms of sympathetic overactivity. It has little place in treatment, except as a last resort in patients who have been unable to tolerate several other drugs. It should never be prescribed if the patient's compliance is in any doubt, and specific warning must be given about the danger of stopping the drug suddenly.

Labetalol blocks both α- and β- adrenergic receptors, and is a relatively new introduction to clinical practice. In theory it should have a hypotensive effect additive to that of a β-blocker alone, due to its α-blocking action, but I have been unable to find any published study which shows this to be so. It causes side-effects more often than the β-blockers, and it has still to be established that it has any useful place in the long-term treatment of hypertension. It is valuable in hospital practice when rapid blood pressure reduction is needed, and can be used either orally or intravenously for this purpose.

Reserpine has been abandoned almost completely in Britain, partly because of its central depressant side-effects, and also because of studies suggesting a possible association with breast cancer. In fact the link with breast cancer has not been substantiated in subsequent studies, and reserpine remains in wide use in the United States and some countries in Europe. When given in low doses it is effective, easy to use, and inexpensive, and there is perhaps a case for its wider use in Britain.

Alternative drug regimens

Patients who cannot take a β-blocker because of contra-indications or side-effects present considerable difficulty in management, and indeed they are a constant reminder of the invaluable role the β-blockers

Table 3 Drugs known (or suspected) to block the action of antihypertensive agents

Non-specific interactions	Specific interactions
oestrogens	*tricyclic antidepressants* (e.g.
corticosteroids	imipramine, amitriptyline) and
carbenoxolone	*sympathomimetics* (e.g. phenylpropanolamine)
indomethacin	in cold cures, decongestants, etc
phenylbutazone	antagonise:
sodium bicarbonate	bethanidine
(other Na-containing drugs)	guanethidine
liquorice	debrisoquine
ergot derivatives	clonidine

have come to play in the treatment of hypertension. A thiazide diuretic is the obvious first choice, and I add methyldopa when another drug is needed. If a third drug is required prazosin is more suitable than hydralazine, as it causes less tachycardia in the absence of a β-blocker.

Resistant hypertension

DIFFERENTIAL DIAGNOSIS

About 10 per cent of patients remain uncontrolled despite a regimen of three drugs at full dosage, and they are defined arbitrarily as having resistant hypertension. There are two ways of tackling this situation—the wrong way and the right way. The wrong way is to embark on a series of empirical changes of treatment with no real attempt to get at the root of the problem. The right way is to approach the patient with resistant hypertension with an explicit differential diagnosis. The appropriate steps needed to confirm the diagnosis and the correct line of management then follow logically. The causes of apparent resistance to treatment are as follows:

1. Drug interactions
2. Non-compliance
3. Secondary hypertension
4. False tolerance
5. True drug resistance – by exclusion.

Drug interactions are not the commonest cause of resistance, but they are the easiest to diagnose if the possibility is remembered. The drugs which are known to block the action of antihypertensive agents are shown in Table 3. The first and simplest step when dealing with resistant hypertension is a detailed review of all treatment, including over the counter preparations. When a potential interaction is present the offending drug should be stopped if at all possible. The possibility of interactions that have not been reported should also be borne in mind.

Non-compliance. Although this term has been criticised because of its 'master-servant' implication, non-compliance remains a useful shorthand to describe irregular tablet-taking for any reason. Non-compliance is remarkably common (Sackett et al, 1975), and there can be little doubt that it is the most important cause of treatment failure. Poor compliance may be caused by *non-comprehension*, when the patient does not understand the instructions; *persistent errors*, when he does understand what to do; or by *deliberate non-compliance*. Non-comprehension and forgetfulness can often be eliminated by the first step in management, which is to simplify the treatment regimen as much as possible and provide clear instructions. When the blood pressure remains uncontrolled despite this, non-compliance may be revealed by skilful questioning. However, it cannot be emphasised too strongly that doctors are very bad at diagnosing compliance or non-compliance accurately by intuitive assessment. The doctor who relies on his judgement will overlook non-compliance when it is present and, worse, will label patients as non-compliant when they are in fact taking their tablets regularly. The label tends to stick for ever.

The simplest way to assess compliance in ordinary practice is the tablet count. A known excess of tablets is prescribed, the patient is asked to bring his tablets with him at each visit, and the remaining tablets are counted. Provided the patient has only one source of tablets, he must be non-compliant, either deliberately or in error, if he returns too many tablets. A correct count does not of course *prove* compliance, as the determined patient can easily falsify the returns.

The management of non-compliance remains difficult even when it is diagnosed. Errors may be tackled by repeated careful instruction, in writing if necessary, or by having the treatment supervised as a last resort. The reasons for deliberate non-compliance should be explored with the patient. A change of treatment may help if side-effects are the cause. Some patients will yield to further explanation of the nature of hypertension and its consequences, and of the reasons for treatment. There remains a group of patients who will not follow treatment for reasons that are unknown. It is important to remember that partial control of the blood pressure is better than no treatment at all, and many of these patients can be persuaded to take very simple treatment, but not a complex regimen.

Doctors rarely attempt to diagnose non-compliance formally, either in general practice or in hospital. Perhaps they feel that it is too time-consuming, but it does not seem nearly as futile as the alternative, which is to continue adding drug after drug while the patient takes no treatment at all.

Secondary hypertension. After non-compliance and drug interactions have been excluded as best possible, the patient should be investigated further aiming to exclude renal hypertension, renal artery stenosis and phaeochromocytoma. A rapid-sequence IVP is generally sufficient to exclude renal artery stenosis, but renal arteriography should be considered in young patients with severe resistant hypertension even when the IVP is normal, as about 20 per cent of patients with renovascular hypertension have a normal IVP.

False tolerance. All the antihypertensive drugs in common use except the diuretics and β-blockers tend to expand the plasma and extracellular fluid volumes. On occasion this volume expansion is sufficient to reduce or abolish the antihypertensive action of the drug, and this phenomenon has been termed false tolerance. False tolerance is seen particularly with drugs of high potency such as minoxidil and the postganglionic adrenergic blockers (bethanidine, guanethidine and debrisoquine), but it occurs also with drugs of moderate potency such as hydralazine, prazosin or methyldopa. It may be present despite treatment with conventional doses of a thiazide diuretic. Weight gain or ankle swelling may suggest this possibility, but false tolerance can be present without any clinical evidence of fluid retention.

The fourth drug: frusemide or spironolactone
From the description of false tolerance given above it is clear that it cannot be diagnosed or excluded clinically. As false tolerance is a relatively common cause of treatment resistance (Ramsay et al, 1980), all compliant patients who remain uncontrolled on a full regimen of three drugs should have a trial of the appropriate treatment, which is to add either frusemide or spironolactone to the regimen. The response is often a substantial fall in blood pressure and in body-weight. Frusemide should be used when renal impairment is present (serum creatinine $>130\mu$mol/litre), but otherwise the choice between frusemide and spironolactone is unclear. The initial dose of frusemide is 40mg daily, and of spironolactone 100mg daily. The dose should be increased according to tolerance until weight loss of one kilogram is attained before abandoning the manoeuvre as ineffective. Patients having this treatment need close clinical and biochemical monitoring which is usually best achieved in a hospital clinic.

Drugs of high potency
When there is no urgency the effect of different drugs of moderate potency (hydralazine, methyldopa, prazosin, labetalol) may be tried in turn before moving on to a drug of high potency. Patients with severe resistant hypertension are at considerable risk from vascular complications, and one of these drugs should be added immediately if frusemide or spironolactone fails to produce a response.

POST-GANGLIONIC ADRENERGIC BLOCKERS
Many doctors are familiar with bethanidine, guanethidine, and debrisoquine, and a few seem reluctant to give them up. They cause postural and exercise hypotension, failure of ejaculation, diarrhoea, and a fall in glomerular filtration rate. It often proves impossible to control the recumbent blood pressure without causing disabling postural symptoms. They should be reserved for patients with resistant hypertension, and even here minoxidil is clearly preferable in men, and in women with renal impairment.

Minoxidil is a potent vasodilator which has only recently become available for prescription, but it has been used widely in resistant hypertension for some time. It often succeeds where all else has failed, and it causes very few subjective side-effects. Like hydralazine it causes reflex sympathetic stimulation, and comcomitant treatment with a β-blocker or, less effectively, with a centrally-acting drug, is necessary. Minoxidil treatment is associated with two particular problems. The first is its marked tendency to promote fluid retention, and virtually all patients need treatment with a loop diuretic such as frusemide, often at high doses. In fact the effect of frusemide alone should always have been tried first, as discussed above. The second problem is excess hair growth, and the pronounced increase in facial hair is particularly unacceptable to ladies. It is for this reason that I still prefer to try a post-ganglionic adrenergic blocker first in women, provided renal function is not impaired.

Captopril inhibits the conversion of angiotensin I to the potent pressor substance angiotensin II, and this is one mechanism for its powerful hypotensive action. It has some serious toxic effects and is not yet generally available, but it may prove to have a valuable role in resistant hypertension.

Total failure of treatment
A few patients remain uncontrolled despite treatment which is admirably planned and executed. This is usually due to persistent non-compliance or inability to take tablets, and not to true drug resistance. Most doctors have met the patient who reacts adversely to every antihypertensive drug, often with the same side-effect to drugs of widely differing properties. Some patients, particularly older patients with severe vascular disease, have considerable postural hypotension even without treatment, and it may be impossible to control the recumbent blood pressure without causing disabling symptoms. There is no option but to accept satisfactory control of the standing blood pressure, and there is in fact evidence that this degree of control provides some protection against vascular complications.

SPECIAL SITUATIONS

Hypertensive emergencies

Certain complications of hypertension need urgent hospital admission. These include *accelerated hypertension*, diagnosed by the presence of haemorrhages and soft exudates in the fundi; *hypertensive encephalopathy*, characterised by severe hypertension, altered level of consciousness, focal neurological signs and convulsions; overt *left ventricular failure*; and suspicion of *aortic dissection*. Most of these are fairly obvious emergencies. However, the treatment of accelerated hypertension is still too often delayed probably because these patients may feel and look perfectly well, and the diagnosis depends entirely on careful examination of the optic fundi. It is important to note that papilloedema need not be present – the presence of haemorrhages and soft exudates alone warrants urgent hospital admission. Delay in treatment may lead to a rapid loss of renal function which cannot be recovered, and the ultimate prognosis in these patients is closely linked to the degree of renal impairment in the acute phase.

The main change in hospital practice recently has been a re-definition of the indications for urgent blood pressure reduction. Dramatic falls in blood pressure occasionally cause 'poor perfusion' vascular accidents in the form of stroke, myocardial infarction or blindness. Intravenous treatment is therefore reserved for a few uncommon extreme emergencies, namely hypertensive encephalopathy, fulminant left ventricular failure, eclampsia and phaeochromocytoma crisis. Intravenous diazoxide and labetalol, given in bolus doses, both seem fairly satisfactory in these situations, and there is little to choose between them. Intravenous frusemide is a useful adjunct in some patients. Nitroprusside infusion is more complicated to use and is best reserved for patients who do not respond to the simpler drugs, although it is the choice when rapid fluctuations of blood pressure are expected, for example during anaesthesia. Parenteral treatment is not necessary, and may be harmful, in accelerated hypertension. In these patients the aim is gradual reduction of the blood pressure over 24 hours or so, to a diastolic pressure of 100–110mmHg, using orally administered drugs. There is no standard oral regimen, and no matter what drugs are given a few patients seem to respond poorly, and a few to respond too rapidly. I use oral labetalol, adjusting the dose on a sliding scale according to the diastolic blood pressure as in the section on acute management, as described by Ghose et al (1978), but have not found it entirely satisfactory.

Secondary hypertension

In general the surgical treatment of curable hypertension has proved disappointing when measured against the optimistic expectations of 10 to 20 years ago. For example, patients with *Conn's syndrome* (primary aldosteronism) are managed medically when it is caused by bilateral adrenal hyperplasia rather than an adenoma, when the hypertension proves unresponsive to full doses of spironolactone, and when the patient is unfit or unwilling to have surgery. When these exclusions are added up it is probable that less than half of all patients come to operation, and for the remainder spironolactone is the treatment of choice. This drug invariably corrects the biochemical abnormalities such as hypokalaemia, but it does not always control the hypertension, and conventional antihypertensive drugs may also be needed. High doses of spironolactone often cause side-effects, and addition of a thiazide diuretic will often allow a reduction in dosage. High doses of amiloride are also effective in Conn's syndrome. Enthusiasm for conventional surgical treatment of *renal artery stenosis* has waned with recognition of the rather high peri-operative mortality, the frequent need for nephrectomy (with loss of functioning renal tissue), and the disappointing cure rate. However, interest in renovascular hypertension has been rekindled by a new technique called percutaneous transluminal angioplasty. Briefly, a special catheter with a balloon near its tip is advanced until the balloon is positioned in the stenotic segment of the renal artery. The balloon is then inflated, and the arterial lumen is restored by compression of the stenotic lesion. The technique is simple, inexpensive, and has a very low incidence of complications. The early results are most encouraging, and if the long-term outcome proves satisfactory this will be a welcome advance in treatment. *Unilateral renal lesions* due to parenchymal disease (e.g. chronic pyelonephritis) or ureteric obstruction occasionally cause hypertension, but again the results of surgical treatment have proved disappointing. In general the correct approach is to deal with any renal abnormality strictly on its own merits. Surgical intervention with the specific aim of curing or improving the hypertension should be considered only when the hypertension is resistant to treatment. *Coarctation of the aorta* is managed medically when it is discovered in adult life because the aorta is atherosclerotic and cannot be repaired easily, and because hypertension often persists after surgery. These patients need antibiotic cover for dental treatment to prevent subacute bacterial endocarditis of the aortic valve, which is often congenitally bicuspid.

Hypertension and pregnancy

HYPERTENSION BEFORE PREGNANCY

When essential hypertension is uncomplicated and well controlled the patient who enquires about future pregnancy can be reassured that the chance of successful pregnancy is very high, that pregnancy has no adverse long-term effect on the blood pressure, and that the antihypertensive drugs in common use have no known adverse effect on the fetus. Close supervision will be needed, confinement should be in hospital, and some time in hospital will often be necessary during the pregnancy. It is usually best to continue the patient's customary drug regimen into the pregnancy, as changes of treatment may result in loss of blood pressure control. The exception is perhaps to change any β-blocker in the regimen to oxprenolol, as published experience with this drug during pregnancy is larger than that for other β-blockers. Patients with *any* complication of hypertension, and particularly those with renal impairment or an abnormal ECG, should be referred for specialist assessment and advice before pregnancy.

HYPERTENSION EARLY IN PREGNANCY

Readings above 150mmHg systolic or 90mmHg diastolic are abnormal at any stage of pregnancy. Elevated blood pressure detected in the first 20 weeks of pregnancy usually indicates pre-existing hypertension, most commonly essential hypertension. Phaeochromocytoma should be borne in mind because of its very bad prognosis in pregnancy. There is evidence that treatment of hypertension of early pregnancy with methyldopa reduces the incidence of mid-trimester abortion and perinatal death (Leather et al, 1968; Redman et al, 1976). The aim of treatment is to lower blood pressure to around 130/80mmHg, and oxprenolol or hydralazine may be added to methyldopa if necessary. Patients who were hypertensive early in pregnancy need to be assessed further after pregnancy to determine whether long-term treatment is needed.

HYPERTENSION LATE IN PREGNANCY

Hypertension developing after 20 weeks, is usually due to pre-eclampsia. The mainstays of management are rest, close monitoring of the mother and fetus, and delivery when it is safe to do so. There is general agreement that antihypertensive drugs should be used when the blood pressure rises to 170/110mmHg or higher, to protect the mother. The role of drug treatment in less severe degrees of late hypertension is not established. As a rule patients with pre-eclampsia are treated in hospital, but some obstetricians manage carefully selected patients with mild hypertension (diastolic 90–100mmHg), and no proteinuria, at home with very close supervision. This includes frequent blood pressure checks, daily self-monitoring for proteinuria with Albustix, warning about the premonitory symptoms of eclampsia (headache, visual disturbance, abdominal pain, vomiting), and arrangements for urgent self-admission if problems arise. Eclampsia can develop with alarming rapidity in this type of patient. Methyldopa, hydralazine and oxprenolol are the drugs used most commonly in pre-eclampsia. Diuretics are generally avoided because the plasma volume is already reduced in pre-eclampsia, although there is no evidence that they are harmful.

Hypertension in the elderly

The vigour of any debate tends to be inversely related to the amount of hard evidence available, and it is quite understandable that the management of hypertension in the elderly has stimulated lively controversy. We know very little about the rights and wrongs of treatment, and dogmatic statements are quite out of place (although they can be found easily in the literature). Answers may well emerge soon from studies which are in progress, but meantime doctors must act upon their interpretation of the scanty evidence available. What follows is my interpretation of this evidence.

There are two arguments in favour of treating hypertension in those aged 70 years or more. First, the association between hypertension and vascular disease seems to hold into old age, although it may well be weaker than in middle-age. Secondly, controlled trials of antihypertensive treatment in middle-aged patients have generally shown that the benefits of treatment increase with increasing age. By extrapolation one might expect elderly patients to benefit from treatment. The arguments against treating hypertension in the elderly are centred largely on possible adverse effects of treatment. Older patients are thought to be more susceptible to the side-effects of antihypertensive drugs. This was probably so with the previous generation of drugs, particularly the post-ganglionic adrenergic blockers, but the elderly seem to tolerate the drugs in wide use at present without special problems. There is also concern that reduction of blood pressure in the elderly may actually cause vascular complications. I do not doubt that 'poor perfusion' strokes do occur, but they seem to be unusual pathological curios, whereas strokes occurring in the setting of uncontrolled hypertension are commonplace in the elderly.

I believe that the balance of evidence favours treatment of at least some elderly hypertensive patients. I treat any patient with important complications, such as renal impairment or cardiac failure, regardless of age. I also recommend treatment for uncomplicated patients between the ages of 70 to 79 years if the systolic pressure averages 200mmHg or more, or the diastolic 110mmHg or more. I am reluctant to treat patients above the age of 79 years. A thiazide diuretic combined with a potassium-sparing agent is the cornerstone of treatment, aiming to lower the systolic pressure below 180mmHg and the diastolic below 100mmHg.

LONG-TERM FOLLOW-UP

DEFAULTING

It is clear from the 'rule of halves' and from prospective studies that many hypertensive patients default entirely from treatment and follow-up. No doubt some do so because they are given inadequate information initially, but this is probably not the main cause of defaulting. Patients who have received intensive education about hypertension, and who have been shown to understand it, still default from treatment, and indeed do so just as often as those given only simple information (Sackett et al, 1975). In other words some patients who are in full possession of the relevant facts choose not to have treatment. Their decision can only be accepted, but these patients should be advised to continue with regular blood pressure checks so that they can learn of any change in risk, for example from a further rise in blood pressure.

The information given to patients should be simple, delivered in small doses over the first few visits, and reinforced by repetition. Leaflets and booklets are available, but the doctor needs to satisfy himself that the contents are sound before using any of them. The patient should understand that high blood pressure usually causes no symptoms; that any feeling of ill-health is probably unrelated to high blood pressure; and that the aim of treatment is not to make him feel better, but to keep him healthy. In short, treatment is insurance for the future. Sensible people should not be expected to take treatment for many years without good reason, and they must therefore be told something of the risk of vascular disease without treatment, although they should not be frightened into treatment by exaggeration of the risk. They should know that protection continues only while treatment is taken regularly, and that treatment is usually for life. They should also know that the number of tablets needed is no measure of the seriousness of their situation – only the final blood pressure level counts.

It is now known that invalidism and absence from work increase after hypertension has been diagnosed, even when the hypertension is of mild degree, and active steps should be taken to combat this tendency. Patients themselves, relatives, and even doctors often impose unnecessary restrictions which can be very difficult to break down. The simplest approach is to spell out clearly the few constraints which are essential, namely to take tablets regularly, to have routine blood pressure checks and, when appropriate, to reduce weight and stop smoking. In all other respects life should be entirely normal, and this fact should be emphasised and re-emphasised to the patient.

As patients continue to default despite adequate education some method for detecting and reviewing those who disappear is needed. The vigour of attempts at recall will obviously depend on the severity of the hypertension and the individual predicament of the patient; but it must stop short of intrusion on privacy. A sub-species of defaulter who continues on treatment, sometimes for years, but never presents himself for blood pressure measurements, could be eliminated easily by routine monitoring of repeat prescriptions.

REPEAT ASSESSMENTS

The frequency of visits after the blood pressure has been controlled depends on the individual patient. Those who are uncomplicated and well controlled on simple treatment can be reviewed at three-monthly intervals, while those with borderline or variable readings, or who are doubtfully compliant, need to be seen at shorter intervals. A routine visit involves only measurement of blood pressure and body-weight, and a general enquiry about side-effects, and this could be done perfectly well by trained and supervised nursing or paramedical staff. It is sometimes suggested that certain procedures such as examination of the fundi, or an electrocardiogram, should be repeated at set intervals. In fact they are best repeated only when the results could possibly alter the management. For instance, there seems no point in examining the fundi repeatedly when the blood pressure has been consistently in the normal range. On the other hand a thorough re-evaluation can be very helpful in patients with borderline or variable blood pressure control. If, for example, this revealed an increase in left ventricular voltage or in radiological heart size over a period of observation, there would be no doubt that treatment should be more vigorous.

THE FUTURE

The next few years will hopefully see light cast upon some of the remaining grey areas in the management of hypertension. The value or otherwise of treating hypertension in the elderly will perhaps be clarified, and the evidence for treating mild hypertension, and hypertension in pregnancy, may be firmed up. The availability of effective and acceptable treatment for 80 per cent of hypertensive patients has tended to obscure the unsatisfactory situation for the less fortunate 20 per cent, who are not controlled by a diuretic and β-blocker. Comparative studies of the various 'third drugs' available are badly needed and, as it is already clear that none of them is entirely satisfactory, the search for new and better drugs must continue. We can also look forward to comparative studies of different drug regimens using mortality and morbidity, and not simply millimetres of mercury, as the end points.

Finally, I hope that two questions of fundamental importance will receive serious consideration in the near future. First, are we willing to settle for life-long drug treatment of 10 per cent of the adult population? There is already sound evidence that the need for anti-hypertensive drugs could be reduced substantially by effective attention to obesity, salt intake and perhaps alcohol consumption, and there are suggestions that other dietary factors such as caffeine may also be important. There is a very strong case for diverting more effort and resources towards these aspects of management. Secondly, how can we get treatment to the majority of hypertensive people who are not under medical care? At the present rate of progress case-finding through general practice will take a very long time. What can be done meantime? One obvious answer is to disseminate information about hypertension, and the need for routine blood pressure checks, to the general public. The populace seems fairly well informed about the supposed dangers of factors such as cholesterol and physical inactivity, when there is no hard evidence that they will actually benefit from this knowledge. On the other hand they seem much less aware of hypertension, although its consequences are universally recognised to be common, important and preventable. The time is surely right to redress the balance.

REFERENCES

Anonymous (1980). Antihypertensive drugs, plasma lipids and coronary disease. *Lancet*, **2**, 19.

Armitage, P., Fox, W., Rose, G. A. and Tinker, C. M. (1966). The variability of measurements of casual blood pressure. II survey experience. *Clinical Science*, **30**, 337.

Atkinson, A. B. and Kellett, R. J. (1974). Value of intravenous urography in investigating hypertension. *Journal of the Royal College of Physicians of London*, **8**, 175.

Batchelor, J. R., Welsh, K. I., Mansilla Tinoco, R., Dollery, C. T., Hughes, G. R. V., Bernstein, R., Ryan, P., Naish, P. F., Aber, G. M., Bing, R. F. and Russell, G. I. (1980). Hydralazine-induced systemic lupus erythematosus: influence of HLA-DR and sex on susceptibility. *Lancet*, **1**, 1107.

Berglund, G., Andersson, O. and Wilhelmsen, L. (1976). Prevalence of primary and secondary hypertension: studies in a random population sample. *British Medical Journal*, **3**, 554.

Berglund, G., Wilhelmsen, L., Sannerstedt, R., Hansson, L., Andersson, O., Sivertsson, R., Wedel, H. and Wilkstraud, J. (1978). Coronary heart disease after treatment of hypertension. *Lancet*, **1**, 1.

Bing, R. F., Russell, G. I., Thurston, H. and Swales, J. D. (1980). Hydralazine in hypertension: is there a safe dose? *British Medical Journal*, **2**, 353.

Committee of Principal Investigators (1980). WHO co-operative trial on primary prevention of ischaemic heart disease using clofibrate to lower serum cholesterol: mortality follow-up. *Lancet*, **2**, 379.

Davidson, C., Thadani, U., Singleton, W. and Taylor, S. H. (1976). Comparison of antihypertensive activity of beta-blocking drugs during chronic treatment. *British Medical Journal*, **2**, 7.

Engelman, K. (1977). Phaeochromocytoma. *Clinics in Endocrinology and Metabolism*, **6**, 769.

Ghose, R. R., Mathur, Y. B., Upadhyah, M., Morgan, W. D. and Khan, S. (1978). Treatment of hypertensive emergencies with oral labetalol. *British Medical Journal*, **2**, 96.

Hart, J. T. (1980). *Hypertension*. Library of General Practice, Volume 1. Churchill Livingstone, Edinburgh, London and New York.

Hypertension Detection and Follow-up Program Co-operative Group (1979 a, b). Five-year findings of the hypertension detection and follow-up program. *Journal of the American Medical Association*, **242**, 2562 and 2572.

Leather, H. M., Humphreys, D. M., Baker, P. and Chadd, M. A. (1968). A controlled trial of hypotensive agents in hypertension in pregnancy. *Lancet*, **2**, 488.

Marshall, A. and Barritt, D. W. (1977). Drug compliance in hypertensive patients. *British Medical Journal*, **2**, 1278.

Marshall, A. J., Roberts, C. J. C. and Barritt, D. W. (1976). Raynaud's phenomenon as side-effects of beta-blockers in hypertension. *British Medical Journal*, **1**, 1498.

Morgan, T., Adam, W., Gillies, A., Wilson, M., Morgan, G. and Carney, S. (1978). Hypertension treated by salt restriction. *Lancet*, **1**, 227.

Ramsay, L. E. (1979). Alcohol use and hypertension. *Practical Cardiology*, **5**, 27.

Ramsay, L. E. (1980). Diuretic and β-blocker in hypertension – then what? *Journal of the Royal College of Physicians of London*, **14**, 249.

Ramsay, L. E., Ramsay, M. H., Hettiarachchi, J., Davies, D. L. and Winchester, J. (1978). Weight reduction in a blood pressure clinic. *British Medical Journal*, **2**, 244.

Ramsay, L. E., Hettiarachchi, J., Fraser, R. and Morton, J. J. (1980). Amiloride, spironolactone, and potassium chloride in thiazide-treated hypertensive patients. *Clinical Pharmacology and Therapeutics*, **27**, 533.

Ramsay, L. E., Silas, J. H. and Freestone, S. (1980). Diuretic treatment of resistant hypertension. *British Medical Journal*, **281**, 1101.

Redman, C. W. G., Beilin, L. J., Bonnar, J. and Ounsted, M. K. (1976). Fetal outcome in trial of antihypertensive treatment in pregnancy. *Lancet*, **2**, 753.

Reisin, E., Abel, R., Modan, M., Silverberg, D. S., Eliahou, H. E. and Modan, B. (1978). Effect of weight loss without salt restriction on the reduction of blood pressure in overweight hypertensive patients. *New England Journal of Medicine*, **298**, 1.

Report by the Management Committee (1979). Initial results of the Australian Therapeutic Trial in mild hypertension. *Clinical Science*, **57**, 449.

Report by the Management Committee (1980). The Australian Therapeutic Trial in mild hypertension. *Lancet*, **1**, 1261.

Sackett, D. L., Haynes, R. B., Gibson, E. S., Hackett, B. C., Taylor, D. W., Roberts, R. S. and Johnson, A. L. (1975). Randomised clinical trial of strategies for improving medication compliance in primary hypertension. *Lancet*, **1**, 1205.

Steptoe, A. (1977). Psychological methods in treatment of hypertension: a review. *British Heart Journal*, **29**, 587.

Taguchi, J. and Freis, E. D. (1974). Partial reduction of blood pressure and prevention of complications in hypertension. *New England Journal of Medicine*, **291**, 329.

Veterans Administration Co-operative Study Group on Antihypertensive Agents (1970). Effects of treatment on morbidity in hypertension. II. Results in patients with diastolic blood pressure averaging 90 through 114mmHg. *Journal of the American Medical Association*, **213**, 1143.

Veterans Administration Co-operative Study Group on Antihypertensive Agents (1977). Propranolol in the treatment of essential hypertension. *Journal of the American Medical Association*, **237**, 2303.

Chapter 3 Chronic bronchitis and emphysema

P. B. ANDERSON MA, BM, BCh, MRCP

INTRODUCTION

Chronic bronchitis is defined in clinical terms as excess production of mucus, presenting as persistent cough and sputum production for more than three months of the year for three consecutive years. Expectoration is the essential point but before chronic bronchitis can be diagnosed as the sole cause of the expectoration, other causes of chronic expectoration such as bronchiectasis must be excluded.

Emphysema on the other hand is defined in pathological terms as dilatation of air spaces distal to the terminal bronchioles, with destruction of their walls. In clinical practice chronic bronchitis is very often associated with emphysema and it is therefore practical to have a combined approach as regards treatment.

The United Kingdom has the highest incidence of chronic bronchitis and emphysema in the world. Symptoms attributable to chronic bronchitis and emphysema may be found in 17 per cent of men and eight per cent of women aged 40 to 64 years. In 1974 25 000 deaths in England and Wales were due to these conditions. In addition about 1000 deaths were due to pulmonary heart disease of which chronic bronchitis and emphysema cause the major proportion. It is probable that chronic bronchitis and emphysema are a contributory factor in deaths certified due to other forms of heart disease or to pneumonia. Chronic bronchitis and emphysema cause the loss of over 30 million working days each year.

A small number of individuals with emphysema (0.5 to 2 per cent) have a deficiency of serum antiproteolytic activity. This defect is genetically determined (Eriksson, 1964) and inherited as an autosomal recessive. Deficiency of alpha$_1$ (α_1)-antitrypsin alone may not be sufficient to cause emphysema and smoking is an important contributory factor. Chronic bronchitis co-exists in many patients.

Three patterns may be distinguished in patients with chronic bronchitis on the basis of symptoms:

1. Simple chronic bronchitis: the patient has a chronic productive cough but no shortness of breath or airflow obstruction.
2. Complicated chronic bronchitis or mucopurulent chronic bronchitis: in addition to a chronic productive cough, the patient experiences episodes of infection characterised by an increase in sputum and by sputum purulence.
3. Chronic obstructive bronchitis: in which airflow obstruction has become established and the patient is wheezy and dyspnoeic.

GENERAL MANAGEMENT

Stopping smoking

Smoking is the single most important factor in the development of chronic bronchitis and emphysema. Air pollution, occupation and social class are further aetiological factors. Not all smokers develop chronic bronchitis nor do all individuals with mucus hypersecretion necessarily progress to chronic obstructive bronchitis with airflow obstruction. The most important measure in the management of chronic bronchitis and emphysema is for the patient to stop smoking.

There is a steady gradual decline in respiratory function with advancing age but non-smokers rarely develop clinically significant airflow obstruction. Many smokers behave similarly but others develop airflow obstruction of varying severity. Stopping smoking will not affect the respiratory function of a non-susceptible smoker. A susceptible smoker who stops smoking will not regain lost function but the subsequent rate of loss of function will approximate to the normal loss with age (Fletcher and Peto, 1977) (Fig. 3/1).

Stopping smoking will reduce cough and sputum and will reduce the rate of deterioration of respiratory function and limit the severity and development of disability.

It can be immensely difficult to stop smoking and a firm but sympathetic approach is necessary. The need to stop should be carefully explained in terms of the benefit to health and survival. Explanation of the

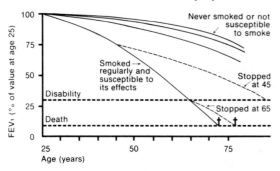

Fig. 3/1 Risks for various men if they smoke (Fletcher and Peto, 1977). Lines illustrate the effect of smoking and of stopping smoking on the FEV_1. Other smokers may not be susceptible and the decline of FEV_1 is that which occurs with age only. Other susceptible smokers will have different rates of loss and will reach disability at different ages. (Reproduced by kind permission of the author, editor and publisher, *British Medical Journal*, 1, 1645–8.)

economic advantages may also be helpful. Even the well-motivated patient may find stopping most difficult because of psychological dependence and nicotine addiction. Reinforcement and repeated encouragement are helpful. Much depends on the patient's own will power. Some do respond to a progressive reduction in cigarettes but the tendency is for consumption to increase again and patients should be told to stop completely. The benefit to an elderly person of stopping completely is, however, debatable but a reduction will produce a worthwhile symptomatic improvement. Recently a nicotine-containing chewing gum (Nicorette) has become available in the United Kingdom as an aid to stopping smoking: gum containing 2mg or 4mg is available. The effectiveness of the gum is yet to be proved, as it potentially has a powerful placebo effect. The nicotine is bound to an ion exchange resin and is released slowly during chewing. Nicotine release depends on the vigour and rate of chewing and nicotine is then absorbed through the buccal mucosa. Nicotine is not released if the gum is swallowed and nicotine swallowed and absorbed is metabolised in the first passage through the liver.

The gum should be used in smokers wanting to stop. Initially, the 2mg gum should be prescribed; the aim being to relieve withdrawal symptoms, the patient resorting to the gum when the urge to smoke is strong and to provide a substitute oral activity. The rise in nicotine level is considerably slower than after a cigarette and relief of symptoms is therefore proportionately slower. It is important that the gum is chewed slowly to avoid excessive salivation and irrita-

tion. The gum should be chewed for a while and then held in the cheek followed by a further period of chewing. Most smokers use about eight pieces of 2mg gum daily. The rare individual using 15 or more pieces should be given the 4mg gum. After three or four months the consumption should be reduced gradually. Those who have not stopped smoking completely after a month probably will not benefit from continuing on the gum.

Blood nicotine concentrations are only half those achieved by smoking and other harmful substances such as carbon monoxide and smoke components are not present. Use of the gum is probably less likely to be harmful than continuing smoking in vascular disease, in thromboembolic disease, in peptic ulceration and to the fetus. Caution is advisable however in those who are pregnant or with vascular disease (Russell et al, 1980; Raw et al, 1980).

TREATMENT OF SYMPTOMS

Cough and sputum

Cough productive of sputum is the essential symptom of simple chronic bronchitis and mucopurulent bronchitis and is the result of hypersecretion. When normal quantities of secretions are produced (about 100ml daily) they are cleared without coughing. Stopping smoking may result in an improvement. In general, cough suppressants are not indicated for what may be called 'useful cough' but may be used if cough is persistent and irritable, particularly when it disturbs or prevents sleep. Then a linctus containing antihistamines such as diphenhydramine (Benylin) or codeine as a linctus or tablet may be given. The antitussive effects of codeine are mediated centrally and the effects from an antihistamine are largely the result of sedation; either of these may therefore also depress ventilation. On occasion the cough may be non-productive and persistent, causing distress and interfering with many activities. In these circumstances the inhalation of nebulised lignocaine is effective (Howard et al, 1977).

Mucolytics have been shown *in vitro* to reduce sputum viscosity but have been disappointing in clinical use. The two most used mucolytics are bromhexine (Bisolvon) 8mg or 16mg three or four times daily and S-carboxymethylcysteine (Mucodyne) 15ml or two capsules t.d.s.

Wheezing and dyspnoea

A proportion of chronic bronchitics eventually become wheezy and dyspnoeic (chronic obstructive bronchitis). The airflow obstruction results from a combination of mechanisms (Table 1).

Table 1 Mechanisms of airflow obstruction

Mucosal oedema and glandular hypertrophy
Secretions within the lumen
Muscular bronchoconstriction
Distortion of the airways

Wheezing is a feature of many other conditions, particularly bronchial asthma. It is important to distinguish between them because prognosis and treatment differ. The differentiation between chronic bronchitis and late onset asthma (cryptogenic asthma) may be particularly difficult. Reversible airflow obstruction is by definition asthma but some chronic bronchitics do have significant reversibility when tested with bronchodilators. This can cause great semantic problems but practically they can be regarded as either having co-existent asthma or as bronchitics with a reversible component.

Table 2 contrasts some clinical features of asthma and chronic bronchitis helpful in their differentiation.

Significant reversibility implies an improvement of 15 per cent or more from baseline values of peak flow rate (PEFR) or forced expiratory volume in one second (FEV_1). An asthmatic would be expected to improve to at least 70 per cent of the predicted. It should be remembered that sputum production is a feature of asthma and does not necessarily indicate the presence of chronic bronchitis.

Atopy, that is allergy to common environmental materials demonstrated by positive skin prick tests, can be a useful pointer to asthma but atopics can also develop chronic bronchitis. Twenty-five to 35 per cent of unselected populations can be found to have positive skin tests and many may be asymptomatic (Davies, 1979). Sputum eosinophilia has long been known to occur in chronic bronchitis and has again been reported recently (McHardy et al, 1980). Thus it is by no means a firm indication of asthma.

Bronchodilators

All patients with chronic bronchitis and/or emphysema deserve a trial of a bronchodilator, preferably the response being monitored by a simple measurement of respiratory function such as the PEFR. PEFR can be measured using the mini-Wright peak flow gauge (Airmed Ltd, London) which is reliable and inexpensive. The response to a bronchodilator may be tested by giving a dose from a metered-dose inhaler, for example 200 micrograms salbutamol (Ventolin) with PEFR measured before and 20 minutes after the dose.

Bronchodilators currently available belong to three groups: the β- sympathomimetics, the xanthines and parasympatholytic (atropine-like) agents.

Beta (β)-sympathomimetics

Historically the first member of this group to be used therapeutically was adrenaline followed by the synthetic isoprenaline. Both are still available in metered-dose inhalers (e.g. Medihaler-Epi, Medihaler-Iso etc). Although effective bronchodilators their action is short, lasting only for between half and one hour. This is because of rapid inactivation by the enzyme catechol-O-methyl transferase (COMT). A further disadvantage is that they are not selective in their action, stimulating both the β-receptors of the heart (β_1-receptors) and of the bronchi (β_2-receptors). Their use can therefore cause tachycardia and there is the potential of their producing serious ventricular arrhythmias such as ventricular tachycardia or fibrillation, particularly if the dose is exceeded. The short duration of action predisposes to abuse as the patient seeks relief as the wheezing tends to recur. The introduction of the newer β_2 selective sympathomimetics has made adrenaline and isoprenaline obsolete in the general treatment of bronchoconstriction and they should no longer be used.

Similarly the β_2-sympathomimetics have rendered ephedrine obsolete. Ephedrine is found in a large number of preparations including Amesec, Asmapax,

Table 2 Features distinguishing chronic bronchitis from asthma

Asthma	Chronic bronchitis
Greater variation in wheezing	More persistent wheezing
Nocturnal wheezing disturbing sleep	Wheezy, tight chest on waking
Specific allergic precipitating factors	Chronic sputum production
Often early onset	Rarely occurs before 40
Often non-smoker	Rarely occurs in non-smokers
Significant reversibility	Less response to bronchodilators

Table 3 Dosages of β_2-sympathomimetics

	Inhaler	Tablets
Salbutamol	$200\mu g$ (2 puffs) 4–6-hourly	2mg or 4mg t.d.s. or q.d.s. Spandets 8mg 12-hourly
Terbutaline	$500\mu g$ (2 puffs) 6-hourly	5mg 8-hourly
Fenoterol	$400\mu g$ (2 puffs) t.d.s. or q.d.s.	—
Rimiterol	$400\mu g$ (2 puffs) Max. 24 puffs/24 hours	—

Expansyl, Franol and Tedral. Amesec, Franol and Tedral also contain a barbiturate, a group of drugs which should not be used in chronic bronchitis or emphysema (see later).

The β_2-sympathomimetics available in the UK are salbutamol (Ventolin), terbutaline (Bricanyl), fenoterol (Berotec) and rimiterol (Pulmadil). Rimiterol has a much shorter duration of action (about an hour, being inactivated by COMT) than the others, which act for between four and six hours. In general the remainder have similar properties in equivalent dosage but fenoterol may have a somewhat longer action than terbutaline or salbutamol. The doses are shown in Table 3.

It is rational to give bronchodilators by inhalation, for high levels are then achieved where needed in the bronchi with minimal blood levels. The relief of bronchospasm with an inhaled β-sympathomimetic is rapid, starting within a minute or two and reaching a maximum in 10 to 20 minutes. The bronchodilatation after an oral dose of a β-sympathomimetic occurs much more slowly and is of smaller magnitude. There is also evidence that the duration of action of an inhaled dose is greater. Bronchodilatation after an oral dose is only achieved with high blood levels leading to a much greater incidence of side-effects, particularly tremor.

An inhaler can be used regularly to give effective prophylactic therapy for wheezing instead of an oral bronchodilator, with the added advantage of also being available for 'rescue' relief of wheezing. It is imperative that patients are shown how to use inhalers and their technique should be checked at intervals. Incorrect technique is otherwise common. Despite careful supervision some, particularly in the older age groups, never learn to co-ordinate activation of the aerosol and inspiration. In order to overcome this difficulty a spacer device has recently been introduced (Bricanyl Spacer) but its effectiveness is yet to be proved.

For those who cannot learn to use an inhaler correctly, the alternatives are to resort to oral therapy or salbutamol Rotacaps from a Rotahaler. The latter device gets round the problem of co-ordination with inspiration but demands dexterity to assemble and to cut the capsule. Capsules are available containing 200 micrograms or 400 micrograms of salbutamol.

Maximal bronchodilatation will be obtained with an inhaler alone and giving a β-sympathomimetic orally in addition will not produce further benefit but will greatly increase the frequency of side-effects.

OTHER ROUTES OF ADMINISTRATION

During the treatment of exacerbations of chronic bronchitis in hospital other routes of administration of β_2-sympathomimetics are used. Salbutamol or terbutaline may be given by continuous intravenous infusion or by nebulisation. Either technique is effective and there is probably little to choose between them. However, an ill, severely obstructed patient may not, at times, be able to use a nebuliser, particularly if previously unfamiliar with the technique.

A drug solution may be nebulised either by a stream of gas at an appropriate flow rate or by ultrasonic vibration produced by a piezo-electric crystal. The gas flow may be provided by a cylinder or by a compressor. Such devices may produce a continuous or an intermittent flow, usually achieved with an intermittent positive pressure breathing (IPPB) technique triggered by the patient on inspiration. These IPPB devices are much more costly and complex than the simple compressors which are now available. IPPB has the advantage that, being triggered, the drug is not wasted because of nebulisation continuing during the expiratory phase. Overall it is doubtful whether IPPB is more effective than simpler systems, although it may be in severely obstructed individuals.

In all cases it is important that the nebuliser unit is properly matched with a compressor of appropriate flow and pressure characteristics. The doses used are much larger than used from metered-dose inhalers (5mg or 10mg salbutamol or terbutaline q.d.s.) and there is a correspondingly higher incidence of side-effects.

There is little evidence as yet to support the domiciliary use of this technique, although preliminary reports (Connelan and Wilson, 1979) suggest it may be of benefit in some patients with severe emphysema. Further investigations into indications, efficacy and equipment are required. Domiciliary nebulisers are not indicated at present and their use must await the answers to these and other questions concerning the safety, servicing and provision of equipment.

Salbutamol injection 500 micrograms subcutaneously or intramuscularly, or 250 micrograms slowly intravenously, may be given to relieve acute episodes of bronchospasm. Alternatively terbutaline in similar dosage may be given.

SIDE-EFFECTS

The commonest side-effect of β_2-sympathomimetics is tremor. It usually occurs with oral treatment but may occasionally be seen after standard inhaler dosage. Tachycardia may also occur but is less than that seen with the non-selective β-stimulators and is a reflex tachycardia in response to peripheral vasodilatation.

CONTRA-INDICATIONS

Isoprenaline and other non-selective β-adrenergic agonists are contra-indicated in acute coronary insufficiency and hyperthyroidism. Special care is required in diabetes and hypertension. The β_2-selective drugs, particularly when a metered-dose inhaler is used in standard dosage, do not have any contra-indications but should be used with caution in hyperthyroidism.

Selective β_2-agonists can be given with cardioselective β-blockers but since selectivity is always relative only, the combination is better avoided.

Xanthines

The bronchodilators theophylline and aminophylline (theophylline in combination with ethylenediamine) belong to this group. These drugs can be shown to increase the concentration of cyclic adenosine monophosphate (3'5' cAMP) by inhibition of the enzyme responsible for its breakdown, phosphodiesterase. Cyclic AMP is an intracellular messenger and an increase in levels leads to bronchodilatation due to smooth muscle relaxation.

The usefulness of this group of drugs is to some extent limited by their narrow therapeutic margin. In order to produce bronchodilatation plasma levels of $10-20\mu g/ml$ must be achieved. Higher levels result in centrally mediated nausea and vomiting, headache and excitation. The xanthines may also cause nausea, vomiting and dyspepsia due to a direct gastric irritant effect. The occurrence of side-effects is minimised by the use of the newer slow-release preparations of aminophylline (Phyllocontin) and theophylline (Nuelin SA) which produce smoother blood levels, avoiding the peaks extending into the toxic range which may follow a dose of a non-controlled release preparation.

It is important to increase the dose gradually to avoid toxic effects, and ideally levels should be measured. Toxic effects can usually be avoided with care. Phyllocontin is available as 225mg and 100mg (paediatric) tablets. The maximum dose is 450mg b.d. and if side-effects occur, it is often useful to tailor the dose by means of the paediatric tablet. Nuelin SA is available as 250mg and 175mg tablets allowing similar flexibility.

Theophylline is 90 per cent metabolised by the liver and the remaining 10 per cent is excreted unchanged in the urine. Any condition impairing liver function, e.g. cirrhosis and congestive cardiac failure, will prolong plasma half-life and lead to higher than expected plasma levels and an increased risk of toxicity. Smoking reduces the plasma half-life of theophylline because of an increased rate of liver metabolism possibly due to liver enzyme induction. Smokers may therefore require a larger dose than non-smokers to achieve satisfactory theophylline levels.

The introduction of modern formulations has made obsolete the older preparations such as aminophylline B.P. with their higher incidence of gastric irritation and unpredictability in terms of the plasma levels achieved. Similarly they should replace the use of aminophylline suppositories with their propensity to produce rectal irritation.

Aminophylline intravenously (250–500mg given over five minutes) is useful when there is an acute exacerbation of wheezing both for its bronchodilator and respiratory stimulant effects. Given too rapidly hypotension may occur and a β-agonist given parenterally may be preferable. Parenteral administration of aminophylline or β-agonists is often associated with a fall in arterial oxygen tension (PaO_2) and if possible should be accompanied by controlled oxygen therapy.

Parasympatholytics

Atropine and related substances have been used since ancient times for the relief of bronchospasm. The systemic effects of atropine have limited its use, although combinations with sympathomimetics have been available (Brontisol, Brovon, PIB etc). With the better understanding of the role of the parasympathetic via the vagus in the maintenance of normal bronchial tone, interest in this group of drugs has increased. The recent introduction of the atropine-like drug ipratropium bromide in a metered-dose inhaler (Atrovent) has provided an additional means of relieving airflow obstruction. Ipratropium bromide has a similar duration of action to the β-sympathomimetics but with a somewhat slower onset. Ipratropium may be particularly effective in chronic bronchitis and response may occur when β-agonists have failed. The normal dose is two puffs (40 micrograms) six-hourly but it is worth trying up to four puffs four-hourly.

Only a very small proportion of the inhaled dose is absorbed and even massive doses have not caused tachycardia or other systemic symptoms. So far no deleterious effects on sputum consistency have been demonstrated. Patients should be advised to ensure that the inhaler is not discharged near or into the eyes.

Combination therapy

As previously discussed there is no point in prescribing both oral and inhaled β-stimulants. There are theoretical advantages in combining a β-stimulator and a xanthine drug, in that their modes of action are different yet complementary. The xanthines work at least in part by increasing cAMP by inhibition of phosphodiesterase, whereas the β-stimulants increase the formation of cAMP by increasing the activity of the enzyme adenylcyclase. *In vitro* experiments have suggested synergism between the two drug groups but clinically only additive effects have been found. Combination is, however, logical and may also allow a similar degree of bronchodilatation at lower individual doses and therefore with fewer side-effects. The best combination is a β-sympathomimetic inhaler and a slow-release xanthine allowing a 'rescue' capability as well as background bronchodilatation.

Similarly it is logical to combine a β-sympathomimetic and ipratropium both by inhaler, as again they have different modes of action. It has been shown (Fig. 3/2) that in severe chronic bronchitis further improvement in respiratory function could be achieved in this way than when either drug was given alone.

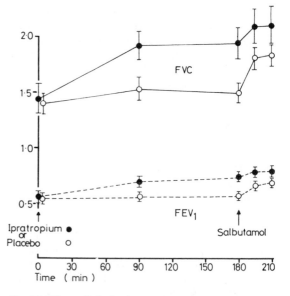

Fig. 3/2 Effects of inhaling ipratropium 80 micrograms or placebo followed by salbutamol 200 micrograms (Douglas et al, 1979). FEV_1 and FVC had risen significantly 180 minutes after ipratropium; salbutamol also produced significant increases in FEV_1 and FVC maximal at 30 minutes. After ipratropium the FEV_1 was significantly greater than after salbutamol. Salbutamol inhaled after ipratropium resulted in significantly higher FEV_1 and FVC than either drug alone. (Reproduced by kind permission of the author, editor and publisher, *Thorax*, **34**, 51–6.)

Steroids

Steroids have a very limited place in the treatment of chronic bronchitis and emphysema and must not be used indiscriminately or without some means of objective assessment of response.

If a substantial degree of reversibility has been demonstrated in response to a bronchodilator (>20 per cent improvement in FEV_1 or PEFR) or marked spontaneous variations in airflow obstruction have been observed, a trial of steroids should be instituted. This should consist of 40mg prednisolone daily for up to four weeks with objective assessment at the beginning, during and at the end of the period. Assessment should be by respiratory function testing and/or a simple exercise test. The five-minute walking test, in which the distance the patient can walk in five minutes is measured, is a convenient method of testing exercise ability. The patient walks at his chosen pace and may stop for as long or as often as he wishes, the clock continuing during his pauses.

Steroids should only be continued if an improvement of at least 20 per cent is observed and the dose should then be reduced to the minimum at which the gain is maintained. In these steroid-responsive individuals it may be possible to reduce oral steroids without a reduction in respiratory function by introducing an inhaled steroid, beclomethasone dipropionate (Becotide) or betamethasone valerate (Bextasol).

Emphysema may from time to time be incorrectly diagnosed when the true diagnosis is chronic asthma. A trial of steroids under proper conditions may then clarify the diagnosis and produce a valuable and rewarding therapeutic response.

A suggested treatment scheme is shown in Table 4.

Table 4 A treatment scheme for airflow obstruction

Inhaled β_2-agonist or ipratropium
Combine
add
Xanthine
add
Steroid

TREATMENT OF COMPLICATIONS

Acute exacerbations

The majority of acute exacerbations of chronic bronchitis are the result of infections. In some studies as many as 60 per cent of all exacerbations have been shown to be associated with demonstrable virus infection. Bronchitics probably suffer the same number and type of respiratory virus infections but are at greater risk of developing lower respiratory tract involvement. Secondary bacterial infection is probably responsible for most of the symptoms and complications.

The bacterial pathogens responsible for the majority of infective acute exacerbations are *Streptococcus pneumoniae* (Pneumococcus) and *Haemophilus influenzae* (May, 1975).

The sputum becomes purulent in the majority of acute exacerbations. However, there may be just an increase in quantity and/or viscidity of the sputum associated with an increase in wheezing and dyspnoea without sputum purulence.

Acute bronchitis in the healthy patient is generally a mild and self-limiting illness. In contrast the consequences may be much more serious in the chronic bronchitic who has little or no respiratory reserve. Central cyanosis, severe dyspnoea or oedema would be indications for admission to hospital.

ANTIBIOTICS

An ever increasing and bewildering variety of antibiotics become available each year. As regards the treatment of acute exacerbations of chronic bronchitis, no evidence exists that more recent and much more expensive additions such as the cephalosporins have any advantage over longer established drugs.

Long-term chemoprophylaxis does not appear to be justified, for although the duration of acute exacerbations may be reduced, the number may not be affected (Medical Research Council, 1966). However, a reduction in the number of exacerbations with chemoprophylaxis was found when the individuals had experienced more than one exacerbation per winter (Johnston et al, 1969). Ensuring that antibiotics when appropriate are given early in the illness is probably more important in limiting the duration of illness (Malone et al, 1968). This can be achieved by providing the patient with a reserve supply of antibiotics. The patient must be carefully instructed to take a full course and be taught to recognise an infective episode. Purulence of the sputum is in itself not necessarily an indication for antibiotics.

Infection is not the primary cause of chronic bronchitis and repeated courses of antibiotics will not abolish the characteristic increased production of mucus. If infections are so numerous that frequent courses of antibiotics are prescribed, continuous antibiotics are worth a trial.

Since the majority of infective exacerbations are due to *Pneumococcus* or *Haemophilus influenzae* and further information from sputum culture rarely modifies management (Paterson et al, 1978), routine culture is not necessary. Sputum should be examined if it remains purulent after one week's treatment or if an unusual organism is suspected. Suitable antibiotics active against Pneumococcus or Haemophilus are:

OXYTETRACYCLINE

Treatment is effective and cheap with 500mg six-hourly. Calcium ions however bind with tetracycline to form a poorly absorbed compound and for maximum absorption tetracyclines should be taken between meals and *not* with milk.

Changes in intestinal flora resulting from the action of unabsorbed drug may lead to loose bowel motions or even frank diarrhoea. Monilial infections of the mouth or vagina may occur, again secondary to the disturbance in the natural flora after long-term use. Rarely photosensitisation and other skin rashes may be seen.

Tetracyclines can induce catabolic effects and lead to a rise in blood urea and are contra-indicated in renal failure and should be avoided in the elderly. They should not be used in pregnancy or early childhood because they cause enamel hypoplasia, cusp malformation and pigmentation of the primary dentition.

A potential disadvantage is that the group is bacteriostatic and eradication of infection may not be achieved in more advanced chronic bronchitis, when the defence mechanisms of the respiratory tract are defective. The group however is active against *Mycoplasma pneumoniae*.

AMPICILLIN
Ampicillin has the advantage of being bactericidal. A dose of 500mg six-hourly is often effective but 1g six-hourly may be required to eradicate Haemophilus.

As with other broad-spectrum antibiotics, moniliasis or diarrhoea may occur. Two types of skin rash may arise, an urticarial rash which usually indicates penicillin hypersensitivity and an erythematous maculopapular rash generally specific to ampicillin.

More recently amoxycillin (Amoxil) has been introduced. This has a similar spectrum of activity to ampicillin but need only be given three times a day, is better absorbed, may cause less diarrhoea and skin rashes and may penetrate better into sputum. Amoxycillin 250mg t.d.s. is as effective as ampicillin 500mg q.d.s. Neither drug should be used when there is a history of penicillin hypersensitivity.

CO-TRIMOXAZOLE
This is a useful alternative particularly in ampicillin or penicillin sensitivity. It is effective at two tablets twice daily, although, because of differences in sputum penetration, the ratio of component concentrations (sulphamethoxazole and trimethoprim) reached is not ideal.

Common side-effects include nausea, vomiting, glossitis, skin rashes and, rarely, blood dyscrasias. Co-trimoxazole should not be used in pregnancy.

A long-acting sulphonamide, sulfametopyrazine (Kelfizine W), has been advocated for prophylactic use in chronic bronchitis, one tablet being taken weekly. There is as yet little evidence as to its efficacy and it has the disadvantage of being relatively expensive. Moreover the prolonged half-life would be a difficult problem were hypersensitivity to arise.

VACCINES
Vaccination against influenza is generally recommended for those with chronic bronchitis. Undoubtedly influenza epidemics can produce a heavy toll in this section of the community, yet in a recent study (McHardy et al, 1980) during which there were two epidemics, influenza virus was seldom isolated in relation to exacerbations. Other viruses particularly rhinoviruses may be more important and influenza vaccination may therefore have little effect on the number of exacerbations.

A pneumococcal vaccine (Pneumovax) is now available for prophylaxis of pneumonia. It is being investigated as to any protective effects regarding acute infective exacerbations of chronic bronchitis.

Cor pulmonale (pulmonary heart failure)

Chronic bronchitis with emphysema is the commonest cause of this syndrome. It is recognised clinically by the presence of central cyanosis, right ventricular hypertrophy, a raised jugular venous pressure, hepatomegaly and peripheral oedema. It is important to exclude other causes of heart failure such as hypertension or ischaemic heart disease. Cor pulmonale was the commonest cause of heart failure seen in acute admissions to hospital in the industrialised north of England in the 1950s and 1960s. It has been reported to be the commonest cause of death in chronic bronchitis and emphysema (Howard, 1974).

The treatment of cor pulmonale demands an understanding of the patho-physiology and an appreciation that hypoxia is the key underlying factor. Hypoxia causes pulmonary arteriolar vasoconstriction which leads to pulmonary hypertension and eventually right ventricular hypertrophy.

The concept that in time the right ventricle fails and oedema appears is an over-simplification. Elevations in pulmonary artery pressure do occur, particularly in acute exacerbations and on exercise. However, these are relatively mild. The right ventricular mechanics are often surprisingly normal and the fluid retention seen in right-sided heart failure is often absent in cor pulmonale. There is evidence from weight changes and isotope studies that the oedema is more the consequence of fluid redistribution. The emphasis has therefore moved from treatment orientated to heart failure towards that of the hypoxia and its metabolic sequelae.

The therapeutic objectives are therefore the alleviation of oedema and hypoxia and in addition management of infective episodes and airflow obstruction as previously discussed.

OEDEMA
The first episode of oedema may occur insidiously but is not infrequently precipitated by an infective episode. More than mild degrees of oedema, particularly when associated with infection and an acute exacerbation of respiratory failure should be treated in hospital because

controlled oxygen therapy is then the most important aspect of management (see below). Initially, one of the powerful loop diuretics is usually required. Treatment should be started with frusemide (Lasix 80–160mg daily) or bumetanide (Burinex 2–4mg daily), the dose being adjusted according to response. Potassium supplements should be given or, alternatively, one of the potassium-sparing diuretics, for example triamterene (Dytac 100–200mg daily). Adding a potassium-sparing diuretic rather than potassium supplements has the advantage of potentiating the diuresis and reducing the total number of tablets to be taken. Spironolactone (Aldactone-A) is an alternative but produces more side-effects (nausea, jaundice and painful gynaecomastia). A potassium-sparing diuretic and potassium supplements should not be used together because of the risk of hyperkalaemia. With resolution of the oedema, the dose of diuretic should be reduced progressively and it may sometimes be possible to substitute one of the longer-acting thiazides such as cyclopenthiazide 0.25–0.5mg daily or bendrofluazide 5–10mg daily.

The role of digoxin in cor pulmonale has long been debated and with the modern understanding of the causation of oedema, digoxin is only indicated for arrhythmias. Digoxin should not be used routinely, for digoxin-induced arrhythmias are potentiated by hypoxia.

OXYGEN

In chronic respiratory failure and cor pulmonale, sensitivity to carbon dioxide as a respiratory stimulant is diminished. Hypoxia then becomes the main factor controlling ventilation rather than the arterial carbon dioxide tension ($PaCO_2$) as in normals. Giving oxygen to relieve hypoxia can remove this hypoxic drive causing hypoventilation, and paradoxically a fall in PaO_2 and rise in $PaCO_2$, carbon dioxide narcosis and acidosis. Oxygen must be given at *low* concentrations using either a low concentration mask (e.g. Ventimask) or nasal cannulae at a low flow rate (nasal cannulae and a flow of 2 litres/minute oxygen gives an inspired concentration of approximately 30%). Higher concentrations are dangerous and must not be used. This technique of low concentration oxygen enrichment, the flow rate being titrated by monitoring the arterial blood gases, has been called controlled oxygen therapy.

Although the mortality in acute episodes of cor pulmonale has improved with the introduction of broad-spectrum antibiotics, powerful diuretics and controlled oxygen therapy, the long-term prognosis has not and mortality remains high at 68 per cent five years from the first appearance of oedema. The reason for the poor outlook is the persisting hypoxia.

Over the last decade attempts have been made to correct the hypoxia by giving low concentration oxygen at home for many hours a day. The oxygen has been given mainly at night both to inconvenience the patient as little as possible and also to minimise the fall in PaO_2 known to occur at night. Long-term oxygen therapy has been shown in uncontrolled trials to reduce elevated pulmonary artery pressure, admissions to hospital and improve well-being. Oxygen must be given for at least 12 hours and probably 15 hours a day (Anderson et al, 1973; Stark et al, 1973; Leggett et al, 1976; Howard et al, 1977). This is expensive by currently available methods (cylinders, liquid oxygen) but oxygen concentrators are being evaluated and could make such domiciliary long-term therapy practicable. Oxygen used in this way seems to reduce the decline in PaO_2 (Fig. 3/3), lower or prevent pulmonary artery pressure from rising (Fig. 3/4) and may reduce mortality to one half (Howard et al, 1977). A multicentre controlled trial under the auspices of the Medical Research Council has recently been completed (Report of the Medical Research Council Working Party, *Lancet*, 1981). The patients had chronic bronchitis or emphysema with irreversible airway obstruction, severe arterial hypoxaemia, carbon dioxide retention and a history of oedema. They were randomised to

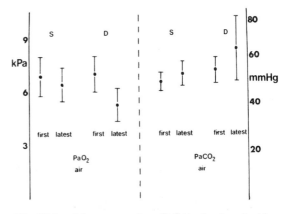

Fig. 3/3 Arterial oxygen tensions (PaO_2) and carbon dioxide tension ($PaCO_2$) in surviving (S) and deceased (D) patients, on long-term oxygen therapy (Howard et al, 1977). The initial PaO_2 of survivors and deceased was similar but the $PaCO_2$ of those who died was higher initially. The PaO_2 did not deteriorate significantly in the survivors but there was a marked deterioration in PaO_2 in those who died. A small but significant rise in $PaCO_2$ occurred in the survivors but there was a much more marked rise in those who died. (Reproduced by kind permission of the author, editor and publisher, *Le Poumon et le Coeur*, **33**, 45–8.)

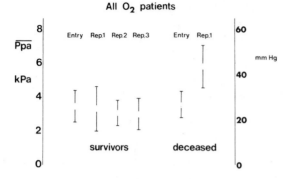

Fig. 3/4 Pulmonary artery pressure and long-term domiciliary oxygen therapy (Anderson, unpublished observations). The mean pulmonary artery pressure (P$\overline{\text{pa}}$) of 40 patients given 12 or 15 hours oxygen daily is shown at entry to the study and at later intervals. P$\overline{\text{pa}}$ was similar initially for those who survive and those who have died. However, the P$\overline{\text{pa}}$ did not change in the survivors but rose significantly in the deceased patients

oxygen therapy (2 litres/minute via nasal cannulae for 15 hours daily) or to a control group. Mortality in both men and women was reduced over three years. The time spent in hospital because of exacerbations of respiratory failure and the work attendance were not affected by oxygen therapy.

There is so far no evidence that long-term oxygen produces benefit in other causes of chronic hypoxia and it must be given for long periods in the day to produce any physiological improvement. Most of the prescriptions for oxygen at present are for intermittent, casual use. Used in this way oxygen is little more than an expensive placebo and this practice can only be deplored. Oxygen should never be prescribed lightly, for there are potential hazards in terms of fire risk and carbon dioxide narcosis.

RESPIRATORY STIMULANTS

These have only a limited place in therapy. Nikethamide (Coramine) should no longer be used. Doxapram (Dopram) is safer, being less likely to cause convulsions and is more effective. Its main use is as an adjunct to controlled oxygen therapy when it is given by intravenous infusion, but it can also be given as a bolus to stimulate respiration acutely. The commonest side-effect is a sensation of perineal warmth. Tachycardia, hypertension and dizziness may also occur. Other sensitisers of peripheral chemoreceptors which can be given orally are currently being evaluated.

DRUGS CONTRA-INDICATED IN CHRONIC BRONCHITIS AND EMPHYSEMA

All drugs with respiratory depressant effects should be avoided particularly in those with chronic respiratory failure. These include *all* hypnotics, sedatives and tranquillisers. The narcotic analgesics should be used with great caution preferably only when means of artificial ventilation are immediately available and certainly with a drug for their reversal to hand (e.g. naloxone (Narcan) 0.4mg IV repeated as necessary). Potentially fatal respiratory depression may follow commonly used drugs such as dihydrocodeine (DF 118) or prochlorperazine (Stemetil). Beta-blockers may cause airflow obstruction and are best avoided.

THE FUTURE

The development of oxygen concentrators enabling larger numbers of patients to be treated, promises more effective management of chronic respiratory failure. Research is proceeding in the field of drugs to lower pulmonary vascular resistance in hypoxic pulmonary hypertension, although this is still at a preliminary phase. An alternative approach to the problem of breathlessness, particularly when out of proportion to the loss of pulmonary function as in emphysema, is by attempts to suppress the sensation itself with drugs such as diazepam, and this may be an exciting development.

Undoubtedly the prevention of chronic bronchitis by health education programmes to reduce smoking and in the control of atmospheric pollution are the most important measures required to limit morbidity and mortality. Nevertheless, established cases will continue to present considerable problems for the health services for many years.

REFERENCES

Anderson, P. B., Cayton, R. M., Holt, P. J. and Howard, P. (1973). Long-term oxygen therapy in cor pulmonale. *Quarterly Journal of Medicine*, **42**, 563–73.

Connellan, S. J. and Wilson, R. S. E. (1979). The use of domiciliary nebulised salbutamol in the treatment of severe emphysema. *The British Journal of Clinical Practice*, **3**, 135–6.

Davies, R. J. (1979). Chronic lung disease. Allergic lung disease. *British Journal of Hospital Medicine*, **22/2**, 136–50.

Douglas, N. J., Davidson, I., Sudlow, M. F. and Flenley, D. C. (1979). Bronchodilatation and the site of airway resistance in severe chronic bronchitis. *Thorax*, **34**, 51–6.

Eriksson, S. (1964). Pulmonary emphysema and alpha₁-antitrypsin deficiency. *Acta Medica Scandinavica*, **175**, 197–205.

Fletcher, C. M. and Peto, R. (1977). The natural history of chronic airflow obstruction. *British Medical Journal*, **1**, 1645–8.

Howard, P. (1974). The changing face of chronic bronchitis with airways obstruction. *British Medical Journal*, **2**, 89–93.

Howard, P., Cayton, R. M., Brennan, S. R. and Anderson, P. B. (1977). Lignocaine aerosol and persistent cough. *British Journal of Diseases of the Chest*, **71**, 19–25.

Howard, P., Anderson, P. B. and Brennan, S. R. (1977). Oxygen therapy for hypoxaemia in association with chronic bronchitis. *Le Poumon et Le Coeur*, **33**, 45–8.

Johnston, R. N., McNeill, R. S., Smith, D. H., Dempster, M. B., Nairn, J. R., Purvis, M. S., Watson, J. M. and Ward, F. G. (1969). Five-year winter chemoprophylaxis for chronic bronchitis. *British Medical Journal*, **4**, 265–9.

Leggett, R. J., Cooke, N. J., Clancy, L., Leitch, A. G., Kirby, B. J. and Flenley, D. C. (1976). Long-term domiciliary oxygen therapy in cor pulmonale complicating chronic bronchitis and emphysema. *Thorax*, **31**, 414–18.

McHardy, V. U., Inglis, J. M., Calder, M. A., Crofton, J. W., Gregg, I., Ryland, D. A., Taylor, P., Chadwick, M., Coombe, D. and Riddell, R. W. (1980). A study of infective and other factors in exacerbations of chronic bronchitis. *British Journal of Diseases of the Chest*, **74**, 228–39.

Malone, D. N., Gould, J. C. and Grant, I. W. B. (1968). A comparative study of ampicillin, tetracycline hydrochloride and methacycline hydrochloride in acute exacerbations of chronic bronchitis. *Lancet*, **2**, 594–6.

May, J. R. (1975). The chemotherapy of chronic bronchitis. *Hospital Update*, **3**, 1, 217–23.

Paterson, I. C., Petrie, G. R., Crompton, G. K. and Robertson, J. R. (1978). Chronic bronchitis: is bacteriological examination of sputum necessary? *British Medical Journal*, **2**, 537–8.

Raw, M., Jarvis, M. J., Feyerabend, C. and Russell, M. A. H. (1980). Comparison of nicotine chewing gum and psychological treatments for dependent smokers. *British Medical Journal*, **281**, 481–2.

Report to the Medical Research Council by their Working Party on Trials of Chemotherapy in Early Chronic Bronchitis (1966). Value of chemoprophylaxis and chemotherapy in early chronic bronchitis. *British Medical Journal*, **1**, 1317–22.

Report of the Medical Research Council Working Party (1981). Long-term domiciliary oxygen therapy in chronic hypoxic cor pulmonale complicating chronic bronchitis and emphysema. *Lancet*, **1**, 681–5.

Russell, M. A. H., Raw, M. and Jarvis, M. J. (1980). Clinical use of nicotine chewing gum. *British Medical Journal*, **280**, 1599–602.

Stark, R. D., Finnegan, P. and Bishop, J. M. (1973). Long-term domiciliary oxygen in chronic bronchitis with pulmonary hypertension. *British Medical Journal*, **3**, 467–70.

Chapter 4   Asthma

R. A. L. BREWIS MD, FRCP

The development of a relatively small number of new treatments in the past 12 years or so has brought about a complete revolution in the management of asthma and in the results achieved. The future may well see further 'break-throughs' and the introduction of even more effective treatments but, even without further pharmacological advance, there is today great potential for improving the lot of most asthmatic individuals which could be realised by encouraging the more rational application of the treatments already in existence. There must be few areas in medicine where a little expertise and attention to the detail of long-term drug management are productive of such obvious improvement in patients' well-being.

The management of asthma has many similarities with the management of diabetes. In both conditions the prime aim is to make the patient independent, as unrestricted as possible, and able to adjust his own treatment appropriately so as to avoid short-term crises which may threaten life and employment. In both conditions the treatment is commonly required throughout life. Patients with both disorders need to be expert in their own management, partly to protect themselves from misleading advice from medical and non-medical individuals who are casually or temporarily involved in their care. There are certain technical skills to be taught in both conditions. It follows from the above that doctors treating asthma become involved in an educational process. Proper guidance, particularly early on in contact with a patient, takes time – merely issuing a prescription for whatever drug is perceived to be most needed is not enough. The remarks which follow summarise some of the points which one clinician feels to be important in the management of asthma and, except for the following section, are geared to the management of the adult. It is taken for granted that the adult asthmatic patient does not smoke.

CHILDHOOD ASTHMA

Space does not allow a detailed review of the drug management of asthma in childhood, but a few features of current practice are worth noting.

In very young children (before about 18 months) there is an important lack of responsiveness to both β-agonist and theophylline bronchodilator preparations however administered. Compressor-driven nebulisers have found increasing use in recent years for the administration of β-agonists to small children with severe asthma. This method of delivery is especially valuable before the age when a child can use pressurised or powder-based inhaled preparations, but even after that age the nebuliser may be found useful in an exacerbation. Regular treatment with inhaled cromoglycate or regular oral (slow-release) theophylline preparations provide good suppression of otherwise regular asthma and are roughly equal in effectiveness. Inhaled steroid aerosol treatment is a highly effective regular prophylactic but tends to be reserved for children who have not achieved satisfactory control with regular cromoglycate and/or theophylline. The powder form of beclomethasone (Becotide Rotacaps) can be managed from between three and five years; older children find the pressurised form more convenient.

Oral corticosteroids may be required to restore control during a severe exacerbation or, equally importantly, when chronic severe asthma has led to a severe functional defect which may be tolerated uncomplainingly and be unaccompanied by any dramatic signs. As in adults the aim is to use oral corticosteroids in short courses promptly when control with regular prophylactic measures breaks down. In severe asthma, parents should be empowered to initiate such a short course if unacceptable delay is to be avoided. In those few children requiring long-term steroid administration to control severe asthma alternate-day administration is finding increasing favour as a means of minimising side-effects.

The importance of proper understanding on the part of patient and parents can hardly be overstated. From a very early age the child should feel involved in and, with increasing age, increasingly responsible for his treatment. Gratifying benefits follow from positively encouraging full normal activities. Most children with asthma can take part in sport and some can excel if sufficient attention is paid to protective medication. Swimming is particularly well tolerated.

For a detailed discussion of the management of childhood asthma the reader is referred to an article by Landau (1979) and a neighbouring paper on related clinical pharmacology by Weinberger et al (1981). The use of bronchodilator drugs in childhood is well reviewed by Milner (1981).

ADULT ASTHMA

Patient's initial understanding

Before turning to the practicalities of treatment for asthma it is worth ensuring that the patient has some reasonable understanding of the nature of asthma. Enquiry may reveal the most surprising ideas of what happens inside the chest or throat and very muddled ideas about causation (as well as firmly fixed notions about certain treatments). Particular patients require different degrees of detail but all should understand that there is a real change in calibre of the bronchial tubes and that cough, wheeze, tightness and thick sputum are all part of the same process and are managed by the same means.

The extent to which external substances may or may not be important needs to be sensibly discussed and it may be necessary to reassure the patient that asthma is not the consequence of emotional disturbance.

Individuals who have developed regularly troublesome asthma relatively recently after previously normal health require a particularly patient and unhurried discussion of their position before treatment is recommended. Such individuals are often seeking some treatment which will, at a stroke, restore them to the state they were in some months earlier. In this situation the concept of regular self-medication is likely to be rejected – or tried only tentatively and stopped because of 'side-effects': the patient remaining dissatisfied, believing that his requirement has just not been recognised by the doctor. This is an important cause of apparent failure of the standard treatments. It is therefore essential to show that the wish is understood completely and to indicate that there is, at present, no procedure or treatment that can fulfil it. It is generally unwise to predict whether or not the future may hold a return to their former state but it may be helpful to refer to the likelihood of a fluctuating course – good phases and bad phases – with the confident forecast that they can become expert at controlling and containing the bad phases with the proper use of available treatments.

Allergen avoidance and desensitisation

Much has been written in the past on these subjects and in this brief review only a few comments are relevant. Most patients who are sensitive to important external allergens know this already. House dust (mite) and grass pollen are the commonest aggravating agents. It is difficult to do more than common sense suggests by way of avoiding grass pollen and even the most assiduous measures to reduce the house-dust mite population have disappointingly little effect. Pets are not often sources of relevant allergen unless it is already obvious to the patient. Desensitisation treatment is very unreliable compared with regular suppressive treatment and it carries a very small but important risk of severe hypersensitivity reactions. It follows from the above that there is only rarely an indication to carry out skin tests. Aspirin hypersensitivity is an important phenomenon causing severe attacks of asthma which may be delayed by half an hour or so after consumption of aspirin so that the cause may be overlooked. It occurs in perhaps 10 per cent of adult asthmatics and the risks of aspirin should be discussed with every patient and avoidance advised unless the patient is known not to be sensitive. Hypersensitivity to aspirin is particularly likely to accompany adult onset asthma without extrinsic features and with nasal polyposis. Aspirin-sensitive individuals should be warned not to take any anti-rheumatic agents as the many new non-steroidal anti-inflammatory drugs can also precipitate attacks. Subjects who demonstrate aspirin hypersensitivity also react to tartrazine dyes which are widely used as colouring agents in soft drinks (especially orange juice), soups, confections and tablets, usually to produce a yellow or orange colour.

DRUG MANAGEMENT OF ASTHMA

The availability of effective drugs means that a fairly standard approach to the management of asthma can now be adopted. Some modification is, of course, required to match the severity of the disorder and it may be helpful to review drug management in circumstances of increasing severity.

Assessment of the severity of asthma

The patients's own account of the severity of his symptoms will usually reflect both severity and progress but some individuals are very stoical and this can result in even experienced observers misjudging the severity. Simple ventilatory tests such as peak expiratory flow rate (PEFR) or inspection of a forced expiratory (FEV_1) spirogram are an essential aid to assessment. As there is often a very large diurnal variation in the readings measurements are principally of value in making the clinician aware of just how severe the airways obstruction is at the time rather than offering a definitive guide to progress. If frequent measurements (two to four times daily) are made by the patient in his own home then a reliable record of progress is obtained (see below). Usually adequate information can be obtained by supporting isolated measurements with the responses to a few key questions. The important questions are: (1) 'How is your chest during the night?' and a note is made of the number of times sleep is interrupted by cough and wheezing dyspnoea in one week and (2) 'How long does it take your chest, in the morning, to become as clear as it is going to become?', the question is usually answered easily and the answer recorded in minutes or hours. Other items like exercise tolerance, loss of schooling or work and the level of bronchodilator usage provide further pointers to progress.

Patients with infrequent minor symptoms who have never exhibited severe asthma

Many individuals in this category will require no treatment at all for much of the time. Exacerbations may be triggered by respiratory infections or the individual may exhibit exercise-induced asthma. Very commonly the only treatment required is a bronchodilator. A bronchodilator aerosol used strategically when significant wheezing and tightness develop is the most effective treatment. It is essential that the patient understands, first, how to use a pressurised aerosol properly and, secondly, the limits to frequency of usage.

The patient with mild asthma requires less exhaustive training than an individual with perpetual symptoms and life-threatening attacks but he does need to understand that the correct response to worsening asthma, which does not respond to his bronchodilator aerosol, is not to progressively increase the dose – but rather to attend his doctor who will consider the use of reserve treatment. The patient should know that the principal reserve treatment is a short course of prednisolone (or equivalent). When an exacerbation of asthma apparently follows acute respiratory infection antibiotic treatment is generally either irrelevant or of peripheral importance. The patient should expect to receive a short course of prednisolone rather than an antibiotic – or at least in addition to an antibiotic.

Exercise induced asthma (EIA)

This phenomenon which is universal in children with asthma is also quite common in younger adults. When it is the principal or sole manifestation of asthma it may be quite puzzling until it is recognised. EIA comprises the development of bronchoconstriction after a period of some minutes of vigorous exercise which persists for many minutes after exercise – much longer than the usual hyperpnoea during recovery from exercise. Historically the ready induction of wheezing dyspnoea after exercise has probably been responsible for the traditional pattern of discouraging activity in asthma, with affected children 'being excused from games' at school. There is rarely any need for such restriction now. EIA may be largely suppressed by prior administration of a bronchodilator aerosol or prior administration of cromoglycate (Intal); sometimes both are required for optimal control. With these simple measures many young people prone to asthma are capable of excelling in athletic pursuits. Reference to this is often helpful and encouraging – especially in the case of parents who, consciously or unconsciously, may have been discouraging activity to avoid aggravation of symptoms.

Patients with regular asthma who have never exhibited severe asthma

One of the most useful indicators of regular asthma is the presence in the morning of a sensation of chest tightness which takes a perceptible time to clear. If this is a matter of minutes it is generally acceptable to the patient without special measures being necessary, but if it persists for an hour or more then regular prophylactic treatment will generally be worthwhile. A second indicator of 'regular' asthma is nocturnal asthma. The patient commonly blames cough for interruption of sleep rather than wheezing. If the patient is woken regularly at night then regular prophylactic treatment is generally indicated. Nocturnal attacks, even if mild and promptly resolved by a bronchodilator aerosol, are a marker of unstable control. Some individuals have 'regular' mild asthma for only part of the year or for some weeks after respiratory infections. A third indicator of regular asthma is the level of consumption of bronchodilator aerosol. If the patient requires a replacement for a pressurised aerosol (200 dose nominal content) every two to three months this represents very modest use and regular prophylactic treatment is probably not needed. On the other hand if a replacement is required every three to four weeks then regular prophylactic treatment will probably bring about gratifying improvement in the control of symptoms. The term 'prophylactic' is used here to indicate regular suppressive medication with either a topical steroid preparation or sodium cromoglycate taken in the form of an aerosol by inhalation.

CROMOGLYCATE

Sodium cromoglycate (Intal) came into use in the late 1960s and has an impressive record of safety. Its role in stabilising sensitised mast cells is widely understood by clinicians and this elegantly demonstrated finding has tended to cast cromoglycate in the role of a treatment reserved for those with extrinsic features. However, some patients without these features are satisfactorily controlled by cromoglycate. In extrinsic asthma and in children, asthma is usually readily controlled by either cromoglycate or steroid aerosol treatment and it is unhelpful to argue that one treatment is better than the other. Patients with persistent symptoms and severe disease are often found to be unresponsive to cromoglycate but responsive to treatment with a steroid aerosol. The reverse situation (failure of steroid aerosol with success of cromoglycate) is seldom seen and, when it is, it is usually attributable to poor co-ordination in the use of a pressurised aerosol. In adult patients most clinicians use a steroid aerosol from the start as it is more reliably followed by successful control.

The usual requirement is one capsule of sodium cromoglycate (20mg) four times daily but many patients find satisfactory control can be achieved with one or two capsules. It is essential that the patient grasps three important points about treatment – its preventive function, the need for regular treatment and the lack of any immediate effect. Cromoglycate should be given in the form of plain powder. There is a compound capsule available containing a mixture of cromoglycate and isoprenaline and patients using this tend to become confused about its purpose so that it is best avoided. It is useful for the patient to keep his bronchodilator inhalation separate from his prophylactic treatment partly because the intensity of bronchodilator usage is a helpful signal to doctor and patient indicating the possible need for alternative measures. It is important that the patient should be shown how to use the inhaler (Spinhaler) – preferably by the doctor – and that the doctor should witness the patient using it (see below).

STEROID AEROSOLS

These agents may be regarded as the hinge-pin of the modern management of asthma. Virtually all patients with regular asthma who are not already well controlled by cromoglycate will show gratifying improvement or complete suppression of their asthma with regular medication with steroid aerosols. The few exceptions are those who are totally opposed to the idea of inhalant treatment, those who are unable to perform the necessary manoeuvre and a small group of extremely severe asthmatics who are relatively resistant to corticosteroid treatment however it is administered. It is sensible for all patients with severe asthma requiring regular oral corticosteroid treatment to be also taking a steroid aerosol in at least standard dosage. This is in order that it can be continuously demonstrated that the oral corticosteroid is really necessary despite the best use of the aerosol route.

The principle underlying steroid aerosol treatment is that very small doses of highly topically active corticosteroid may have an effect equivalent to much larger doses administered orally. The well known side-effects of systemic administration are totally avoided with aerosol steroid preparations used in standard dosage. The only side-effect seen is oro-pharyngeal candidiasis. This is most likely to arise when above-standard dosage is employed, with antibiotic treatment, in elderly subjects and in those with dentures. It is easily controlled by antifungal agents and treatment should not be interrupted. The complication can be largely avoided by taking the aerosol before meals or by rinsing the mouth after inhalations.

The most widely used steroid aerosol preparation is beclomethasone dipropionate (Becotide) which is available in a pressurised inhaler giving a metered puff of 50 micrograms. There is a further steroid aerosol preparation available in similar form giving a metered puff of 100 micrograms of betamethasone-17-valerate (Bextasol). Beclomethasone dipropionate is also prepared in dry powder form inhaled from a capsule by means of a simple breath-actuated device (Rotahaler). Two strengths are marketed, 100 micrograms and 200 micrograms, which are in practice roughly equivalent in effect to one and two puffs respectively from the pressurised preparation. The powder form is best reserved for those who are found to be unable to inhale efficiently using the more convenient pressurised device. Proper coaching in the use of all aerosols is essential (see below). The patient must understand the preventive role of the steroid aerosol and should not expect any immediate relief from an inhalation. If the actual inhalation causes coughing or if the patient has wheezing or chest tightness when a dose is due, a bronchodilator aerosol should be used a few minutes before the dose is taken. The need for regular treatment must be stressed and, as the usual requirement is two puffs four times daily, it may assist the patient's memory if treatment before meals is recommended. Many individuals achieve satisfactory control of symptoms with twice-daily or even once-daily inhalation but the requirement for regular usage remains for as long as treatment is in use. If asthmatic symptoms are completely controlled for several weeks the patient should be encouraged to reduce systematically the number of inhalations in the day at weekly intervals. It will usually be found that the re-appearance of morning tightness of more than transient duration or the return of nocturnal cough and wheeze serve as useful indications of the lowest tolerable dosage. Further reduction will certainly be accompanied by more troublesome asthma and in some by a proneness to abrupt attacks. The doctor's aim should be to encourage the patient to carry out occasional systematic testing of the requirement for regular treatment while avoiding any impression that it is important to 'try to get off inhalers' or that failure to withdraw treatment represents addiction, weakness of character or a grave outlook. Acceptable control of asthma should remain the first priority.

It is important that the patient should understand that steroid inhalation may be ineffective during an exacerbation when a short course of oral corticosteroid (see below) will usually be indicated. For the same reason a steroid aerosol should not be introduced alone during an exacerbation of other than mild severity. The patient will almost certainly be disappointed by the lack of benefit and this will seriously undermine confidence in the preparation. One of the commonest reasons for hospital referral of patients whose asthma has failed to respond to standard measures is rejection (or disguised under-use) of steroid aerosol treatment because it proved ineffective when it was (inappropriately) introduced for the first time during a severe exacerbation.

USE OF INHALERS
The effectiveness of treatments administered by inhalation is greatly increased by proper training in the technique of inhalation. It is generally insufficient merely to provide a prescription for the medication and to hope that the patient will learn its proper use. A significant proportion will fail completely through either misunderstanding, apprehension or incoordination. The demonstration of inhalation is probably best done by the doctor and ideally he or she should inhale the genuine preparation rather than a dummy. In the case of the dry powder preparations it is especially important for the doctor to inhale the powder rather than merely pretending to do so. As well as demonstrating proper technique the doctor by this means also conveys confidence in the preparation and in its safety. The patient should be observed using the aerosol. Where performance is poor it may be worth training a relative to coach the patient. Where performance with a pressurised aerosol is hopeless and does not improve then the dry powder inhaler (Rotahaler) should be tried. The inhalation technique

is easier and little co-ordination is required but some clumsy individuals who find inhalation difficult also find loading of the inhaler difficult. In the case of bronchodilator inhalation it is worth trying a spacing device developed for use with a pressurised terbutaline aerosol (Spacer-inhaler; Bricanyl). The metered aerosol dose is pre-discharged into a small box-like extension of the mouthpiece and the patient inhales the aerosol from this as soon as possible afterwards. Precise synchronisation of the inspiration with discharge of the aerosol is no longer important. It is worth checking the technique of inhalation later in the long-term management of patients with asthma when this is less than adequately controlled. Some individuals develop ineffective habits such as inhaling through clenched teeth, discharging into the mouth and inhaling through the nose (especially smokers) or trying to discharge two quick puffs into a single inhalation. Good inhalation technique with a pressurised aerosol can be made even more effective by inhaling vigorously through the widely-opened mouth with the mouthpiece held just outside the lips.

ORAL CORTICOSTEROID TREATMENT
Another important cornerstone in the management of patients with more than mild asthma is training in the use of a *self-initiated* short course of prednisolone (or equivalent). This is essential for patients who have had previous hospital admissions or who have had other expressions of life-threatening asthma and it is very desirable for those taking regular steroid aerosol treatment. A short course of oral steroid should be started early in an exacerbation of asthma rather than late. This is because it is more effective started early, unnecessary distress is avoided, and the total dosage of the short course can generally be much less. An early start will only be achieved by training the patient to initiate treatment. The reasons for this conclusion are as follows: (1) Most patients defer seeking help from their doctor in an exacerbation whatever they are told; (2) Individual doctors are less available than formerly and (3) If the patient's regular doctor is not available his deputy is highly unlikely to initiate steroid treatment on first acquaintance with the patient and very likely to give either an antibiotic or a bronchodilator as a first measure. There is a widely held view that it is an act of treachery to start an asthmatic on the 'slippery slope' of taking steroids for asthma and doctors still tend to hold back from being the first to give such treatment. The understandable desire to protect the patient from side-effects has resulted in steroid treatment being regarded by many as a 'last resort' treatment so that it is given only when the patient has had severe asthma for

many days. The experience of former years was that it was regularly difficult to withdraw oral steroids from patients with severe asthma because of troublesome recurrence of symptoms. However, since the advent of steroid aerosols it is uncommon for this to be the case. If after satisfactory control of asthma a short course of prednisolone cannot be withdrawn then the individual has particularly severe asthma or, alternatively, the aerosol treatment is inadequate either in dosage or efficiency of administration. If there is a real need for long-term oral corticosteroid treatment this requirement will only become evident after many weeks or months of careful attention to the detail of the supporting treatment.

The short course. A short course of oral steroid treatment is a safe procedure carrying much less hazard than poorly controlled asthma. The patient must understand the clear distinction between the known hazards of long-term treatment in high dosage and the negligible risks of a short course of the same drug. It should be understood that the drug is not addictive and furthermore that its efficacy is not dulled by previous exposure to it (both of these points are significant worries which are commonly harboured by patients and they require to be articulated and neutralised). The patient who is to be trained to initiate his own short course of steroids needs precise guidance firstly, on how much to take and, secondly, on the indications for starting. Advice must be accompanied by a written summary because the need for a short course may not arise for many months after the training interview. The 'instructions' and the steroid tablets should be kept together in the same place.

How much? Individual requirements naturally vary but a few general points may be noted. If the short course is started promptly in an obvious exacerbation then the total requirement will tend to be less than when the start of treatment is delayed. It is common to find that very short courses are effective (for example 20mg of prednisolone on the first and second days, 10mg on the third and fourth days and then nothing). Ultra-short courses such as this emphasise the temporary nature of the treatment and do not alarm the patient, family or doctor. Experience with the individual patient may show that a bigger starting dose or a more protracted course is required. The dose should not be reduced from the initial level until definite improvement is noted and treatment with a steroid aerosol should be continued throughout the episode. Adrenal suppression is not a problem with short courses of prednisolone. Several weeks of regular steroid consumption

are required before clinically appreciable effects accompany abrupt withdrawal. The only reasons for including a step-wise reduction in dosage in the recommended course are first, that a smaller dose is usually effective once improvement has begun and, secondly, it allows warning of a continuing tendency to severe asthma.

When? The indications for starting a short course of oral corticosteroid must be readily recognisable by the patient and they must also be sufficiently early features of an exacerbation to allow it to be aborted promptly. A number of indications have been found to meet both requirements. The patient is advised to start a short course if *any one* of the following six circumstances is encountered:

1. Severe wheezing is unrelieved by a bronchodilator aerosol ('inhaler doesn't work').
2. Cough and wheezing interrupt sleep at night either repeatedly or for a long period leading to tiredness the following day through lack of sleep ('terrible nights').
3. Morning symptoms, instead of being brief, last for many hours before the day's optimum is reached ('morning tightness lasts till lunchtime').
4. Wheezing dyspnoea prevents the patient from moving about to carry out normal daily tasks ('immobilised').
5. Progressive deterioration occurs over several days so that the above features are clearly inevitable ('getting worse day by day').
6. An emergency intravenous injection is given by a doctor.

Any exacerbation of asthma severe enough to require intravenous bronchodilator treatment is severe enough for a short course of oral corticosteroid to be started. Some doctors, notably casualty officers working in accident and emergency departments, omit this if there is early improvement after the injection. Severe asthma may then recur a few hours later or perhaps the following night.

The vast majority of patients admitted to hospital as emergencies because of severe asthma will have crossed most of the six thresholds mentioned above a day or two before admission and hardly any of these will have initiated appropriate treatment with oral corticosteroids. It is usual for patients admitted to hospital to have had clear features of deteriorating asthma for one week.

It is difficult to assert that most asthmatic deaths would be avoided by prompt self-medication because there are certainly examples of sudden fatal asthma developing on a background of apparently complete control of asthmatic symptoms. However, experience has shown that well-trained patients with severe or volatile asthma are able to avoid hospital admission whereas a high proportion of those admitted are, by comparison, untrained. In some centres a policy of self-admission to hospital by patients with asthma has been evolved. Patients who recognise the development of severe asthma make their own arrangements without waiting for a prior visit from their own doctor. The need for this arrangement is probably limited to a very few patients and training in prompt self-initiation of short courses of oral corticosteroid means that most severe asthma is adequately terminated outside hospital.

The level of consumption of prednisolone is readily controlled by the doctor prescribing only one or two short courses at a time and personally checking all prescriptions for replacement. In practice excessive self-medication is very unusual in trained patients and undue postponement of a short course is a more common error of treatment. It is then helpful to tell patients that, when in doubt, it is better to start a short course and for it to turn out to be a 'false alarm' – than to delay unnecessarily. The inexperienced patient should consult his or her doctor soon after starting the course. Sufficient tablets for one short course should always be held in reserve.

PATIENT EDUCATION

It is very important that all patients with asthma understand that there are three sorts of treatment for asthma:

1. Treatment to *relieve* asthma
2. Treatment to *prevent* asthma
3. *Reserve* treatment for severe asthma.

There is only a small proportion of patients who cannot be trained to organise their own short-term relief, regular prevention and, where necessary, their own short course of prednisolone. The patient with severe or regularly troublesome asthma needs to understand more than 60 pieces of information relating to his treatment so that, as well as spending time with the patient, the doctor needs to exploit every available aid to memory and understanding. Techniques derived from the worlds of education and salesmanship are as relevant as purely medical skills in this context. I have found the drawing of a diagram (Figs. 4/1(a) and (b)) to be the most helpful and effective way of conveying and recording information. The diagram is built up anew for each patient and the arrangement remains constant so that it can be repeated or added to if necessary. I

have *not* found it helpful to give patients a photocopied ready-made diagram for a number of reasons: only a proportion will read it; the doctor cannot monitor understanding if they do read it and, even if the doctor reads through the prepared scheme with them, there is a tendency for attention to wander to part of it that is not under discussion. If a new diagram is prepared every time attention is forcibly directed to the new part being added as it builds up and instruction is slowed to a manageable pace by the need to write each item clearly. The diagram can also be varied slightly to suit the individual – omitting detail in those of limited understanding – including names of drugs familiar to the patient etc. The specially prepared sheet also has more authority than a mass-produced item which the patient is inclined to regard as not necessarily applying to him/her in some respects. The diagram is made on ordinary A4 paper and the layout is as shown in Figures 4/1(a) and (b). Provided the patient is attentive and receptive, reference is made to oral bronchodilators, antibiotics and other treatment that may be encountered in future even if he/she is not using them at the time. Severe asthmatics should understand that during a severe exacerbation commencement of an antibiotic alone or of an oral bronchodilator will not terminate the episode.

THE UNRESPONSIVE PATIENT

A few patients have unacceptably severe asthma despite the measures described above. The first steps in any attempt to help such individuals are to check that the steroid aerosol is being used regularly and that the technique of inhalation is good. If inhalation using a pressurised aerosol is faulty then the Rotahaler version should be used. Supervised training in aerosol use is particularly important in the patient who is experiencing poor control of symptoms.

The next step should be to determine the degree of improvement that the patient is capable of by initiating a course of oral prednisolone which under these investigative circumstances should be of rather higher dosage and potentially of longer duration than the self-administered short courses described above. It is very helpful if the patient undertakes regular measurements of the peak flow rate (PEFR) during this therapeutic trial. Observations should preferably be recorded four times daily using an inexpensive peak flow gauge. A number of things may be revealed, for example it may be found that the asthma is abolished but returns when oral prednisolone is withdrawn or that asthma is truly trivial or that it is severe and unresponsive to prednisolone etc.

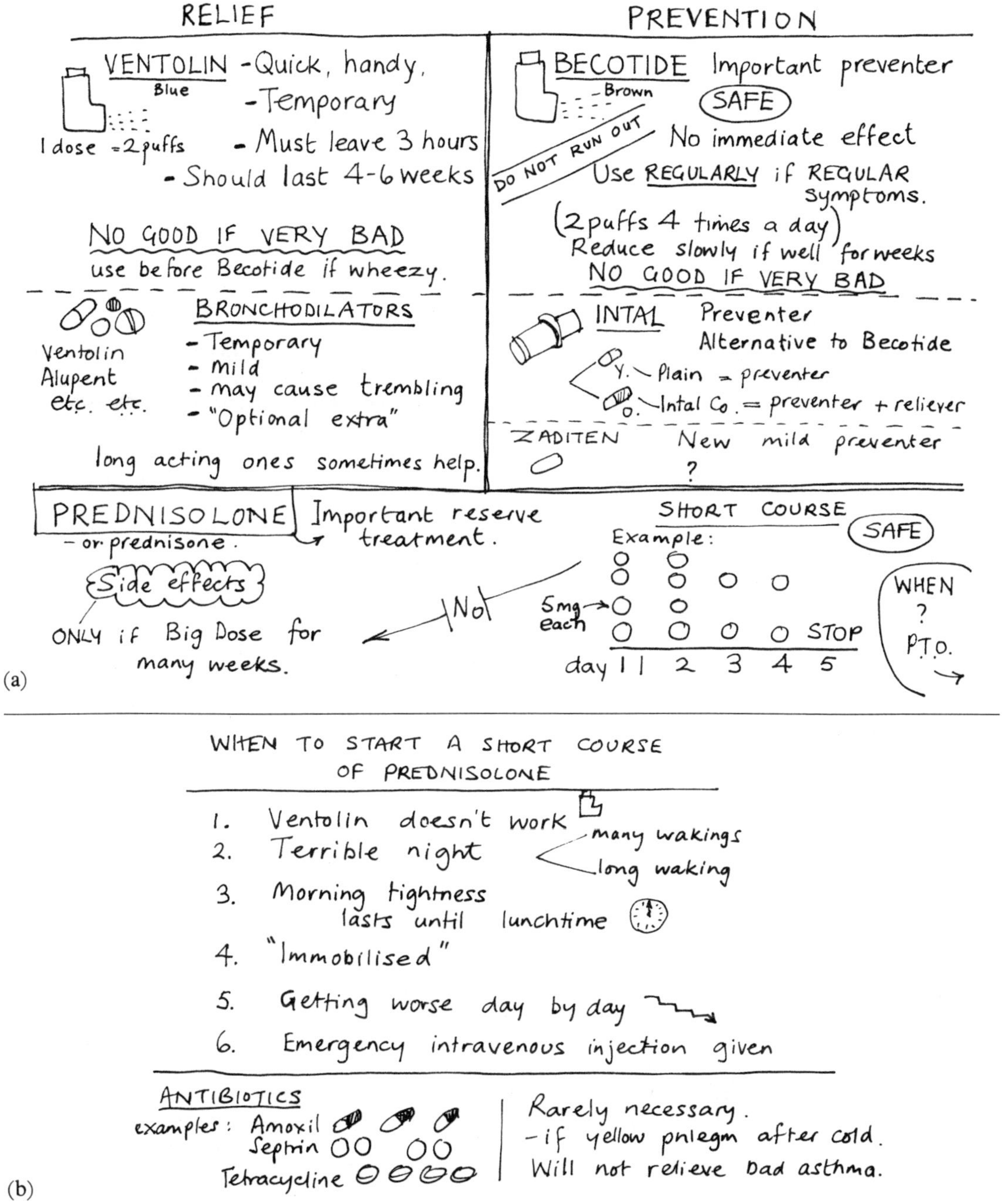

RELIEF | PREVENTION

VENTOLIN – Quick, handy,
Blue
  – Temporary
I dose = 2 puffs – Must leave 3 hours
  – Should last 4-6 weeks

NO GOOD IF VERY BAD
use before Becotide if wheezy.

BECOTIDE Important preventer
Brown
(SAFE)
DO NOT RUN OUT No immediate effect
Use REGULARLY if REGULAR
symptoms.
(2 puffs 4 times a day)
Reduce slowly if well for weeks
NO GOOD IF VERY BAD

BRONCHODILATORS
Ventolin – Temporary
Alupent – mild
etc. etc. – may cause trembling
  – "Optional extra"

long acting ones sometimes help.

INTAL Preventer
Alternative to Becotide
Y. – Plain = preventer
O. – Intal Co. = preventer + reliever

ZADITEN New mild preventer
?

PREDNISOLONE | Important reserve
– or prednisone. treatment.

Side effects

ONLY if Big Dose for
many weeks.

No

5mg each

SHORT COURSE
(SAFE)
Example:

WHEN
?
P.T.O.

day 1 1 2 3 4 5 STOP

(a)

WHEN TO START A SHORT COURSE
OF PREDNISOLONE

1. Ventolin doesn't work
2. Terrible night — many wakings
   — long waking
3. Morning tightness
   lasts until lunchtime
4. "Immobilised"
5. Getting worse day by day
6. Emergency intravenous injection given

ANTIBIOTICS
examples: Amoxil
  Septrin
  Tetracycline

Rarely necessary.
– if yellow phlegm after cold.
Will not relieve bad asthma.

(b)

Fig. 4/1(a) and (b) The layout (both sides) of a diagram used
to assist the training of patients. A fresh diagram is prepared
for each patient so that the content can be varied to suit the
individual's requirements and understanding: the general
arrangement remains constant

If asthma is still unacceptable after ensuring optimal use of a steroid aerosol and an optimal starting point for treatment then the following measures may be tried:

a. Higher dosage of steroid aerosol
Some patients who are not controlled using a steroid aerosol in standard dosage may find benefit from doubling the dose (four puffs of beclomethasone four times daily; total dose 800 micrograms daily). At and above this dosage tests of pituitary-adrenal responsiveness may show some impairment but clinical evidence of hypercorticoid side-effects is not encountered. Oropharyngeal candidiasis is more likely to occur at this higher dosage. It is worth trying the effect of a higher dosage of steroid aerosol in patients who inhale poorly from a pressurised aerosol and who are also too clumsy or impatient to load capsules into the Rotahaler. The bigger inhaled dose compensates for the wastage incurred through bad technique.

b. Long-acting theophylline preparations
There are now a number of slow-release preparations of theophylline and its analogues available and one of these may prove a useful addition to the basic treatment outlined. An example is Phyllocontin containing 225mg of aminophylline in slow-release formulation; one or two tablets twice daily. Such a measure may be particularly appreciated when interrupted nights or morning tightness are still an unacceptable feature.

c. Treatment of bronchial infection
If poor response to standard treatment is accompanied by continued production of purulent sputum improvement may follow antibiotic treatment (amoxycillin if the individual is known not to be sensitive to penicillins; alternatively a tetracycline or co-trimoxazole).

d. Check over-use of bronchodilator aerosol
Improved control of asthma may sometimes be achieved by persuading the patient to use less bronchodilator aerosol. Excessive use of aerosols may aggravate asthma and this effect seems to begin when the individual is consuming a whole pressurised canister (nominal content at least 200 inhalations) in under 10 days. Males aged between 15 and 25 seem more prone to this problem than other groups. Clinical impression suggests that the phenomenon is less common than was the case before the introduction of selective β_2-stimulant aerosols, cromoglycate and steroid aerosols. The usual reason for over-use of a bronchodilator aerosol is under-use of a steroid aerosol or cromoglycate.

e. Trial of ketotifen
Ketotifen is an oral antihistamine. Convincing response to this drug is rare.

f. Longer-term use of systemic corticosteroids
The need for longer-term use of systemic corticosteroids becomes evident gradually by the patient showing a tendency to relapse repeatedly when short courses are withdrawn despite close attention to the points outlined above. A continuing requirement for oral steroid treatment is particularly likely to be found in patients with allergic bronchopulmonary aspergillosis, those who have already been on continuous oral treatment for more than 15 years, and some aged patients who are unable to use aerosol preparations but who obtain control of otherwise intolerable asthma on a modest dose of prednisolone. Apart from this last group it is sensible for all patients on long-term systemic corticosteroid treatment to be taking regular aerosol steroid treatment at the same time so that their oral intake may be continuously shown to be necessary despite the best use of the aerosol route.

Continuing systemic steroid therapy is usually given in the form of a divided twice daily dose of prednisolone by mouth. Intelligent patients may experiment and find improved control or a lower requirement if a single dose is taken in the evening or morning. Significant reduction in the risk of side-effects (including adrenal suppression) can be achieved by giving treatment on alternate days in a dose roughly equivalent to double the daily requirement. This may prove successful, particularly in children with moderate asthma who are unable to use aerosols. Unfortunately it is often accompanied by unacceptable asthma on alternate days and the regimen has found widest use in other conditions less volatile than asthma. Patients requiring long-term oral prednisolone can be encouraged to explore the effect of gradual reduction in dosage from time to time if asthma is well controlled – the aim being to ensure that the minimum tolerable dose is being taken. Even small reductions are worthwhile and 1mg tablets can prove convenient. Hectic variation in dosage on a day-to-day basis should be avoided. Patients on long-term prednisolone should be trained to initiate a short-term increase in dosage to cover severe asthma and the indications for such an increase should be clearly understood and preferably written (see above). The need to increase the dose of (or to re-start) prednisolone during severe intercurrent illness should also be understood; this requirement may persist for two to three years after withdrawal of systemic steroid treatment.

There is no evidence that other corticosteroids offer

a lower risk of steroid side-effects than prednisolone when equivalent disease-suppressing doses are compared. In children the use of ACTH or tetracosactrin (Synacthen) by long-acting injection three times weekly may carry some advantage through reduced tendency to suppress growth. There are, however, disadvantages which include the discomfort of the injection, uneven control of asthma and a tendency of the nurse or parent to give a constant injected dose instead of varying it so as to administer the minimum compatible with adequate control. Only a few children with very severe asthma should require long-term steroid treatment. There is no advantage in using ACTH or tetracosactrin in adults. Steroid side-effects are still produced and are more difficult to predict because of variable adrenal response to the drug. Adrenal suppression is of course avoided but this is a spurious advantage because the high level of endogenous cortisol secretion induces pituitary suppression so that the same problem of reduced pituitary-adrenal responsiveness tends to accompany withdrawal after long-term use.

g. Nebulised bronchodilator treatment

Bronchodilator drugs, notably salbutamol, may be delivered by inhalation with the use of a mask containing a nebulising device. Several masks are now available. A small electrically powered compressor or, alternatively, a cylinder of oxygen or compressed air is required to drive the nebulising mechanism. The domestic use of this technique has proved most helpful in young children and those who find pressurised aerosols unacceptable as well as ineffective during an exacerbation. Cromoglycate can be delivered effectively by the same means.

ACUTE SEVERE ASTHMA

Acute severe asthma which is not rendered tolerable over a period of a few minutes following inhalation of a bronchodilator aerosol may require treatment with an intravenous agent and aminophylline is still the most widely used preparation. An initial injection of 250mg (small adult) to 500mg (large adult) is usually given slowly over about three minutes. A short course of oral corticosteroid should always be commenced even if asthma is rendered tolerable by intravenous aminophylline. Measurement of peak flow rate may not be possible but it is worth attempting and may be quite illuminating revealing the asthma to be more or less critical than expected. It may be useful to leave a peak flow gauge with the patient to check progress when the patient is to be left at home apparently re-

covering after the intravenous injection. When severe asthma is not rendered tolerable within 20 minutes or so after intravenous aminophylline a dangerous situation exists and admission to hospital should be arranged promptly. It is difficult to define 'tolerable' in this context and much depends upon the patient's usual state, his experience and his/her indication of progress; the following are features of dangerously severe asthma: cyanosis, interrupted speech at rest, tachycardia over 120 per minute, pulsus paradoxus of over 15mmHg, continuing fear and absolute immobility. It is sensible for an injection of hydrocortisone hemisuccinate 100mg to be given intravenously as soon as this situation is recognised but no early effect should be expected and arrangements for urgent admission to hospital should still proceed.

The outstanding hazard of critically severe asthma is hypoxia and oxygen should be administered in high concentration and not with a 'dilute' Venturi type of mask which is now the type most widely available. Sometimes panicking patients will not tolerate a mask touching the face and nasal cannulae may be tried instead.

The management of acute severe asthma in hospital is outside the scope of this review but it centres upon keeping the patient adequately oxygenated and hydrated until corticosteroid and bronchodilator treatments take effect. Once survival is secure and the patient is calm and distractible, advantage must be taken of the opportunity to review the patient's understanding of his condition and of his treatment. The events leading up to the admission should be reviewed and the importance of intervention with an *early* short course of prednisolone emphasised. The technique of inhalation should also be scrutinised. Time spent on this phase is extremely important and, ideally, several sessions with doctor and patient seated together are required – merely giving the patient a bag of 'discharge drugs' as he leaves hospital is quite inadequate. It is naturally desirable that the manner of the explanation and supporting written matter should be consistent between all members of a hospital team and the family practitioner should receive full details of what has been proposed. The specific indications for self-initiation of a short course of prednisolone should be included in correspondence. Some doctors are opposed to the idea of the patient starting his own short course and this proposal requires to be sensitively discussed where difficulties arise. Usually the security offered by the patient being provided with only a small number of prednisolone tablets provides the necessary reassurance.

The reader will recognise that this account of the drug management of asthma reflects the personal views and practices of one clinician and some apology for a rather didactic presentation may be due since other approaches which vary somewhat from that described may be equally effective. No apology is offered, however, for the heavy emphasis on the importance of the patient understanding and, as far as possible, regulating, his own treatment; this is the key to achieving calmness, confidence and the minimal disturbance of normal life.

REFERENCES

Landau, L. I. (1979). *Paediatric Clinics of North America*, **26**, No 3, 581.

Milner, A. D. (1981). Bronchodilator drugs in childhood asthma. *Archives of Disease in Childhood*, **56**, 84.

Weinberger, M., Hendeles, L. and Ahrens, R. (1981). *Paediatric Clinics of North America*, **28**, No 1, 47.

BIBLIOGRAPHY

Austen, K. F. and Lichtenstein, L. M. (Eds) (1973). *Asthma; Physiology, Immunopharmacology and Treatment*. Academic Press, New York.

Lichtenstein, L. M. and Austen, K. F. (Eds) (1977). *Asthma; Physiology, Immunopharmacology and Treatment* (Second International Symposium). Academic Press, New York.

Clark, T. J. H. and Godfrey, S. (Eds) (1977). *Asthma*. Chapman and Hall, London.

Recommended reading for the literate and enquiring patient

Lane, D. J. and Storr, A. (1979). *Asthma; The Facts*. Oxford University Press, Oxford.

Chapter 5   Children with neurological disorders

GWILYM HOSKING MB, MRCP, DCH

SEIZURES

Seizure disorders in children are common with approximately seven per cent of children having at least one febrile or afebrile seizure before the age of five years.

Children have a wide variety of different seizure types with many being confined to relatively specific ages. Thus, infantile spasms are grouped almost entirely around the second half of the first year of life and febrile seizures typically affect the child between nine months and five years of age.

Not only are there seizure types that are confined to children but children differ from adults in being less 'static' beings. They grow and they mature and with this their seizures and the management of their seizures alters.

With the child it can be argued that the aims of the treatment of a seizure disorder are to prevent seizures, or at least reduce their frequency and severity; but with this to ensure that development is allowed to continue. It could be simply stated that there is no difficulty in stopping seizures with anticonvulsant medication in the majority of patients, but the cost of slavishly doing so may be that one is left with an overdrugged 'zombie'. Compromises are at times necessary. It may be that in a small proportion of patients there has to be an acceptance of a number of seizures occurring when the alternative will be heavy medication – with sedation, behaviour problems, and learning disabilities – but complete freedom from seizures.

Careful behavioural studies of children on anticonvulsant therapy have revealed clearly that the incidence of behavioural and learning disorders, with medication, is of major concern. This problem is also not necessarily dose related. Some exhibit behavioural problems on doses of drugs that are hardly considered therapeutic. What may be revealing, as well as worrying, is the improvement in behaviour and learning that becomes so obvious in some children when anticonvulsant medication is removed.

In recent years much has been learnt about the pharmacokinetics of anticonvulsant therapy – mainly through the measurement of serum levels of anticonvulsant drugs. With this has emerged the tenet that therapy of any child with a seizure disorder should be commenced on one drug only. Combinations at the outset of therapy are never indicated, even though, in some, it may become necessary later.

On the question of the measurement of anticonvulsant serum levels certain advantages and disadvantages of this facility should be considered. The advantages are that the differing metabolism of patients may give rise to varying patterns of handling of the drug(s) in question, the interaction of different combinations of drugs when they are used can be appreciated if their serum concentration is known, and finally compliance can be assessed. The disadvantages are that so-called therapeutic levels are difficult to judge and children do not like blood tests. While the measurement of serum levels of drugs may be very helpful, it is not a routine test and, most particularly, it is not the aim of therapy necessarily to achieve the 'therapeutic' drug level.

In the patient on more than one anticonvulsant, interaction between the differing drugs may occur. The most important interactions between drugs takes place at the cellular level in the liver. The activity of hepatic-drug-metabolising enzymes can be enhanced or inhibited by a drug. Enhancement occurs as a result of stimulation of enzyme production, and will lead to increased degradation and excretion of another drug and a lowering of the plasma level.

Inhibition of one drug may occur because another inactivates some of the enzymes involved in the metabolism of the other. This may result in an increase in the level of the other drug.

Overall, the interaction of one anticonvulsant with another does not present major therapeutic problems, although some important interactions have been experienced. Sulthiame (Ospolot) is a major inhibitor of enzyme activity, and it has been suggested that this drug has no intrinsic anticonvulsant properties but acts by enhancing the efficacy of the anticonvulsants already given. This particularly relates to the administration of phenytoin (Epanutin). Greatly elevated levels of serum phenytoin may arise from the concomitant administration of sulthiame. Carbamazepine (Tegretol) also interacts with phenytoin by reducing its half-life so that with this combination there may be a lowered serum phenytoin. Phenobarbitone has a more complex interaction. Initially, it may have an inhibiting action on enzyme function, therefore elevating serum levels of other anticonvulsants, but later will have the reverse effect. Just how significant this might be clinically is open to question.

Over and above drug interaction at enzyme level, certain combinations are generally undesirable because some of their side-effects may be additive. The combination of primidone and phenobarbitone may produce both sedation and behavioural disorders. Benzodiazepines, when combined with other anticonvulsants, can also be responsible for sedative side-effects.

With most anticonvulsants it is preferable, at the time of the initiation of therapy, that the drug is introduced gradually over a period of about two weeks. This will minimise the chances of side-effects.

The duration of therapy is a difficult area in which to be dogmatic. Many suggest that therapy should continue for four to five years after the last seizure and that removal should not coincide with puberty. This author believes that consideration to the withdrawal of therapy can be given when a child has been free of seizures for two years, although in agreement with others, should not coincide with removal at the time of puberty. The two year recommendation has to be weighed against the form of epilepsy and the initial response to treatment. With the tonic-clonic epilepsies that respond rapidly to the institution of therapy, withdrawal after two seizure-free years may well be successful, while the child with myoclonic epilepsy who was difficult to stabilise on therapy is less likely to cope without therapy after two years. Withdrawal must always be slow, as a sudden cessation of therapy – even in the child who no longer needs therapy – may precipitate seizures or even status epilepticus. This particularly applies to withdrawal of phenobarbitone.

Those in clinical practice and involved with the treatment of large numbers of children with seizures rapidly develop preferences for drugs with which they are familiar and for which they have some faith as to their efficacy and the low level of their side-effects. This author does not escape the bias that arises out of his personal experience!

Phenobarbitone

Of the anticonvulsants still in use this has the longest history, having been first described in the treatment of epilepsy in 1912. Phenobarbitone has potent anticonvulsant activity in a number of seizure disorders in childhood, excepting infantile spasms, petit mal epilepsy, myoclonic epilepsy and photosensitive epilepsy. However, in spite of its efficacy there is a high incidence of side-effects. At least 50 per cent of patients on treatment suffer from learning disorders, related to the administration of this drug. In a smaller, but still significant proportion of children, major behavioural disorders may occur. Thus, the use of this drug is limited because of the side-effects.

Phenobarbitone has a long half-life and can be given in a single daily dose, most preferably in the evening. The dose related to body-weight is predictable in the serum levels that will be achieved and there is an acceptable margin between its therapeutic response and its toxicity. The recommended dosage is 4–5mg/kg/day in a child with a weight of up to 20kg. With this the estimated therapeutic serum level is between 64 and 172 μmol/litre (15–40 μg/ml).

The remaining indications for the use of phenobarbitone, in the opinion of this author, is in the neonatal period. Its anticonvulsant properties in this age group are beyond dispute and the incidence of significant side-effects is low.

It has been shown that the continuous administration of phenobarbitone, in adequate doses, will reduce the incidence of recurrent febrile seizures. While this may be true it has also to be recognised that the high incidence of side-effects has reduced compliance and acceptance of this treatment. The administration of phenobarbitone in the 'at-risk' child at the onset of a fever is valueless.

While it is felt that phenobarbitone does have significant anticonvulsant action it can no longer be considered a first line anticonvulsant because of the high incidence of its side-effects.

Phenytoin (Epanutin)

This drug also has a long track record, being first introduced in 1938. For many years this drug has been 'the' first-line drug in the treatment of many of the seizure disorders. Again there can be no doubt as to its effectiveness but major concerns do exist over its side-effects.

The margin between the therapeutic level of this drug and its toxic levels in the body is very narrow. Unlike other anticonvulsants *saturation* occurs very readily. With this there is not a linear relationship between the dose and the serum levels. Very small increases in dose may produce dramatic and worrying increases in serum levels.

The side-effects that occur are, broadly speaking, considered under acute and chronic.

The acute toxic effects of phenytoin include nystagmus, ataxia and tremor, together with worsening control of seizures. Phenytoin can cause seizures if given in too high a dose. With all of this there may be an encephalopathy manifesting itself with mental dulling, behavioural disorders, dystonia and choreo-athetosis.

Among the chronic toxic effects are behavioural and learning disorders that often are insidious and not obvious. Clinical experience has heightened concern over the effects of phenytoin. Comments made by parents and teachers over behaviour and learning capabilities after coming off the drug indicate all too clearly that the child's performance while on medication was sub-optimal. While behaviour and learning dysfunction under medication is worrying enough there is the other long-term specific side-effects from the administration of phenytoin. Gum hypertrophy occurs in a number of children and may be unsightly and require active dental therapy. Hirsutism and thickening of subcutaneous tissues may combine to produce major cosmetic problems which are highly significant in the female.

Macrocytosis is commonly reported and, rarely, aplastic anaemia with the long-term administration of phenytoin. The role of folate deficiency caused by phenytoin therapy is an ongoing question. The administration of folic acid to patients on phenytoin has been claimed to improve their mental state, but some have advocated caution with its administration because it is thought to aggravate seizure control.

Metabolic bone disease – rickets and osteomalacia – seems to be associated, not only with the administration of phenytoin, but also phenobarbitone and primidone. These bone changes are probably due to vitamin D deficiency from drug induction of liver enzymes involved in the hydroxylation of vitamin D in the liver.

Phenytoin is effective in the treatment of tonic-clonic seizures, partial seizures with complex symptomatology (psychomotor or temporal lobe attacks) and partial seizures of a Jacksonian type.

Recommended dosages are between 5–6mg/kg/day in a child with a weight up to 30kg and therapeutic serum levels are between 20–80μmol/litre (5–20μg/ml). Some check on the serum level of phenytoin is advisable because of the narrow margin between the therapeutic and the toxic level. With the long half-life associated with this drug it may be given as a single daily dose.

Carbamazepine (Tegretol)

This drug is still probably best known for the treatment of trigeminal neuralgia and less well known as a first-line anticonvulsant with a low incidence of side-effects.

There is a wide margin between the therapeutic and the toxic levels. Rarely allergic skin rashes, initial drowsiness and apathy, ataxia and transient leucopenia occur. Depressant activity is infrequent.

Carbamazepine is effective in the management of the majority of patients with tonic-clonic seizures and those with simple or complex partial seizures. It is ineffective in the treatment of petit mal absences and myoclonic epilepsy.

Claims have been made that carbamazepine has some psychotropic activity and behaviour may be improved in those medicated with this drug. On the other hand, it may well be that the absence of the depressant effects so often seen with phenytoin and phenobarbitone suggests this benefit.

Carbamazepine has a relatively short half-life and in most children it should be given three times a day at a dose of approximately 2mg/kg/day after gradually working up to that level over a period of two weeks. The optimum serum level appears to be between 25–42μmol/litre (6–10μg/ml).

Benzodiazepines

The benzodiazepines are widely used for both hypnotic and anxiolytic effects. For more than 10 years the efficacy in the treatment of some forms of epilepsy has been more widely recognised.

Diazepam (Valium) is effective intravenously in the emergency treatment of prolonged seizures or status epilepticus. It is also effective given rectally but ineffective intramuscularly. For maintenance therapy of seizure disorders its use is limited by the tolerance that rapidly develops and sedation, frequently at therapeutic levels.

Nitrazepam (Mogadon) may be an effective treatment in many children with myoclonic epilepsy – whether manifesting as infantile spasms or with later onset. While generally well tolerated the dose will inevitably be limited by the sedative effect. In most patients twice- or thrice-daily doses are employed, starting at 1.25mg. Even in quite young children remarkably high doses may eventually be attained with no definite indications of sedation.

Clonazepam (Rivotril) is one of the newest benzodiazepine drugs used in the treatment of epilepsy. The action is longer than nitrazepam and diazepam and tolerance is said not to occur often. Nevertheless, the side-effects described with the other benzodiazepines – particularly sedation – can certainly still occur and in this author's experience there is a high incidence of behavioural disorders. Another side-effect in babies and younger children may be salivary or bronchial hypersecretion.

The anticonvulsant effectiveness of clonazepam is towards a wide range of seizure disorders excepting the petit mal forms. It should be started gradually, working up to daily doses of 0.5–1mg in infants, 1–3mg in young children and 3–6mg in older children of school age.

Sodium valproate (Epilim)

This is one of the newest anticonvulsants that before being introduced in the United Kingdom had been used widely in Europe. It differs widely in structure from the other anticonvulsants and is effective towards a number of differing seizure disorders.

Side-effects are relatively uncommon but do include gastro-intestinal upsets, transient alopecia, and elevations of liver enzymes. Gastro-intestinal problems are common when the drug is introduced and may be minimised by administration on a full stomach. Sedation is uncommon.

Sodium valproate is effective in a high proportion of patients with tonic-clonic, myoclonic, photosensitive, and petit mal seizures. It would appear that the drug is less effective in partial seizures with complex symptomatology, than carbamazepine.

Because sodium valproate acts as a microsomal enzyme inhibitor transitory elevations of phenobarbitone and phenytoin levels may occur if it is used in combination with these drugs.

The dose of sodium valproate may be between 20–60mg/kg/24 hours with higher doses being used in some children difficult to control. Therapeutic levels appear to be between $300–600\mu mol/litre$ $(50–100\mu g/ml)$.

Originally it was thought that the half-life of sodium valproate was short so that thrice-daily doses were needed. More recent evidence suggests to the contrary and a single daily dose may be as effective as divided doses. If all the drug requirements are given at once many patients will require an enteric-coated preparation in order to avoid gastro-intestinal side-effects.

Ethosuximide (Zarontin)

This is the drug of choice for petit mal epilepsy at a dose of approximately 20mg/kg/24 hours. Once-daily administration is satisfactory therapeutically, but the incidence of gastro-intestinal side-effects appear increased with a single daily dose. Overall, side-effects with ethosuximide are uncommon but are gastro-intestinal when they do occur.

Corticosteroids are, from time to time, used in the treatment of some severe epilepsies, although usually for short periods only. The infantile spasms syndrome appears resistant to therapy with most anticonvulsants except the benzodiazepines (and possibly sodium valproate) but frequently is responsive to corticosteroids or daily ACTH.

A ketogenic diet may, with cream or medium triglycerides (MCT), be resorted to in children with difficult to treat seizures – particularly the myoclonic variety. The services of a dietician are essential and most often it is necessary for the diet to be commenced during a few days in hospital.

In the overall management of a child with a seizure disorder, consideration must be given to help parents cope with seizures when they occur at home.

This author is disenchanted with prophylaxis against febrile convulsions and favours careful immediate advice on the management of the seizure and the administration of an anticonvulsant by parents if necessary. Rectal diazepam at an agreed dose of 0.5mg/kg can be reliably administered after instruction by the majority of parents. Alternatively, parents can be supplied with paraldehyde that their general practitioner can give when he arrives. A glass syringe is not necessary if the solution is given within 30 minutes of being drawn up into the syringe. Recommended doses of paraldehyde would be either 0.1ml/kg/dose or 1ml/year of age/dose given intramuscularly into the lateral aspect of the thigh. No more than 5ml should be injected into any one side to avoid the risk of a sterile abscess.

The same recommendations can be made for children with afebrile seizures that may be (dangerously) prolonged.

It must never be assumed that the treatment of epilepsy is simply a question of finding the right drug at the right dose. Careful diagnostic evaluation is essential, together with equally careful monitoring of the efficacy and the presence or absence of drug side-effects.

MIGRAINE

This is one of the commonest paroxysmal disorders in childhood (and adults). All too often doctors and others deny that this disorder can affect a child.

For many, making the correct diagnosis is therapy enough. In a small proportion, short-term prophylaxis has to be considered after examining the possibility of certain foods aggravating the frequency of attacks.

There are two drugs that may be effective in prophylaxis – diazepam and clonidine (Dixarit).

In the presence of superadded stress in the migrainous child diazepam, at a dose of between 1–2mg twice daily given over a period of two months, may be helpful towards breaking the vicious circle.

Clonidine may similarly be used at a dose of 25–50 micrograms twice daily.

Although this author may recommend at times the use of these two drugs, he will be the first to admit that the 'proof' of their efficacy is lacking and the placebo effect may well be the reason why they work – when they work.

The treatment of acute attacks of migraine should be with the early administration of simple mild analgesics. If vomiting is an early and major problem in the attack, analgesics together with an anti-emetic may have to be given by suppository.

SPASTICITY

The treatment of the spastic child is predominantly physical supplemented at times by surgery to joints which have contractures.

In the presence of severe spasticity even skilled and frequently administered physiotherapy may not be able to mobilise a limb. Consideration then needs to be given to the use of a muscle relaxing agent. Diazepam has been, and still is, employed for this purpose. Unfortunately, it would appear that for adequate muscle relaxation the dose has to be so high that drowsiness occurs. Probably more effective and with a lower incidence of sedative side-effects is baclofen (Lioresal). Extensive experience has been gained in the use of the drug in adults with spasticity – particularly from multiple sclerosis. Many children, but not all, with cerebral palsy benefit from the use of baclofen in doses that range from 5–10mg twice or thrice a day. While baclofen may be capable of decreasing spasticity, it is important that function is carefully monitored when treatment is instituted. In some, their spastic leg is an effective 'prop' and a decrease in spasticity will deprive them of that. In practical terms it is recommended that the child on this drug therapy should be under the close supervision and observation of an appropriately experienced physiotherapist.

THE HYPERACTIVE CHILD

The restless, overactive child with a short attention span may be either of normal intelligence or be significantly retarded. Into whichever group the child may fall, the short attention span will inevitably impair the ability to learn and to relate to the environment. Such children need careful evaluation by a psychologist in order to identify their learning capacity and any specific area of difficulty. Even with careful evaluation and the provision of appropriate psychological and educational remediation, a small hard core of children remain who should be considered for drug therapy.

In the first instance, the possible side-effects of drugs that are already being given (particularly anticonvulsants) must be considered. Next consideration should be given to the short-term administration of drugs specifically aimed at modifying behaviour.

In the restless, hyperactive child a paradoxical reaction to drugs is very frequently observed. Sedative drugs may be stimulants and stimulant drugs sedative. It is this latter observation that may from time to time be exploited therapeutically. Two amphetamine drugs have been used in treatment.

Dexamphetamine (Dexedrine) at a dose of between 2.5–5mg twice daily (with the second dose being given in the middle of the day) may have very beneficial results in the overactive child – particularly the child with normal intelligence.

Methylphenidate (Ritalin) at a dose of between 5–10mg twice a day may achieve similar results.

In general, therapy should be continued for some months with attempts made to remove therapy from time to time in the hope that the behaviour will remain satisfactory without therapy.

THE MENTALLY HANDICAPPED CHILD

There is virtually no role in the primary management and care of the retarded child for drug therapy.

The side-effects of drugs with the treatment of epilepsy in the retarded child must always be remembered – particularly phenobarbitone and phenytoin. The paradoxical action of drugs that are normally sedative must be known. On the other hand, the equally paradoxical action of stimulant drugs referred to above may be helpful.

In conclusion, it must be emphasised again, that in all the above conditions the prescription of drugs must never become a substitute for the sensitive evaluation and management of the child – and his family.

BIBLIOGRAPHY

Laidlaw, J. and Richens, A. (eds) (1976). *A Textbook of Epilepsy*. Churchill Livingstone, Edinburgh.

O'Donohue, N. V. (1979). *Epilepsies of Childhood*. Postgraduate Paediatric Series (ed Apley, J.). Butterworths, London.

Chapter 6 The adult epileptic

M. P. TAYLOR FRCGP

INTRODUCTION

To have epilepsy may have shattering implications for the individual and family, disrupting life and ambitions. On the other hand, if accurately diagnosed and effective drug therapy instituted, life can be normal or near normal – that is, of course, if the medication itself does not create incapacitating side-effects.

Drug side-effects cannot be totally avoided but it is intolerable that they should have to be endured through a mistaken diagnosis, and this happens. On the other hand to have the unusual, perhaps disabling, seizures of psychomotor epilepsy without the dramatic signs and symptoms of grand mal may be to fail to achieve either a true diagnosis of epilepsy or the benefits of seizure control.

It can be said at the present time that there is much room for improvement in the drug management of epilepsy. It is important to get both diagnosis and treatment right at the start.

THE ADULT EPILEPTIC

Epilepsy can begin at any age but for three-quarters of sufferers it begins in childhood or adolescence. Since epilepsy is by definition a tendency to recurrent seizures and this is an indication for anticonvulsant therapy, then most adults with epilepsy will have been diagnosed in childhood or adolescence and started on therapy. The prevailing fashions in medication at the time of the original prescription may well persist like a fossil record, or have been added to, together with any attendant advantages or disadvantages.

The adult epileptic will be one in 300 of the adult population, he or she will be on the list of a NHS general practitioner who will have 12 to 15 other patients with epilepsy, one-third under the age of 16. Since true petit mal is rare after childhood most adult epileptics will be subject to generalised tonic-clonic seizures, many with focal or partial seizures or evidence of focal onset.

The numbers of sufferers make it impossible for a hospital-based neurological service to supervise all anticonvulsant drug therapy. It must therefore be done in the main by the general practitioner.

The practitioner faced with deciding what medication to prescribe for a patient newly diagnosed with epilepsy, or what changes to make in the regimen of a patient already on anticonvulsants but whose control is unsatisfactory, naturally seeks for simple rules and decision pathways. Effective anticonvulsants have been available for many years and traditional regimens have evolved usually based on multiple drug therapy, either as an initial decision because of the belief that the effects of anti-epileptics were additive, or in response to repeated seizures. Advances in the past few years, in particular in understanding the pharmacokinetics of anticonvulsant drugs and the ability to monitor serum levels, have called into question time-honoured regimens. Polypharmacy is seen to be less effective than carefully judged treatment with one drug, and to be the cause of considerable morbidity from drug side-effects and interactions.

It is no longer regarded as good practice to start treatment with more than one drug, a second may be added in certain circumstances, but it is not normally acceptable to add a third and certainly not a fourth. Why is this so? Are there any simple sensible rules to be followed? How much do practitioners need to know? Firstly, we need to know the problems in order to avoid them, and secondly, the possibilities in order to reach out and help our patients to achieve them.

Problems

Numerous problems have been identified by both doctors and patients in the management of epilepsy and in the use of anticonvulsant drugs. While most would agree that accurate diagnosis should be the basis for treatment in one survey (Jeavons, 1975), of 470 patients attending epilepsy clinics 20 per cent were identified as not having epilepsy. Misdiagnosis was considered to have the following major causes: inadequate history taking; the occurrence of clonic movements or incontinence; the existence of a family history of epilepsy; previous febrile convulsions or an abnormal EEG, and perhaps the most fundamental of all, insufficient knowledge of the nature of epilepsy.

Among the many problems encountered by patients with regard to their general practitioners are: failure to explain the cause of epilepsy, failure to explain the cause of seizures and failure to explain the purpose of anti-epileptic drugs, polypharmacy in response to repeat seizures, and ignorance of blood level monitoring.

Hopkins and Scambler (1977), in a survey of adults with epilepsy on the lists of 17 general practitioners, identified: inadequate communication of the diagnosis, inadequate medication and follow-up supervision unrelated to patient need. They observed: 'anticonvulsant treatment is conservative both in choice and quantity of drug and half of those having generalised seizures monthly or more frequently are probably undertreated. Continuing medical supervision seems random, half of the few still attending hospital clinics have rare seizures, while some of those with very frequent seizures do not see even their general practitioners for months at a time'.

Possibilities

It has been a general view that, although widespread practice, polypharmacy was unsatisfactory as it had led to increased risks of toxicity and drug interaction. When drug serum level measurements became available it led to both a better understanding of the pharmacokinetics of anticonvulsants, especially showing the wide variation of serum levels between patients on the same dosage of drugs, and also showing a significant relationship between improved seizure control and optimum serum levels of anticonvulsant.

Having established that where two drugs were being taken, improvement in control was associated with optimum levels of at least one drug, it was then demonstrated that 76 to 88 per cent of new patients could be controlled with a single drug (Shorvon et al, 1978). Later it was shown (Shorvon and Reynolds, 1979) that polypharmacy could be reduced in chronic epilepsy with a reduction to a single drug in 72 per cent of patients with improvement in seizure control in 55 per cent, plus a striking improvement in mental functioning in 55 per cent.

AUDIT OF CARE

Audits in general practice, although varying in their conclusions, support the view that there is considerable potential for improvement in the management of epilepsy.

In one practice of 6,500 patients (Taylor, 1980) doubts were expressed about the diagnosis in three patients; of 35 patients considered to be suffering from epilepsy careful adjustment of dosage of anticonvulsants led to improvement in seizure control in 27 per cent. This was associated with a reduction of polypharmacy in 24 per cent. Some patients were tolerating chronic drug toxicity and frequent seizures, both generalised and partial, unknown to the family doctor.

Improvement in general well-being as a result of reducing polypharmacy was marked in several patients. The overall improvements were considered to be due, not simply to more effective prescribing, but also to a better understanding of the nature of epilepsy and the purpose of medication by patients. This could not have come about without a preceding improvement in understanding and knowledge on the part of the doctors. A great deal was learned from detailed understanding of the individual patient's problems.

The following case histories illustrate in individual human terms most of the common problems in epilepsy management and in drug treatment in particular.

Case history no. 1

Margaret was 15 years old, had just returned home from school and was sitting watching television. What happened next was described by her mother. Suddenly she stiffened, lost consciousness, became blue, her breathing became noisy and she developed violent generalised jerking movements which lasted for a few minutes. She became limp, pale and sweaty and was unrousable for about ten minutes. On regaining consciousness she was confused, had no recollection of what had happened, she went off to sleep and when she awoke she complained of headache, soreness of the jaws and the insides of her cheeks, and she had petechial haemorrhages around her eyes. A diagnosis of epilepsy was feared and Margaret's general practitioner referred her to a neurologist to confirm this. She had a full neurological examination, skull x-ray and EEG. These were normal. A diagnosis of grand mal epilepsy was made and treatment was advised with phenytoin 100mg three times a day, together with diazepam 5mg twice a day since this had already been prescribed for episodes of acute anxiety and panic the previous year. Margaret was having difficulties at school, both socially and academically, although a year or two before she had high academic achievements associated with a high IQ.

After a few weeks of treatment with phenytoin Margaret became ataxic and developed a widespread rash. This was attributed to phenytoin (Epanutin) which was stopped and replaced by her general practitioner with sulthiame (Ospolot) 100mg b.d. Despite this the ataxia persisted and after a further week Margaret complained of headaches, pins and needles in the arms and legs and was noted to be hyperventilating. The situation was discussed with a second neurologist who advised discontinuing sulthiame and withholding further medication unless there were further seizures; he suggested that clonazepam (Rivotril) should be held in reserve since this drug had an anxiolytic effect in common with other benzodiazepines. In fact, the day after the sulthiame was discontinued Margaret had her second tonic-clonic seizure, and medication with clonazepam was started. Over the next few months there were no further seizures. However, Margaret appeared lazy and sleepy, was difficult to get up in the mornings and exhibited aggressive and irritable behaviour with loss of inhibition. On hearing of this, the neurologist advocated changing from clonazepam to sodium valproate (Epilim) 200mg t.d.s. whereupon she had a withdrawal seizure. Margaret's behaviour improved remarkably, but her hair became thin. This caused her natural distress, and although she continued on the drug over the next year or two, she nevertheless reduced the dose to 200mg daily while remaining seizure-free. Soon after she was 18 years of age she discontinued medication.

At the age of 19, still seizure-free and off medication, she purchased a motorcycle, had her first driving lesson, but a few minutes afterwards had a tonic-clonic seizure. She resumed medication with sodium valproate but took this in diminishing dosage, eventually discontinuing it over the following year, when she had a further tonic-clonic seizure. On this occasion, however, she was aware that something was wrong beforehand in that she had a sensation of 'going backwards and slowing down' beforehand. She accepted the need for regular medication. She is now well and seizure-free on 600mg of carbamazepine daily which does not cause her any side-effects.

COMMENTARY ON CASE No. 1

Margaret had had a classical tonic-clonic seizure. The onset was sudden, there was a good description by a witness and the post-ictal symptoms of drowsiness, headache and stiffness were typical. There could be no confusing this event with a syncopal attack, even though in the latter jerking or twitching and even incontinence of micturition may follow cerebral anoxia.

There was, as is usual, overwhelming pressure to confirm or refute the diagnosis and, to prevent further fits, the referral to a neurologist was almost ritual. Such referral may be appropriate but it must be emphasised

that the diagnosis of epilepsy is a clinical one, an epileptic seizure is an event, a combination of signs unperceived by the patient, and a possible history of other additional symptoms. Tests and investigations may elucidate the cause of an individual's seizures and this may help in determining treatment but tests do not confirm or disprove the diagnosis. The diagnosis is clinical and a witness' account is invaluable.

Epilepsy is by definition a tendency to recurrent seizures. Margaret had only one and statistically had a 50 per cent chance of a further seizure over the subsequent three years. The decision to start anticonvulsants after a single seizure might nowadays be criticised as could be the first choice of phenytoin for a young girl; although an effective anticonvulsant, phenytoin has an acknowledged tendency to cause, among other things, hirsutism, thickening of features and acne.

Margaret had ataxia as a side-effect of phenytoin. The dose of 300mg was perhaps too high for her, there was no need to give this drug three times daily, and it would have been better to have started on 200mg daily. However, the development of an allergic rash made the question of its suitability and dosage academic. Interestingly, her ataxia persisted when sulthiame (Ospolot) was taken, presumably because this drug, which is known to inhibit the metabolism of phenytoin, delayed the fall in her serum phenytoin level. Hyperventilation and paraesthesiae are well described side-effects of sulthiame.

Stopping the sulthiame was followed by a withdrawal seizure and the next anticonvulsant, clonazepam (Rivotril) also caused troublesome side-effects, especially sedation and aggressive behaviour, and the hurried changeover to sodium valproate (Epilim) precipitated a further withdrawal seizure.

She remained well and seizure-free on sodium valproate despite the dose she unilaterally opted for because of hair thinning. Was she well controlled on this small dose or was the pattern of her epilepsy simply one of infrequent generalised seizures and was an important part of her life disrupted more by her treatment than her illness? Certainly three of the drugs given singly caused side-effects, there was allergy to one, possible interaction between two, and most of the seizures were due to sudden drug withdrawal. Her last described seizure had evidence of focal onset.

Case history no. 2

Robert began to have 'attacks' at the age of 17 or 18. Most of these occurred in the late evenings or during sleep. In them Robert experienced an acid taste in his mouth and within seconds lost consciousness. His wife reported that he made chewing movements prior to becoming unconscious. In his records he was variously described as suffering from blackouts, minor seizures, petit mal and temporal lobe epilepsy. An EEG showed a focus in the left temporal lobe.

For a time he appeared to be helped by the then standard dosage of phenytoin 100mg, phenobarbitone 30mg each three times a day. He began to have up to four attacks per night and occasionally he would thump his wife a number of times and wander out into the street in his pyjamas. Over the next few years, while attending hospital regularly, he continued to have seizures and exhibited bizarre behaviour which was attributed to psychiatric deviation. His anticonvulsant cover was changed and added to. By the time he was 25 years old he was taking phenytoin 100mg t.d.s. (Epanutin), primidone (Mysoline) 250mg t.d.s. and pheneturide (Benuride) 100mg t.d.s. At the age of 26 he was admitted to hospital with status epilepticus and tonic-clonic seizures were described for the first time. He was discharged from hospital with his medication unchanged. After this the frequency of his tonic-clonic seizures increased and therefore his pheneturide was increased to 200mg q.d.s. One month later he was described as having two fits each day, mainly at night time. His pheneturide was increased to 400mg t.d.s. and three months later he was re-admitted to hospital with status epilepticus. He was discharged on the same therapy and, when reviewed at the neurological outpatients three months later Robert reported that he had had relatively little trouble until the previous month when he had had 14 'blackouts'. He associated this with the fact that his wife had had a baby and the hospital doctor agreed with him and decided to leave his medication unchanged on the basis that 'if his attacks were emotionally precipitated then they should settle down with time and a little reassurance'. This was provided and arrangements were made for his further review in three months. In fact, he was reviewed earlier and seen by a different registrar and he, since Robert appeared to be having three minor attacks a day, added sodium valproate (Epilim) 200mg b.d. to his regimen. By January 1977 Robert was taking phenytoin 100mg t.d.s., primidone 250mg t.d.s., pheneturide 200mg t.d.s. and sodium valproate 200mg t.d.s. He was still having frequent attacks mainly at night. He expressed himself tired of travelling a long way to the hospital and seeing a different doctor each time and was discharged back to his general practitioner, described as being 'comparatively well despite brief attacks almost each night'.

In the weeks ahead his condition varied but he might sometimes have 13 major seizures in 24 hours, less during the day than in the night. He was often quite confused, inco-ordinated and muddled for days, and it was quite impossible to have an intelligible conversation with him at these times. On average he was having several generalised tonic-clonic seizures a week, and in addition he also had seizures which did not always proceed to generalised seizures. During these he was observed by his doctor, he appeared confused as if drunk, was noted to smack his lips and made repetitive movements with the right arm and leg.

Clearly life could not be much worse for Robert and his family, and so it was decided to attempt to simplify his treatment, reduce drug toxicity and try to achieve better seizure control on a smaller number of drugs. On the grounds that phenytoin was probably the most potent anticonvulsant and sodium valproate the least toxic, the former was maintained in a dosage of 300mg t.d.s. and sodium valproate was increased to 1200mg a day; the pheneturide was stopped and the primidone gradually withdrawn. Over the next six months, although he improved in general well-being, he was still having up to three generalised seizures per week. Drug serum levels, now available, indicated that he was probably taking adequate dosage of valproate, but serum phenytoin was noted to be always in the subtherapeutic range, and the dose of phenytoin was therefore increased to 400mg a day and because he had difficulty in remembering his mid-day tablets his anticonvulsants were prescribed morning and at night.

For the next six months he continued to have two to three seizures a week. His serum level of phenytoin was regularly low and he admitted that he did not like taking tablets and he readily agreed to discontinue his sodium valproate and continue treatment with phenytoin alone, this to be taken in a single daily dose of 300mg which his wife agreed to administer. At first this seemed to reduce his seizure frequency, but then a further run of seizures associated with low serum levels and his admission that he 'scived off taking tablets' led to further exhortation to take his single anticonvulsant regularly. For three months he had only occasional nocturnal seizures. When reviewed by a colleague in August 1980 he had had a run of attacks in the previous few days, his serum phenytoin was only 10mmol/litre and therefore his phenytoin was increased to 400mg a day. Four weeks later he was taken to hospital where he was diagnosed as having acute phenytoin toxicity. His behaviour was described as bizarre and a possible diagnosis of underlying schizophrenia was entertained. Despite this blood levels were not done, he was not admitted but sent home with instructions to leave off tablets for 24 hours and restart on a dosage of phenytoin 300mg daily. Over the next few days he was ill, toxic, ataxic and having several tonic-clonic seizures a day. Treatment with carbamazepine (Tegretol) was started in a dosage of 200mg t.d.s. and slow withdrawal of phenytoin commenced. Over the following four months he had occasional nocturnal seizures, none by day, he felt better and looked better, and his phenytoin was finally stopped in December 1980.

He still has occasional seizures, still occasionally forgets his tablets on a prescribed dose of 800mg a day of carbamazepine.

COMMENTARY ON CASE No. 2

Robert suffers from temporal lobe epilepsy, sometimes called psychomotor epilepsy. Nowadays his seizures would be described as 'complex partial seizures with secondary generalisation'. The EEG findings of a temporal lobe focus were consistent with this. It is not clear what caused his odd behaviour, and some of this might have been psychomotor or partial seizure status. Was he in a post-ictal fugue when he beat his wife and wandered off into the night? Did his medication contribute? At a later date he almost certainly had acute phenytoin toxicity so was he, even at an early stage, suffering from sub-acute phenytoin toxicity?

Robert's initial treatment with phenytoin and phenobarbitone was standard for the time. Later the phenobarbitone was replaced by primidone which is, in fact, metabolised to phenobarbitone. Both phenytoin and phenobarbitone are known to induce the activity of liver enzymes and may, in fact, lead to the reduction of each other's serum level. Does this reduce anti-epileptic activity?

Robert's later management shows increasing polypharmacy in response to repeat seizures and he developed episodes of status epilepticus. Whatever the strength of the case of pheneturide (Benuride) as an anticonvulsant, it is certainly known to influence serum phenytoin levels. Like sulthiame it inhibits phenytoin metabolism causing higher serum levels. Overdosage with some anticonvulsants, notably phenytoin, can cause not only toxic side-effects but an increase of frequency of seizures. Perhaps Robert's worsening state was due to phenytoin toxicity in turn brought about by the increased dose of pheneturide.

When Robert's wife had her baby he had more seizures. Was this because of the stress? Or did he simply forget his tablets when his wife was not there to remind him? And did he then have withdrawal seizures? Either or both could be true.

Although there are serious doubts about polypharmacy leading to improved seizure control, there is no doubt that the toxic side-effects, especially sedation and ataxia, are additive and certainly after the addition of sodium valproate as the fourth anticonvulsant,

Robert's mental state worsened and his seizures continued. In fact, his fits seemed to change and on one occasion, which was observed by his doctor, he was noted to have unilateral motor signs with lip smacking. This has been described in phenytoin encephalopathy. No serum levels were available and this explanation was not considered. In fact it was assumed that the problem was poor control due to polypharmacy and it was decided to simplify his medication.

Reducing the number of drugs was followed by a quite definite improvement in general well-being, despite fairly frequent seizures. Robert was very difficult to weigh up. Was his low serum phenytoin level due to poor compliance? His valproate level was in the therapeutic range. Was he taking valproate regularly but not phenytoin? On the other hand was he a high metaboliser of phenytoin? Poor compliance was held as the most likely explanation and his runs of seizures were thought probably to be due to lapses in medication leading to withdrawal seizures, rather than escape from control. Eventually his phenytoin was increased from 300mg to 400mg. He apparently did as he was advised for he developed acute phenytoin toxicity three or four weeks later. The increase of 100mg was unwise – 50mg would have been better. Serum phenytoin levels are not directly dose-related and small increments in dosage can raise serum levels from subtherapeutic into the toxic range. Why is this so? It was decided that phenytoin, although an effective anticonvulsant, depended upon a degree of sophistication and dedication in the titration of dosage which was beyond the combined efforts of Robert, his wife and the doctor, and therefore carbamazepine as a single anticonvulsant was introduced.

The saga of Robert, of course, is not ended, although he is very much better than he has been for many years. His story can be seen as a tragic, confused mess. The problems he got into were the result of accepted practice, not bad practice. Whatever lessons emerge from this story, and there are many, the main one is the need for continuity of care by the smallest number of doctors with shared aims, a brand of continuity of care which brings the benefits of new knowledge to patients with chronic disease.

THE BASIS OF MANAGEMENT: (1) DIAGNOSIS

From the foregoing it is apparent that, although there are many problems, there are nevertheless many opportunities for improvement in the management of epilepsy. These cover initial diagnosis, doctor-patient communication, drug therapy and continuing care.

The basis of effective management for the individual patient rests upon an accurate diagnosis and an understanding of its implications in his particular life and circumstances. Without an understanding of the nature of epilepsy and of his own fits, the individual patient cannot sensibly adapt his life to his handicap, nor can he see the relevance of his medication and the way in which it must be taken if its purpose and manner of working is not explained. He depends first and foremost upon his doctor to teach him and it is helpful if his doctor has a simple concept of epilepsy and of seizures which he can convey.

Classification

Although it is beyond the scope of this chapter to go into detail about seizure types and types of epilepsy, they must be referred to in outline because of the relevance to prognosis, general management and choice of anticonvulsant. Very full descriptions are available (Laidlaw and Richens, 1976). The 1969 classification put forward by the International League of Epilepsy and accepted by the WHO is rather complicated for clinical application; a newer simpler classification is currently being considered. This builds upon the increased knowledge gained from video-recording of seizures and EEG telemetry, and is more relevant to clinical decision-making especially in deciding drug therapy. Using similar terms a clear and simple account is available in a recent booklet written for patients and relatives, and it is also eminently suitable for doctors (Laidlaw and Laidlaw, 1980).

Epileptic seizures

To doctors an epileptic seizure is an abnormal paroxysmal discharge of cerebral neurones. It can conveniently be described to patients and relatives in terms of *electrical activity* and subsequent events related to a simple explanation of how the brain works.

Epilepsy

To suffer from epilepsy is to have a continuing tendency to epileptic seizures. It is not usually desirable to apply the label of epilepsy, and certainly not to start treatment, on the basis of a single seizure.

As far as general practitioners are concerned, for practical purposes the majority of seizures may be divided into two kinds, generalised seizures and partial (focal) seizures. Many of the latter may become generalised but underlying there is evidence of a focal origin either clinically or from the EEG; it is sometimes, for this reason, referred to as 'symptomatic epilepsy', i.e. symptomatic of a localised area of structural abnormality.

GENERALISED SEIZURES

Generalised seizures fall into two groups: grand mal tonic-clonic seizures, and petit mal absences. In a primary generalised seizure there is no evidence of focal onset. For example, there is no aura, which often precedes typical tonic-clonic fits, and these therefore should be regarded as partial seizures of focal onset which evolve to secondary generalisation and require rather different medication. Petit mal absence is described elsewhere in this book (Chapter 5): it is almost totally a problem of childhood and approximately 30 per cent of children with it will have grand mal attacks at some time. This combination of grand mal with petit mal is termed *primary generalised epilepsy*. Sodium valproate is effective against both of these types of seizure and is the drug of choice when they are present in the same patient.

PARTIAL SEIZURES (Includes those evolving to generalised tonic-clonic seizures)

Table 1 gives a classification of partial seizures. Grand mal with an underlying focal source is commoner than primary generalised grand mal. Many patients have more than one type of seizure. Not uncommonly a patient who one day has an olfactory aura succeeded by a tonic-clonic seizure may on other days experience a brief aura (simple partial seizure) only, or the process may be so rapid that the focal symptom or aura is not perceived. Drugs are more effective in controlling generalised than partial seizures, with the result that a patient on treatment may have very few tonic-clonic seizures but the partial attacks may be more persistent though less likely to become generalised.

In managing an individual patient it is helpful to have a clear understanding of the different types of seizure he experiences. It can become a muddle if

Table 1 Classification of partial seizures

1. *Simple* No impairment of consciousness
   Symptom relates to focus of origin, e.g. motor
   sensory
   cognitive, affective, olfactory, psyche

2. *Complex partial* With impairment of consciousness
   (a) Simple onset or
   (b) Impaired consciousness from onset

3. *Generalised tonic-clonic seizures*
   (a) Evolved from a partial focal seizure
   (b) Spontaneous but EEG evidence of focus

doctor and patient are not agreed about what is an 'attack' and 'of what type'. Attempts to suppress all partial seizures (not secondarily generalised) may lead to drug toxicity and a balance may have to be struck between the two. An occasional absence, or aura, or even a complex partial seizure of psychomotor epilepsy may be preferable to drug side-effects.

THE BASIS OF MANAGEMENT: (2) CHOICE OF ANTICONVULSANT

The value of the many anticonvulsants in use has been established over the years from their empirical use, mainly in combinations, and very few controlled trials have been carried out. Recently the effectiveness of single drug therapy has been established and with this a better idea of which drugs are effective and of their effectiveness relative to each other. There is still disagreement about the relative merits of individual drugs for particular seizures.

Table 2 provides a recent list of first-line anticonvulsants with optimum serum levels (Reynolds, 1978). Phenytoin and carbamazepine have generally been regarded as equally effective against grand mal and partial seizures, but there is increasing support for the use of carbamazepine as the drug of choice for partial seizures, especially complex partial seizures, e.g. temporal lobe epilepsy (*B.N.F.*, 1981).

Phenobarbitone and primidone are also effective, the latter almost certainly due to its metabolism to phenobarbitone. These two drugs and clonazepam (Rivotril) are generally too sedating and prone to cause behavioural disturbance to encourage first choice for chronic use. Sodium valproate, although effective against grand mal, is probably not so effective against partial seizures.

Since most adults with epilepsy will have partial seizures with grand mal or evidence of focal onset, then either carbamazepine or phenytoin are now likely to be prescribed singly as first choice, usually depending upon the preference and experience of the clinician. Both drugs have toxic side-effects but phenytoin gives the most problems in this respect. In addition it has unfortunate consequences for facial appearance for some patients, and its optimum use in more severe epilepsy may require meticulous dose-adjustment to give control while avoiding toxicity. Although more expensive, carbamazepine is probably the drug of first choice in general practice for grand mal with or without focal onset.

Each general practitioner, however, will see only one or two new patients with epilepsy each year and even then may not initiate therapy, although he will be the person best placed to supervise the early stages of medication and it cannot be emphasised too much how important it is to get it right at the beginning.

In providing continuity of care for his 12 to 15 patients the general practitioner has no choice but to cope with the good and bad consequences of past prescribing. He faces the challenge of reviewing his patients on long-term therapy, identifying those suffering from either side-effects, poor control, or both, and then deciding whether to attempt the perhaps hazardous course of simplifying or changing treatment.

THE BASIS OF MANAGEMENT: (3) PHARMACOLOGICAL FACTS

Having made an accurate diagnosis of epilepsy and possibly elucidated the cause and the type and frequency of seizures in an individual, our major concern is to prevent seizures. Drug therapy is aimed at achieving and maintaining an effective concentration of an appropriate anticonvulsant in brain tissue while avoid-

Table 2 First-line anticonvulsants and optimum serum levels (*after E. H. Reynolds, 1978*)

Type of epilepsy	Drug	Optimum serum levels (μg/ml)	(μmol)
Tonic-clonic (grand mal) or partial (focal) ± tonic-clonic	phenobarbitone	15–40	45–105
	phenytoin	10–20	40–80
	primidone	as for phenobarbitone	
	carbamazepine	4–10	15–42
	clonazepam	?	?
	sodium valproate	50–100	300–650
Petit mal	ethosuximide	40–80	280–710
	clonazepam	?	?
	sodium valproate	50–100	300–650

ing adverse effects. The concept of *maintaining* an effective concentration is most important since continuing seizures may in fact be 'withdrawal seizures' due to a sudden drop in drug levels and not loss of 'control' (cf Robert's increased seizures when his wife was in hospital).

Brain anticonvulsant levels correlate closely with serum levels and there is a relationship between seizure control and serum levels of many drugs in use. Serum levels, however, vary widely between individuals on the same dose of drug.

In addition to the fundamental factors of 'if', 'how', and 'when' medication is taken, many other factors influence blood serum levels: they are summarised in Table 3.

Table 3 Factors determining serum anticonvulsant levels

ABSORPTION
DISTRIBUTION – protein binding
METABOLISM – hepatic enzymes
RENAL ELIMINATION

These all influence the plasma half-life and form a necessary guide to:
    Frequency of dosage
    Time to steady serum level
    Minimum intervals for dose adjustment

These factors may be influenced by:
    Age
    Disease
    or Drug interactions

Absorption

Absorption is not the source of many problems with oral preparations in use in the United Kingdom, although phenytoin dosage may vary if the B.P.C. suspension is not well shaken. Intramuscular injections may be more slowly absorbed than oral preparations, as with phenytoin and diazepam or no more quickly, as with phenobarbitone. It is therefore useless to give these drugs intramuscularly in status epilepticus.

Distribution

After absorption, anticonvulsants, like many other drugs, bind reversibly with plasma protein but vary in the extent to which they do so. Free drug concentration in the plasma determines the eventual concentration in the brain and other tissues. Problems may arise if there is competition for protein binding between drugs or if there is a reduced plasma albumin level. In practice problems only arise in drugs which are highly protein bound, i.e. of the order of 90 per cent. Phenytoin is 90 per cent protein bound.

Metabolism

Anticonvulsants are cleared from the plasma by hepatic metabolism to yield metabolites easily excreted by the kidneys; the rate of metabolism varies considerably between individuals and, in practice, this shows up in the wide variation of dosage needed to produce comparable drug serum levels. This is especially the case with phenytoin. A further problem with phenytoin is that liver enzymes become saturated within the range of serum levels associated with effective seizure control, and so quite a small increase in phenytoin dose may, in the absence of resistance from hepatic enzymes, lead to toxic serum levels. Conversely, missed doses may lead to an equally dramatic fall and to withdrawal seizures. The dose of all anticonvulsant drugs should be gradually increased to gain seizure control but extra doses of phenytoin should be very small once near or within the so-called therapeutic range, e.g. 50mg if just below the therapeutic range, 25mg if within it.

Anticonvulsant serum levels

There are advantages in being able to monitor serum levels, there are also disadvantages. It provides a useful check on compliance. Unexpected toxicity on a small dose may be demonstrated to be due to low metabolism, poor control may be seen to be associated with low serum levels despite standard dosage in high metabolisers. Precise logical dose adjustment may then follow to achieve optimum serum levels. There is a real danger that serum levels rather than the patient may be treated, especially if the anticonvulsant dose is directed at achieving levels in the therapeutic range which may lead to unnecessary risk of toxic side-effects. In less severe epilepsy 30 per cent will be seizure-free on a low dose and low serum levels. It is unnecessary to take a larger dose. A further 25 per cent will be controlled if drug levels high in the optimum range are achieved. The top of the range is the point at which most patients have troublesome side-effects, some will have them at lower dosage and yet others may tolerate higher dosage, and for a few it may be worth pressing on past the optimum range.

Enzyme induction

Hepatic metabolism of drugs may be increased or inhibited and either may cause problems. The induction of hepatic microsomal enzymes (increased activity) is brought about by many drugs including anticonvulsants. These are powerful enzyme inducers capable of increasing the metabolism of other drugs and so reducing serum levels. It is important to recognise that anticonvulsants in combination induce each others metabolism. Robert (Case 2) at one stage was on phenytoin, primidone, pheneturide and sodium valproate. Phenytoin and primidone both induce enzymes (the latter after metabolism to phenobarbitone). Pheneturide on the other hand inhibits phenytoin metabolism and raises its level. Sodium valproate is now known to potentiate the side-effects of the first two. Recently, cimetidine (Tagamet) has been found to raise serum phenytoin levels.

Sulthiame (Ospolot) (given to Margaret (Case 1)) also inhibits phenytoin metabolism, as does isoniazid prescribed for tuberculosis and viloxazine as an antidepressant.

Liver enzyme induction may lead to therapeutic failures in other drugs given with anticonvulsants, e.g. griseofulvin prescribed for fungal infection, tricyclic antidepressants and the oral contraceptive pill. Margaret, should she wish to take it would probably be safer on a high dose oral contraceptive preparation.

Adverse effects and drug-induced disease
Some of the commoner adverse effects were experienced by Margaret and Robert. Margaret had ataxia with phenytoin but also a rash and both suffered the common side-effects of sedation and mental dulling. For Robert this was made worse by polypharmacy and Margaret was sleepy and aggressive on clonazepam (Rivotril). Robert suffered acute toxicity with phenytoin – ataxia, hallucinations and increased seizures. Although both are better controlled and well on carbamazepine, this drug too can cause sedation, ataxia and diplopia, especially when first taken. Sodium valproate caused hair thinning for Margaret. It can also cause sedation – especially in combination, behavioural problems, and rarely encephalopathy with increased seizures.

The coarsening of features, hirsuties and gingival hypertrophy associated with chronic phenytoin therapy is now well recognised. Folate deficiency and haematological abnormalities have been associated with long-term use of phenytoin, phenobarbitone and primidone, as have osteomalacia and rickets. Hepatitis has been described with phenytoin and phenobarbitone; and sodium valproate has also been noted to cause liver disease and, rarely, pancreatitis in children.

More relevant to Margaret, when the time came to have children, would be the possibility of teratogenic effects, e.g. hare-lip, cleft palate and heart defects. If she wished to breast-feed she would be reassured to know that the quantities of anticonvulsant in breast milk is unlikely to be harmful.

THE MANAGEMENT OF EPILEPSY
Getting the diagnosis right
The first requirement is an accurate diagnosis based upon a description of the seizure by a witness, plus whatever can be remembered by the patient. For the new patient suspected of having had a seizure, obtaining such a description is the most important thing to be done. I have obtained crucial information by speaking to work-mates and, on one occasion, a driving instructor. It may be equally important for the chronic patient, and if there is no descriptive statement in the records, one should be obtained – invariably something new is learned; and frequently unrecognised partial seizures come to light. A diagnostic label, with no supporting evidence, such as 'grand mal' is of little value to anyone but the person who wrote it. It may be the result of jumping to conclusions and is a poor foundation or justification for a lifetime of medication. A full description of events such as that provided by Margaret's mother (p. 67) is more valuable than any neurological opinion, EEG or brain scan, useful as these may be in identifying any underlying cause or clarifying the type of seizure.

A diagnostic statement
Advice and guidance and drug treatment must be relevant to the patient's particular seizure, to the disorder in his particular life and circumstances, and a diagnostic statement in an extended form is a useful basis for action. It should contain the following information:

> Age and mode of onset
> Types of seizure and frequency of each
> Presumed cause
> Medication
> Associated features
> Social/economic status (and ambitions)

For Margaret (Case 1) this becomes:

'Margaret, aged 22 years, had her first tonic-clonic seizure aged 15, witnessed and described by her mother. No cause was found and there was no evidence of focal onset, although she had attacks of phobic anxiety in the previous years.

'Has suffered side-effects from phenytoin, sulthiame, clonazepam and sodium valproate. Of five seizures three were associated with drug withdrawal.

'Stopped drugs for 18/12 but had further two seizures.

'Now seizure-free on carbamazepine.

'She is an unemployed typist, currently separated from her husband.

'She has mild polyarthritis which interferes with her hobby of painting.'

Teaching the patient about epilepsy and drugs
Compliance in conforming to general advice, for example about driving or leisure activities such as swimming, and the necessity for taking continuous medication, must be based upon an understanding of the causes of seizures, of the dangers, of the purpose of medication and how it works, and what can cause it to fail and what problems this might create.

The effective doctor is a good teacher. It is helpful to have a list of points which should be covered over a number of consultations, depending upon their relevance to the patient at the time (Table 4). A helpful booklet for patients has been referred to (Laidlaw and Laidlaw, 1980) and in addition the British Epilepsy Association provides invaluable literature. Nevertheless, the doctor has the best opportunity to help get it right at the start.

Table 4 Patient education – check list

Fits

What causes fits?	What happens
What causes *your* fits	
What sets them off?	
	Avoiding fits
Dealing with fits –	Single
	Status epilepticus
Rest	
Work	
Recreation	
Alcohol	
Driving – the law	
Marriage	Oral contraception
Children –	Danger of inheriting
	Teratogenic effects

Drugs
How they work

Your drugs
How to take them so that they work

I find it helpful to explain epilepsy in terms of electrical activity, localised bursts causing partial attacks, such as auras or more complicated partial seizures, either occasionally or frequently leading to generalised spread causing a major seizure. I explain what is happening in the individual's own fits and invite discussion about what might set them off:

e.g. tiredness, boredom – loss of sleep
    tension
    menstruation
    alcohol
    TV
    missing tablets

I point out that the opposite may ward off seizures:

activity, involvement, regular rest.

Dealing with fits
Although it is important that close relatives are told what to do by the doctor, the patient ideally needs to be able to explain to a wider circle of acquaintances. Emphasis should be laid on doing as little as possible during a seizure, but insisting upon medical aid for repeated seizures in status epilepticus which is a serious emergency. The advice should be to seek aid if seizures and unconsciousness are continuing for over ten minutes.

Having fits is bad enough without having your teeth broken by the well intentioned, if ill advised, be he layman or doctor, or finding yourself once more unwillingly and unnecessarily in hospital.

Most of the other points in Table 4 are self-explanatory, some are more important than others, and some assume greater importance as life rolls on, e.g. choice of oral contraceptive, decisions about having children.

With regard to pregnancy two main issues arise: the risk of having children who will develop epilepsy and the risk to the developing fetus of drugs. The risk of epilepsy is approximately 1:30 if one parent is affected, less if the epilepsy is due to acquired disease, e.g. trauma. If both parents have epilepsy or there is a strong family history the risks are considerably greater and genetic counselling may be needed. The genetic risk of developing epilepsy itself carries a small risk of fetal abnormality. Drug therapy is associated with congenital abnormality, especially hare-lip, cleft palate and heart defects. Because of polypharmacy there is uncertainty about which drug or drugs are responsible, for both phenytoin and phenobarbitone have been incriminated, and carbamazepine is suspect.

As a general rule the risk of seizures should guide decisions about therapy, and the decision to withdraw anticonvulsants is probably unwise once pregnancy has started.

Starting anticonvulsant therapy

Deciding to start in the face of repeated seizures poses little difficulty, but the single seizure does. It is current practice to await further seizures, of which there is a 50 per cent chance within three years in young adults.

My choice for grand mal, with or without partial seizures, is carbamazepine, followed by phenytoin, sodium valproate and phenobarbitone, in that order.

Whichever drug is selected it is current practice to start with a low dose increasing until seizures are controlled or side-effects appear. However, since 30 per cent of patients are seizure-free on relatively low dosage and a further 25 per cent when serum levels in the optimum range are reached, it is sensible to aim to produce serum levels in the lower part of the optimum range in patients who are seizure-free and, like Margaret, possibly only subject to infrequent fits.

DOSE ADJUSTMENT

Although the patient may need to be seen frequently for many reasons, drug dosage should not be increased at too short intervals. The aim is to produce stable serum levels and knowledge of the half-life of the drug helps judge the intervals (Table 5), and usually four to five half-lives are needed before one achieves steady serum levels.

FREQUENCY OF DAILY DOSAGE

Most anticonvulsants may be given in daily or twice-daily dosage, even drugs with a short half-life such as sodium valproate or carbamazepine. Compliance is said to be better with less frequent dosage. However, to forget a whole day's dosage, e.g. of, say, 300mg phenytoin may have more serious consequences than a single tablet of 100mg. I therefore prefer and advocate twice-daily dosage.

Serum level monitoring is helpful if used wisely and if the laboratory employs satisfactory techniques subject to quality control. Drug dose may be pushed into the so-called toxic range in resistant cases and this may prove successful, but it must be remembered that seizures may increase in the toxic range and that partial seizures are especially difficult to eliminate; so a balance may have to be struck.

Changing therapy

If seizures are not controlled (85 per cent are likely to be) the choice lies between adding a second drug, and either accepting polypharmacy or with the intention of transferring to the second. Since there is evidence that adding a second drug makes little, if any, difference, there can be no objection to changing over completely. Margaret's experience (Case 1) teaches us that the first drug should not be withdrawn suddenly, but very gradually, over many weeks, and not until the new drug is providing serum levels in the optimum range. Stopping the first drug may still lead to withdrawal

Table 5 Pharmacokinetic data

Drug	Serum half-life	Minimum daily dosage intervals	Suggested interval dose adjustment
phenytoin	1–4 days*	daily	3–4 weeks
carbamazepine new	24–46 hours	twice a	2–3 weeks
chronic	8–19 hours	day	
phenobarbitone	2–5 days	daily	4 weeks
primidone		three times a day	4 weeks
sodium valproate	6–10 hours	**twice a day or daily (evening)	2–3 weeks
clonazepam	20–40 hours	twice a day	2–3 weeks
ethosuximide	2½–4 days	daily	4 weeks

*   True half-life in chronic therapy not available
** Despite short half-life a daily dose may be adequate

seizures and the temptation to retreat may be difficult to resist. Withdrawal may also influence the serum level of the new drug if the first was an enzyme inducer.

Reviewing patients on multiple therapy

If, on reviewing established patients on polypharmacy they are found to be well, seizure-free and truly free from side-effects (although they might not appreciate the latter until a drug is withdrawn), they should be left alone, unless there are reasons to consider withdrawal of medication. If side-effects and/or seizures are present, consideration should be given to simplifying therapy despite the fact that there is a risk of withdrawal seizures and, for a small number, a worsening of their epilepsy. For the majority there is the likelihood of better control and reduced drug toxicity.

Confidence should be placed in the drug among those being taken believed to be most effective, ensuring that its dosage is such that its serum levels are in the optimum range before any other drugs are withdrawn. Reduction in dosage should involve one drug at a time, and it is safer to take several weeks between individual dose changes and two to three months to withdraw a drug.

Stopping therapy

After a number of years seizure-free, it may be reasonable to consider withdrawing anticonvulsants altogether. The decision is difficult and weighing the benefits and risks is a matter for individual decision. To be free and whole versus the fear of further seizures is a conflict that has consequences for career and driving if seizures recur.

In making a decision to stop treatment the following should be borne in mind. One in three children with temporal lobe epilepsy become seizure-free, and adults on anticonvulsants, who have been seizure-free since childhood, may reasonably consider withdrawal. The likelihood of relapse, as might be expected, is related to the extent and siting of any organic focal lesion. Consequently, an abnormal EEG, history of very frequent seizures in the past, difficulty in control, evidence of brain damage, or non-febrile seizures at a very early age are all factors associated with likelihood of relapse.

It is current practice to attempt withdrawal after two or three seizure-free years in patients who have had rare seizures. About 30 per cent of this group will relapse within two years. As in changing or simplifying therapy withdrawal should be very slow over several months with each drug, leaving the most potent until last. In fact, effective monotherapy must be the first stage in planned withdrawal.

Seizures during withdrawal may simply be withdrawal seizures and not an indication that the individual would have seizures when totally freed from anticonvulsant effect. It is impossible to tell the difference and it takes courage to persevere in the face of this happening. If repeated seizures or status epilepticus occurs, then a return to anticonvulsants will have to be accepted.

Treatment of status epilepticus

This is a rare medical emergency of repeated generalised tonic-clonic seizures; it is important because it has a substantial mortality rate and may lead to further neurological damage in some survivors. Not infrequently its seriousness is not appreciated by relatives or doctors: repeated seizures lasting longer than ten minutes are an indication for action. Treatment in adults is by intravenous diazepam in a dose of 5–10mg or clonazepam 1mg, given over two to three minutes and repeated if necessary after 30 to 60 minutes. There is a risk of apnoea, possibly greater in children, and ideally means of resuscitation should be available.

An alternative is intramuscular paraldehyde 8–10ml but this takes 30 minutes to act.

Individual anticonvulsants

Full accounts appear elsewhere (Laidlaw and Richens, 1976) especially of the older anticonvulsants. Less comprehensive but up-to-date is the *British National Formulary*, 1981.

CARBAMAZEPINE

This is the drug of choice for tonic-clonic seizures associated with focal or partial seizures. Since up to 68 per cent of adults with epilepsy may have evidence of focal onset (Hopkins and Scambler, 1977) and evidence of focal onset may become apparent in time with patients with grand mal, there are arguments for its use as first choice for all grand mal in adults, with or without partial seizures. Carbamazepine does not work for everybody and it does have side-effects – dizziness, drowsiness, and gastro-intestinal disturbance, especially early in treatment. For this reason it is best started in a dose of 100mg b.d., increased by 200mg daily at a minimum of fortnightly intervals. Serum levels are very variable between individuals and an average daily dose is 600mg, maximum 1200mg. Toxic effects include ataxia and diplopia.

PHENYTOIN

This is an effective anticonvulsant, but problems with toxicity may be a serious problem for some patients. Dose adjustment may be difficult as increasing dosage may lead to a disproportionate rise in serum levels.

Nevertheless, it is a powerful drug which suits and serves many patients well.

Dose: Start with 200mg daily, either in a single or divided dose, adjust no more than once per month. If serum levels are not available and seizures persist, increase to 300mg daily and thereafter increase the daily dose by 50mg each month until seizures stop, or signs of toxicity develop, in which case *stop treatment for two days* and restart on a lower dose, e.g. 25mg less per day.

If serum levels are available (having started on 200mg daily) and serum concentration is less than 8μg/ml (32μmol/litre) increase by 100mg daily; if 8–12μg/ml (32–48μmol/litre) increase by 50mg daily; above 12μg/ml (48μmol/litre) increase by 25mg daily.

Average adult dose is 350mg; maximum 600mg.

PHENOBARBITONE (also primidone)

This is effective against grand mal but not partial seizures. Side-effects are well known, especially drowsiness, mental slowing and occasionally ataxia. It has a long half-life, therefore dosage adjustments have to be four or six weeks apart.

It is started in a dose of 30mg daily, increased to 60mg after a week if drowsiness is not a problem, and then increased by 30mg per day every four weeks. Up to 150mg daily may be required. Upper limits are determined by individual tolerance to side-effects.

SODIUM VALPROATE

This is effective against grand mal but probably not partial seizures. It is the drug of choice for petit mal associated with grand mal. Despite a short half-life, twice-daily dosage is usually effective. The dosage range is 400mg daily to 2.5g.

Its main side-effects are gastric irritation and hair loss. It may cause sedation, especially when used in combination. A rare toxic effect may be encephalopathy. Thrombocytopenia, impaired liver function and pancreatitis (in children) may also occur. Malaise, anorexia and vomiting may precede abnormalities of liver function tests. Some of these adverse reactions have been fatal but most relapse when the drug is stopped.

CONCLUSION

The challenge is to the general practitioner to provide better advice and management for his patients with epilepsy. The opportunities to improve their care over the past few years have increased considerably. Old regimens have been challenged, better use made of established drugs, a few new drugs have appeared, and hopefully others with fewer side-effects will emerge making seizure control safer and simpler.

One is left wondering if some patients with epilepsy might be better off untreated, but which ones? Polypharmacy or irregular erratic therapy may be responsible not only for toxic side-effects, but perhaps more fits than would have occurred naturally.

REFERENCES

Jeavons, P. M. (1975). The practical management of epilepsy. *Update*, **10**, 269–80.

Hopkins, A. and Scambler, G. (1977). How doctors deal with epilepsy. *Lancet*, **1**, 183–6

Shorvon, S. D., Chadwick, D., Galbraith, A. W. and Reynolds, E. H. (1978). One drug for epilepsy. *British Medical Journal*, **1**, 474–6

Shorvon, S. D. and Reynolds, E. H. (1979). Reduction in polypharmacy in epilepsy. *British Medical Journal*, **2**, 1023–5.

Taylor, M. P. (1980). A job half done. *Journal of the Royal College of General Practitioners*, **30**, 456–65.

Laidlaw, J. and Richens, A. (eds) (1976). *A Textbook of Epilepsy*. Churchill Livingstone, Edinburgh.

Laidlaw, M. V. and Laidlaw, J. (1980). *Epilepsy Explained*. Churchill Livingstone, Edinburgh.

Reynolds, E. H. (1978). Drug treatment of epilepsy, *Lancet*, **2**, 721–5.

British National Formulary (1981) Number 2. British Medical Association and Pharmaceutical Society of Great Britain, London.

ACKNOWLEDGEMENT

Grateful thanks are due to Dr J. H. Silas, Lecturer in Pharmacology and Therapeutics, University of Sheffield, for the enlightenment given me in the effective use of anticonvulsants.

Chapter 7 Other chronic neurological disorders

R. W. ROSS RUSSELL MD, FRCP

and J. P. H. WADE MD, MRCP

MIGRAINE

Migraine is the most widespread and the most variable of all neurological disorders. Its effects range from occasional transient painless visual disturbance to severe frequent and disabling headache. There are almost as many theories of causation as there are patients but the underlying abnormality is probably an inherited disturbance of amine metabolism leading to an abnormal variation in the concentration of circulating vaso-active amines which have their effect chiefly on the carotid circulation. The visual aura of classical migraine is due to narrowing (by oedema or vasoconstriction) of the internal carotid or basilar arteries with resulting temporary focal ischaemia. Headache is due to dilatation or inflammation of the vessel wall; it follows the phase of narrowing and mainly affects the external carotid territory.

As with all chronic recurrent conditions treatment must begin with reassurance and explanation. Patients must accept that they have a long-term tendency to headache which usually, though not invariably, becomes less frequent with the passage of time. In some, headache may be provoked by dietary items such as chocolate, cheese or citrus fruits, in others by such disparate factors as contraceptive medication, menstruation or physical exercise but in the majority no precipitating event can be identified and a continuing obsessional scrutiny of the diet for possible allergens is best discouraged.

In the majority of migraine sufferers the first requirement is relief of headache; this is best achieved by a simple, safe and rapidly-acting drug such as aspirin or paracetamol which, if taken early in the attack, often reduces the pain to an acceptable level. If nausea and vomiting are prominent the addition of metoclopramide is useful.

The traditional place of ergotamine in the treatment of migraine is undergoing some revision. This drug, a powerful vasoconstrictor, gives rapid relief of headache to some patients when all other simpler preparations fail. On the other hand, in those patients whose attacks occur frequently the administration of ergotamine appears after a time to lose its effectiveness and may even cause headache as a part of a syndrome of mild chronic toxicity. True ergotism with ischaemic symptoms in the extremities may also occur rarely, but the drug should not be given to those with symptoms of arterial disease or in pregnancy. Ergotamine should therefore be reserved for those patients having occasional severe attacks which are unresponsive to simple analgesics. It is given sublingually or by suppository 1–2mg followed by 1mg two-hourly not exceeding 6mg/24 hours. A more rapid effect can be achieved by subcutaneous injection (0.25–0.5 mg) or aerosol inhalation (0.36 mg per dose). There is little to recommend its use in frequent attacks or as a preventive except in the self-limiting condition of migrainous neuralgia (see below).

Patients with frequent attacks of classical or common migraine, sometimes occurring as often as once a day, should be given prophylactic treatment. Three preparations are available: a beta-adrenergic blocking drug such as propranolol 40–160mg b.d. is particularly useful for middle-aged patients with a recrudescence of migraine or for those who develop migraine for the first time in association with hypertension (Weber and Reinmuth, 1972). Clonidine (Dixarit) is another antihypertensive drug with both central sympatholytic action and a depressant effect on peripheral vascular reactivity; the dose used for migraine (0.05mg twice daily) has no effect on blood pressure but only a minority of patients derive substantial relief. Pizotifen (Sanomigran) is a recently introduced serotonin antagonist for migraine prevention: at a dose of 3mg a day it has few side-effects, has both antihistamine and anticholinergic action and has been shown to be effective in a number of clinical trials (Hughes and Foster, 1971). When migraine or vascular headaches are combined with depression, amitriptyline or the MAO inhibitor phenelzine (Nardil) may give excellent results. These two drugs should not be given together and in the case of phenelzine appropriate dietary restrictions are necessary.

Whether for pharmacological or psychological reasons, it is a common finding in migraine that a new preparation works well for a time but then loses its effectiveness. This makes the management of severe migraine and the evaluation of new drugs a difficult exercise.

In the related condition of *migrainous neuralgia*, more commonly encountered in middle-aged men, and principally involving the facial, scalp and orbital branches of the external carotid artery a different approach is needed. Here the regular daily attacks of severe pain are relatively brief, often occur during the night and usually cease spontaneously after a few days or weeks. Preventive treatment is required and the most effective drugs are ergotamine, 1–2mg nightly, propranolol, 40–120mg a day and, in severe cases, corticosteroids (prednisone, 20–40mg a day). Methysergide is too toxic for general use but may be helpful in patients who are resistant to conventional therapy.

TRIGEMINAL NEURALGIA

The treatment of this protracted and distressing complaint which almost always occurs in the elderly has been transformed in the past few years by the introduction of the highly effective and almost specific remedy, carbamazepine. So rapid and complete is its effect that lack of improvement after a day or two on the drug should provoke a reappraisal of the diagnosis. The paroxysms affect mainly the maxillary division of the trigeminal nerve and characteristic of the pain are its reflex nature (provoked by tactile trigger factors) and its intermittency. The periods of freedom may last for years. The pain is described by patients in various ways; typically it is brief and shock-like but in some there is a duller background burning sensation which lasts for a longer period.

Treatment should begin with a small dose of carbamazepine 300mg per day in divided doses, increasing as necessary until adequate relief is obtained. Some patients tolerate up to 1.5 grams per day but most find that more than 1 gram provokes ataxia and drowsiness especially in the very elderly. While on the drug the paroxysms can be sensed but are no longer painful. Attempts to withdraw the drug should be made every three months but occasional patients insist on continuing the drug indefinitely and they apparently come to no harm. In the rare instances of intolerance to carbamazepine (skin rashes or granulocytopenia), phenytoin may be used instead. Very rarely recourse must still be made to alcohol injection of the trigeminal ganglion or to neurosurgical division of the sensory root: this should only be considered after a full trial of medical treatment.

CEREBRAL TUMOUR

The satisfaction which comes from the diagnosis and surgical removal of a benign cerebral tumour is unfortunately tempered by the knowledge that the majority of tumours cannot be cured in this way. Gliomas, the commonest type of cerebral tumour, infiltrate and replace normal brain tissue causing a local loss of function as well as interfering with the circulation of the cerebrospinal fluid (CSF) to cause raised intracranial pressure. The presence of cerebral oedema around the tumour adds to the mass-effect.

The growth of gliomas is enormously variable; a well-differentiated astrocytoma may be dormant for decades and show progressive infiltration with minimal mass-effect or raised intracranial pressure. On the other hand, the highly malignant glioblastoma and some secondary tumours are characterised by rapid growth, haemorrhage and massive oedema formation and may cause the death of a patient within a few weeks. The microscopic examination of tissue removed at surgery will give some indication of the degree of malignancy. Furthermore during surgery the tumour mass is removed as far as possible to afford an internal decompression and allow space for regrowth.

The aims of medical treatment in those patients in whom tumour cannot be removed are to inhibit the growth of residual tumour, to relieve brain swelling, to prevent epilepsy and to alleviate the symptoms of raised intracranial pressure.

Radiotherapy is highly effective in certain neural tumours such as medulloblastoma and in lymphomatous deposits around the brain. Some glial tumours such as ependymomas and the pituitary adenomas are also sensitive. Radiotherapy is probably beneficial in slow-growing astrocytomas though in all cases recurrence is likely after some years. It is probably ineffective in the highly malignant gliomas or secondary tumours such as bronchial metastases or melanoma. When the lesion is suitable it should be treated with a full dose of radiotherapy to the tumour bed after operation and it may also be necessary to irradiate the spine. For glioblastomas there is at present no very effective treatment although systemic tumour chemotherapy with *x*-radiation is beginning to show worthwhile benefits in terms of survival.

Cerebral oedema, a prominent feature of many malignant tumours, can now be effectively treated with the synthetic glucocorticoid, dexamethasone. This is given initially in a large dose 8–16mg a day reducing to a maintenance dose of 2–4mg per day. This drug has radically altered the long-term management of malignant tumours and patients no longer suffer a protracted period of raised intracranial pressure with fluctuating coma, severe headache and blindness. In rapidly deteriorating patients very large doses of steroids (100–200mg per day) are sometimes recommended but the side-effects are usually unacceptable. Epilepsy, particularly temporal lobe epilepsy, may be difficult to control but best results are obtained with phenytoin and carbamazepine. Headache in tumour patients is due to obstruction of the CSF pathways leading to ventricular dilatation or to a distortion of basal structures especially blood vessels. Involvement of the skull base by secondary tumours may also cause pain. Obstruction may be relieved by surgical measures such as an atrioventricular shunt and dexamethasone treatment is most effective in reducing oedema. If pain is still a problem it may be necessary to use codeine or aspirin and if nausea or vomiting are prominent chlorpromazine and metoclopramide may be added. In the later stages the combination of opiates and chlorpromazine given on a regular four-hourly basis is usually effective in controlling headache.

A difficult problem is posed by patients with tumour but with only minor symptoms since with modern CT scanning the diagnosis of an infiltrating tumour may be established in patients at an early stage. When the sole complaint is of occasional seizures these are easily controlled by anticonvulsant treatment. Even at this stage a glioma is rarely removable by surgery and such patients are best left untreated either surgically or medically until symptoms become more prominent.

The policy of non-intervention may even apply to some benign tumours such as sphenoidal wing meningiomas which are technically irremovable, or to meningiomas or neurofibromas if they occur in elderly or debilitated patients. In this case the tumour may never become large enough to cause serious trouble during the life of the patient and is best left alone.

DRUG TREATMENT OF CEREBRO-VASCULAR DISEASE

In patients who have transient ischaemic attacks (TIA) or who have survived a stroke the prime consideration is to prevent a major infarction. A small minority of patients may have underlying rheumatic heart disease or other cardiac condition, a few may have an unusual form of arterial disease or blood disorder, but the great majority have atherosclerosis, a generalised disorder affecting larger arteries throughout the body but causing symptoms mainly in the heart, brain and lower limbs. An attack of acute ischaemia is usually provoked by thrombotic occlusion at the site of a previous atheromatous lesion.

A TIA or minor stroke is thus a sign of a generalised disease and requires generalised treatment. Long-term follow-up studies indicate that TIAs are followed by a complete stroke at a frequency of approximately five per cent a year, but the risk is greatest in the first few months after TIA. Life expectancy is substantially reduced but as many patients die from myocardial infarction as from cerebrovascular disease.

The principal long-term aims of treatment are (1) to reduce any thrombotic tendency of the blood and (2) to retard or, if possible, reverse the underlying atherosclerosis. Arterial thrombi are formed by platelets, fibrin and blood cells and the initiating event is adhesion and aggregation of platelets to a region of arterial narrowing or ulceration. Various drugs have been found to influence platelet aggregation *in vitro* and *in vivo* and are under clinical trial in patients with TIA. Of these aspirin is probably the most promising and has been shown significantly to reduce the incidence of stroke and death in male patients (Canadian Cooperative Study, 1978). The dose required is at present uncertain but the main beneficial effects can be obtained by as little as 300mg per day. Treatment is usually continued for two years or longer.

Dipyridamole (100mg per day) also affects platelet aggregation by a different mechanism and may find a place as an adjunct to aspirin treatment or in female patients (Sullivan, Harken and Gorlin, 1968). Conventional anticoagulants have been used for some years. They are of proven value in embolism from the heart and, in such patients, life-long treatment is required (Carter, 1965). They are probably of some value in patients with TIA in preventing attacks and in reducing the incidence of stroke but they appear to have no effect on the death rate and have been largely superseded in this group of patients by aspirin.

Heavy cigarette smoking carries an increased risk of vascular occlusion both in the heart and brain though the precise mode of action is unknown. It probably acts as a stimulus to thrombosis rather than to atherosclerosis. It has now been shown that stopping smoking is followed by a reduction in the risk of myocardial infarction within a few months. Since this is a major cause of death in patients with cerebrovascular disease cigarettes should be proscribed entirely in all patients with TIA or minor stroke.

Preventive treatment

Measures aimed at treating underlying atherosclerosis are more controversial since the process is probably far advanced by the time symptoms appear. Of the various risk factors known to be associated with atherosclerosis there is undoubted benefit in the treatment of blood pressure, and probable benefit in the treatment of impaired glucose tolerance and in the surgical removal of carotid artery lesions. There is very doubtful benefit in the treatment of hyperlipidaemia and the evidence on other factors such as haematocrit, obesity, exercise and stress is still under review.

It has long been known that in hypertension atherosclerosis is more widespread, more severe and characteristically affects smaller vessels (Fisher, 1979). Hypertensive patients are known to be more at risk from cerebrovascular disease, both haemorrhagic and thrombotic, and the incidence of vascular disease is directly related to the height of the blood pressure (either systolic or diastolic). What has now become clear is that these effects are reversible and that by lowering blood pressure the incidence of cerebrovascular disease may be reduced. This was first shown in those patients who had survived a minor stroke (secondary prevention) but more recently it has been shown also in patients who are hypertensive but have no cerebral symptoms (primary prevention) (*Lancet*, 1980). It is interesting that myocardial infarction although also due to atherosclerosis is relatively little influenced by antihypertensive treatment.

The level of blood pressure at which treatment should be begun and the level to which it should be reduced depend on the age of the patient and the duration of the disease.

Elderly patients and those with chronic hypertension have a disturbance of those physiological mechanisms, both neurogenic and intrinsic, which regulate blood supply to the brain. They may be unable to tolerate a sudden reduction in blood pressure without fainting, especially if they already suffer from occlusive atheromatous changes in the main cerebral arteries.

Drugs such as propranolol or methyldopa which produce a moderate but 'smooth' reduction in pressure without marked postural variations are the most suitable and the objective should be to treat all those with pressures greater than 160/100 and to reduce it below that level. The addition of a thiazide diuretic may be advantageous provided the haematocrit is not raised. In younger patients or those with shorter-term hypertension it should be possible to achieve more truly physiological blood pressure levels without side-effects.

The tendency of diabetic patients to suffer from vascular disease is well known and is attributed to two factors – the acceleration of atherosclerosis and the development of a specific micro-angiopathy. It is the latter change which is responsible for the characteristic neuropathy, nephropathy and retinopathy of diabetes. Cerebrovascular disease results partly from large vessel occlusion and partly from micro-angiopathy. It has long been known that poorly controlled diabetics tend to develop complications and it is now known from experimental work and from clinical trials that micro-angiopathy can be prevented and even reversed by optimal control (Cahill et al, 1976). There are thus good reasons for attempting to impose strict control of hyperglycaemia using modern methods of self-monitoring of blood glucose by the patient.

Although atheromatous lesions contain fat and although hypercholesterolaemic patients have increased amounts of atheroma and an increased incidence of coronary artery disease, the evidence linking abnormal lipid metabolism with cerebrovascular disease is not strong. Epidemiological surveys show a significant association with hyperlipidaemia only in young men. Furthermore, although cholesterol levels can be lowered by dieting or drug treatment, and although skin xanthomas may become smaller, it has been difficult to show any change in the size of lesions in the vessel wall. In the recent controlled trial of clofibrate in ischaemic heart disease the treated group had fewer myocardial infarctions but this beneficial effect was offset by a higher death rate from other causes (WHO Clofibrate Trial, 1978). There are as yet no trials claiming benefit in cerebrovascular disease (VA Co-operative Study, 1973). At present there is insufficient evidence to recommend long-term dietary treatment or the use of drugs to lower blood cholesterol, except in children with familial hypercholesterolaemia. Public campaigns aimed at altering the eating habits of the nation in order to prevent arterial disease seem unjustified on present evidence.

GIANT CELL ARTERITIS

Giant cell arteritis is a disease of the elderly probably caused by an auto-immune reaction to arterial elastic tissue; there is inflammation, thickening and occlusion of elastic and muscular arteries in various parts of the body. It most commonly affects branches of the external carotid, vertebral and subclavian arteries as well as the aorta itself. Intracranial arteries are not involved but cerebral infarction may result from embolism derived from inflamed neck vessels. The major complication is loss of vision due to occlusion of branches of the ophthalmic artery within the orbit.

Corticosteroids dramatically relieve headache and systemic symptoms and, once treatment is established, they prevent ocular complications. The drug is given initially in high dose (60–80mg a day) the dose being progressively reduced after two or three weeks to a level that will control muscular symptoms and keep the sedimentation rate below 30mm. Patients with a history of peptic ulceration should receive enteric-coated steroid preparations and cimetidine.

After six months an attempt should be made to discontinue steroids but many patients suffer a relapse with further headache and muscle pain, but not with ocular complications. Relapses should be controlled for as long as necessary (sometimes for years) by as small a dose of steroids as possible. Long-term high-dose steroid treatment causes a high morbidity from osteoporosis, infections, muscle weakness and diabetes. These are often worse than the disease itself and such treatment is best avoided.

CHRONIC PAIN IN NEUROLOGICAL DISORDERS

Although often disabling and distressing, chronic neurological disorders are seldom painful. There are, however, a number of conditions mostly involving sensory pathways at various points where pain is the predominant symptom. The best known of these conditions is post-herpetic neuralgia which affects 40 per cent of those with shingles, particularly around the head and neck in the elderly and infirm. There is some evidence that in the acute stage systemic corticosteroids or topical applications of 5% idoxuridine to herpetic skin lesions may lessen the incidence of neuralgia. As the eruption subsides a continuous burning pain in the affected region continues and is often combined with an obsessional and hypochondriacal melancholia and with general physical debility and sleeplessness.

At the onset patients need to be told that the pain will eventually subside although it may last many months, that immediate and complete pain relief is not possible, but that palliation can usually be achieved. An effective safe and inexpensive method of pain relief is counter-stimulation using an electrical skin stimulator or mechanical vibrator. These are thought to act by stimulating inhibitory pathways or by releasing endogenous analgesic peptides. About one-third of patients can be helped by these means during the first year. The patient may not be able to tolerate the stimulation in the affected area but it can also be effective when applied to adjacent regions. Other non-invasive methods interrupt pain pathways. Some produce skin anaesthesia either by Cryogel pack application or pain relieving (PR) spray. Local anaesthetic nerve blocks

are rather unpredictable in their effects both in duration and degree of relief. In general, response is disappointing but occasional patients with pain in the supraorbital region or on the trunk may be helped. Conventional analgesics are curiously ineffective; sedatives such as barbiturates make the pain worse, and strong analgesics induce a state of dependency which must at all costs be avoided. Carbamazepine is often given but is a poor analgesic for general use and may produce cardiac side-effects in elderly patients. In drug treatment, antidepressants, alone or in combination with simple analgesics or phenothiazines, afford the most relief and are particularly helpful when the patient is overtly depressed or has a past history of depressive illness. Of the various phenothiazines, chlorprothixene (Taractan) is the most effective but, because of side-effects, is best used in high dosage for short periods. The combination of amitriptyline and sodium valproate is also worth a trial.

Other painful entrapment neuropathies such as the carpal tunnel syndrome are best treated by surgery but neuralgia of the greater occipital nerve may be treated by counter-stimulation. Intercostal neuralgia also often responds well to this.

A painful neurological syndrome of a different kind is causalgia, a frequent cause of referral to a specialist pain clinic. This can occur at any age, and usually follows from partial damage to a large mixed peripheral nerve such as the median or sciatic. Reflex sympathetic dystrophic pain of a similar kind such as post-myocardial infarction syndrome, shoulder–hand syndrome, or Sudek's atrophy produce pain with similar characteristics. The pain is continuous and burning in quality accompanied by dysaesthesia and hypersensitivity and by skin changes such as atrophy, cyanosis, hyperhidrosis and finger clubbing, possibly due to involvement of sympathetic fibres in the nerve trunk. The most satisfactory method of treatment for these patients is local sympathetic block, either achieved by a local injection, e.g. into the Stellate ganglion or by the technique of intravenous guanethidine infusion of a limb.

The most difficult patients to help are those with a *central* cause for the pain, such as those with vascular lesions in the thalamus, and occasional patients with syringomyelia and multiple sclerosis. Counter-stimulation is well worth trying but often ineffective.

Prominent among the causes of less severe chronic pain is atypical facial pain. This causes continuous unilateral burning discomfort especially in the cheek lasting many hours at a time, and often accompanied by retardation, insomnia and depression. This syndrome is almost always found in middle-aged women and usually responds satisfactorily to tricyclic antidepressants or, if these fail, to monoamine-oxidase inhibitor drugs. The condition is often mistaken for referred pain from dental causes. Referral to a dental surgeon, however, inevitably leads to progressive removal of all remaining teeth and serves only to aggravate the condition.

MULTIPLE SCLEROSIS

Multiple sclerosis is one of the commonest disabling diseases to affect young adults, and the average general practitioner can expect to have on his list one or two patients suffering from it. In most instances the disease pursues a relapsing and remitting course but in some patients it is progressive from the outset. This variable prognosis has led to practical difficulties in mounting adequately controlled trials of drug treatment and there is no conclusive evidence that any of the therapies currently available affect the natural history of the disease.

In some patients multiple sclerosis follows a relatively benign course with little or no disability for many years. Patients presenting with optic neuritis or sensory symptoms are more likely to have a favourable prognosis than those presenting with either brainstem or cerebellar symptoms, although there are many exceptions to the rule. One of the first problems in management is deciding what and when the patient should be told; when the patient is adult it is generally best to reveal the true diagnosis if this is beyond doubt, but in the young, especially after an isolated first attack of optic neuritis, there is little point in telling the patient since multiple sclerosis may never develop or may take many years to do so. When subsequent attacks occur most patients appreciate a full explanation and it is important to emphasise the variable prognosis of the disorder. In established disease informed and open discussion about the condition is almost always welcomed by the patient and relatives. Associations of fellow sufferers such as the M.S. Society play a most valuable part in spreading information and providing group support.

Since young people are often affected many will want advice about whether to marry and have children, and on the subsequent chances of their children inheriting multiple sclerosis. Any patient contemplating marriage should be urged to tell the fiancé the full facts and this can be followed by discussion with both parties. When it comes to having a family, advice will depend on individual circumstances and, although the puerperium carries an increased risk of a relapse, the eventual degree of disability does not appear affected. A familial tendency is noted in about five per cent of patients with multiple sclerosis but no genetic pattern has emerged and, although no precise genetic advice can be given, the chances of a child also developing the condition are low.

Specific treatment
Although there is no cure for multiple sclerosis various drug and dietary regimens are tried by some physicians in the hope of modifying the course of the disease. Adrenocorticotrophic hormone (ACTH) will shorten the duration of an acute relapse but does not prevent further attacks or the progression of the condition. It is commonly prescribed in the dose of 40 units ACTH gel b.d. for one week and then once daily for a further week. It should then be discontinued and patients should not be put on long-term treatment because of the inevitable side-effects. Steroids (prednisolone 40mg a day or dexamethasone 2mg t.d.s.) are probably just as effective and have the advantage of oral administration, but again long-term treatment should be avoided. Immunosuppressive regimens involving cyclophosphamide and azathioprine have been suggested but in the absence of proven efficacy these drugs should be reserved for patients who relapse frequently. Transfer factor is still under evaluation and although some reports have given encouraging reports, further research is necessary.

Gluten-free diet has enjoyed wide popularity following rather unconvincing evidence of its efficacy in inducing remission. There are no sound reasons for supposing that such a diet might modify the disease but no harm comes from trying it, provided the patient does not lose weight excessively. Polyunsaturated fatty acid diets, based on sunflower oil, have also been suggested because some patients with multiple sclerosis have abnormally low blood levels of linoleic acid, and epidemiological evidence has demonstrated a possible correlation between the incidence of the disease and the amount of animal fat taken in the diet. The regimen involves avoiding animal fats as well as taking polyunsaturated fatty acids by mouth and there is some evidence that this may reduce the number of relapses although it will not cure the condition. Many patients seem to find it palatable and helpful.

General measures
It is a common finding that multiple sclerosis deteriorates markedly during intercurrent illness, physical exercise and when the body temperature is slightly increased. Over-exertion should therefore be avoided and bed rest is advisable during any acute relapse. Disturbances of mood often accompany

multiple sclerosis and, contrary to the usual teaching, depression is more frequently observed than euphoria. This is of the reactive type and may respond to anti-depressants.

Spastic paraparesis with or without sensory loss, brainstem or cerebellar signs, are the usual persisting disabilities in multiple sclerosis. Little can be done to improve sensory loss, co-ordination or weakness, but the spasticity which results from interruption of descending motor pathways can be partially relieved. The principles of treatment of spasticity are the reduction of sensory input to the spinal cord, the diminution of reflex activity and spontaneous spasms, the giving of drugs to increase synaptic resistance within the cord, and the development of extensor tonus. Reduction of sensory stimulation varies from such common sense measures as the avoidance of skin irritation or pressure sores and the treatment of urinary infection to the surgical or chemical interruption of sensory nerve roots by intrathecal phenol. As flexor activity diminishes the development of extensor tonus is encouraged by early standing.

Drugs never completely relieve severe spasticity but can be of considerable help in some patients. Baclofen (Lioresal) 10mg or diazepam 2mg is administered twice daily, increasing until maximal effect is obtained. Dantrolene (Dantrium) 25mg b.d. is a drug which acts directly on the muscle fibres and offers a useful alternative. Relief from spontaneous flexor spasms is often gratifying but if too much of the drug is given the legs tend to become flaccid. Intermittent cutaneous electrical stimulation over the lumbar region or upper thigh may also lessen spasticity and improve mobility in some patients.

Disturbances of sphincter control are common in established multiple sclerosis and propantheline (Pro-Banthine) or emepronium (Cetiprin) may help to control precipitancy of micturition. Urinary infection sometimes presents with urgency or incontinence and therefore should be excluded whenever a sudden deterioration in bladder control occurs. When incontinence becomes a persistent problem, permanent catheterisation or, more rarely, the surgical fashioning of an ileal conduit may be undertaken.

Paroxysmal symptoms may occur in patients with multiple sclerosis and are important to recognise because some will respond dramatically to carbamazepine (Tegretol) 200mg t.d.s. (Matthews, 1975). They may take the form of tonic seizures, which are brief and often painful episodes during which the limbs on one or both sides of the body assume a posture reminiscent of tetany. Brief paroxysmal episodes of dysarthria and ataxia or very transient paresis may also occur. Symptoms indistinguishable from trigeminal neuralgia have been reported in young patients with multiple sclerosis and also respond to carbamazepine. These paroxysmal symptoms should not be confused with the painful flexor spasms which many patients complain of, especially during the night. The role of spinal cord stimulation (with electrodes implanted in the epidural space) as a form of palliative treatment in patients with spasticity and disturbed bladder function is currently under evaluation (Read, Matthews and Higson, 1980). Although early results appear encouraging, this facility is not widely available and, of course, does not offer the possibility of cure of the disease.

PARKINSON'S DISEASE

When a diagnosis of Parkinson's disease is made, many patients and their families envisage a rapid descent into both physical and mental incapacity. It is therefore important to explain the nature of the disorder with emphasis on its variable prognosis and the favourable response to treatment. In patients with limited symptoms this may be all that is required but more usually psychological support is supplemented by drug therapy. With the advent of more successful medical treatment, surgical procedures are now rarely undertaken, although they still have a role in certain types of the disorder.

Drug therapy
The introduction of levodopa has radically affected the management of patients with Parkinson's disease but, as with most new drugs, initial enthusiasm has been tempered by an increasing awareness of the side-effects which may occur when the drug is first given or after many years on maintenance therapy (Marsden and Parkes, 1977). Nevertheless, levodopa represents a considerable breakthrough in treatment and when combined with a peripheral decarboxilase inhibitor it is the drug of choice in patients with moderate or severe disability.

In patients with mild symptoms, anticholinergic drugs still have a place in the treatment of Parkinson's disease. There are a large number of synthetic anticholinergic agents available (for example, benzhexol, benztropine, orphenadrine) and all have similar side-effects. None of the drugs is outstandingly effective and having made the decision about which one to try, the initial dosage should be low. As the dose is gradually increased side-effects such as dry mouth, blurred vision, constipation and difficulty with micturition will indicate the limits of tolerance. A specific contra-indication is narrow-angle glaucoma.

Mental changes, with hallucinations and paranoid delusions may occur in a few patients and necessitate a reduction or withdrawal of the offending drug. Although anticholinergic drugs will improve functional capacity in patients with idiopathic parkinsonism, the effects are not dramatic and the most notable feature is some reduction in rigidity.

Levodopa is a dopamine precursor; its development stems from the observation that there is a selective loss of dopaminergic neurones in the basal ganglia of brains from patients dying with Parkinson's disease. When used alone the early side-effects include nausea, vomiting, postural hypotension and cardiac arrhythmias, which can be attributed to the peripheral action of dopamine occurring outside the central nervous system. These unwanted side-effects are reduced when levodopa is given in combination with an inhibitor of extra-cerebral decarboxylase, which blocks the conversion of levodopa to dopamine but does not inhibit the central effect since it cannot cross the blood-brain barrier. Two combined preparations are currently available and it is usual to commence patients on either Sinemet (which contains levodopa and carbidopa) or Madopar (which contains levodopa and benserazide). The use of a combined preparation reduces the incidence of peripheral side-effects without compromising the efficacy of levodopa alone.

Both Sinemet and Madopar are available in two strengths and the preparations are roughly equivalent to five times the dose of levodopa alone. Initial treatment consists of one of the weaker capsules (Sinemet 110 or Madopar 125) given twice daily with weekly increments of one capsule until the more powerful capsules can be substituted. Maximum efficacy is usually obtained with a dose of 400mg to 1 gram of levodopa in combined form. Contra-indications include the concurrent administration of monoamine-oxidase inhibitors and the presence of haemolytic anaemia. Narrow-angle glaucoma should be treated prior to starting the drug. The use of levodopa must be undertaken with caution in patients with a history of ischaemic heart disease especially if there is associated history of cardiac dysrhythmia.

Even when levodopa is prescribed in combined form, side-effects may occur during the introductory phase of treatment and limit subsequent increases in dose. Nausea and vomiting are sometimes troublesome but may be relieved by taking the capsules after meals and by an even more gradual increment in dosage. Postural hypotension, which although less severe than when levodopa is used in isolation, can occur and may restrict dosage.

Psychiatric disturbances can be expected in about a quarter of all patients treated with levodopa or one of the combined preparations. Although these may amount to no more than a welcome improvement in mood, some patients may suffer more profound and occasionally psychotic mental changes with visual hallucinations. All patients should therefore be monitored carefully for the development of mental changes when the drug is introduced. As the dosage is increased mild involuntary movements may become troublesome and usually indicate the limits of tolerance. Facial dyskinesias, which include grimacing, blepharospasm, persistent chewing and alternating protrusion and retraction of the tongue are often the first to appear, but dyskinesia may affect any part of the muscular system. Flexion and extension movements at the ankle, and sustained inversion of the foot are fairly common. Head tremors, spasmodic torticollis and more dramatic involuntary movements of the trunk have also been described and may necessitate a reduction in dosage.

Intolerable involuntary movements sometimes supervene after many years on maintenance therapy and patients on Sinemet or Madopar therefore require long-term supervision with drug adjustments to achieve optimal benefit. There may be a loss of therapeutic efficacy after several years of treatment and a further late complication is the development of the 'on-off' phenomenon which denotes sudden but transient bouts of profound hypokinaesia and unsteadiness. These shortcomings have prompted research into other drugs designed to replace or supplement levodopa.

Bromocriptine, a dopamine receptor agonist, has received considerable attention over recent years and most reports suggest that its efficacy is equivalent to levodopa. In patients displaying the late side-effects of levodopa, bromocriptine may allow levodopa to be reduced or completely withdrawn. The early side-effects are similar and initial dosage should not exceed 5mg a day. Over a period of weeks this can be gradually increased to a maximum of 80–100mg/day although this may prove impossible because of persistent side-effects. It is a useful drug in patients whose response to levodopa appears exhausted and it is of limited benefit in patients displaying the 'on-off' phenomenon. Its use may be broadened when a peripheral dopamine receptor antagonist becomes available since this will reduce the incidence of gastro-intestinal and cardiovascular side-effects (Agid et al, 1979).

Introduced as an antiviral agent, amantadine hydrochloride was accidentally found to have an anti-parkinsonian activity. When given in the dosage 100–200mg daily it leads to a rapid, if modest, improvement in rigidity and hypokinesia. Its effect is often short-lived and tends to diminish after a month or so of continuous therapy, but it represents a useful adjunct to treatment when levodopa dosage is limited by side-effects. The drug may produce mild gastro-intestinal symptoms as well as drowsiness and insomnia, although these side-effects are not usually a serious problem. In addition amantadine occasionally produces ankle oedema and, even more rarely, heart failure.

Many patients with Parkinson's disease develop an associated depression which adds to their functional disability. Imipramine or amitriptyline (75–150mg daily) can be safely used with levodopa and should be prescribed for extended periods when indicated.

In summary, levodopa given in combination with a peripheral decarboxylase inhibitor (Sinemet or Madopar) is an extremely useful drug in patients with moderate or severe disability. The drug is initially given in a low dose, shortly after meals, and the patient should be carefully monitored for signs of intolerance. Dosage can be gradually increased and the limits of tolerance are frequently heralded by the development of involuntary movements. These may occur even when the dosage is small and it is then worth trying amantadine hydrochloride (200mg/day) as an adjunct to therapy. Patients with minor disability can be treated with an anticholinergic drug either alone or in combination with amantadine hydrochloride. Bromo-criptine represents a useful additive to levodopa in patients who develop the late side-effects of sustained levodopa therapy but it is not yet established as an alternative drug of first choice.

If parkinsonian symptoms develop in patients who are receiving phenothiazine medications then levodopa is contra-indicated and the ideal treatment should consist of withdrawing the offending drug. However, if this is unacceptable it is reasonable and often helpful to add one of the synthetic anticholinergic agents.

Surgical measures

Stereotaxic surgery may be contemplated in young patients with unilateral disease, particularly if drug treatment is poorly tolerated or eventually proves ineffective. Many techniques have been used to produce focal lesions in the basal ganglia and the chief benefit is on tremor and rigidity. If bilateral surgery is undertaken, subsequent speech abnormalities and intellectual deterioration may occur and there is therefore no place for operation on elderly patients with generalised disease.

Conclusion

The management of Parkinson's disease is still far from ideal and the treatment of patients with this condition carries some risk and involves regular follow-up. However, evidence is now accumulating which suggests that the use of levodopa leads to a reduction in the mortality rate, which used to be some three times higher in patients with Parkinson's disease than in the general population. Although levodopa may not halt the progression of the disease, most patients may be returned to normal health for two to three years and many remain independent for much longer.

MYASTHENIA GRAVIS

Myasthenia gravis is a disease manifested by muscular weakness which fluctuates in severity and commonly affects the ocular and other cranial muscles. It is caused by circulating antibodies to acetylcholine receptor protein and is associated with other autoimmune diseases, the most frequent of which is hyperthyroidism. Because of its rarity (the prevalence rate in the United Kingdom is about 6 per 100,000 population) many general practitioners will not have been faced with either the problems of diagnosis or management, but it is a disease where close liaison between hospital and general practitioner is vital.

Women are more frequently affected than men and although onset during the third or fourth decade is the most common the disease can present at any age. Patients may give a vague history of intermittent fatiguability involving the cranial muscles with few signs on examination. Ptosis and diplopia are the most common symptoms, and will almost always vary during the course of the day. Difficulties with chewing, talking and swallowing, again with fatiguability, are frequent. When limbs are involved, weakness may appear in any muscle group but the abductors of the shoulder and extensors at the elbow and wrist are more often affected.

Once the diagnosis is suspected, fatiguability should be assessed during the physical examination and a mild ocular palsy for instance can often be accentuated by asking the patient to maintain an upward gaze. Immediate confirmation of the diagnosis can sometimes be obtained by the response to intravenous anticholinesterase drugs. In adults, 1ml of edrophonium chloride (Tensilon), containing 10mg of the drug is given. Two milligrams are first injected and if the patient does not experience any side-effects the remaining 8mg is given and power in specific muscle groups is evaluated. The test is easy to interpret when assessing weakness of the cranial muscles because the response is both prompt and dramatic, but evaluation of limb weakness may on occasion prove difficult. An electromyograph is sometimes necessary to provide confirmation of the diagnosis.

In some centres, serum acetylcholine receptor antibody activity can also be measured and since this antibody is specific to myasthenia gravis it is very useful when the diagnosis remains in doubt. The test is positive in 80 per cent of patients with generalised myasthenia.

Treatment usually starts with either neostigmine or pyridostigmine. Both drugs are antagonists to cholinesterase, the enzyme which normally destroys acetylcholine; neostigmine is available in 15mg tablets (Prostigmin) and pyridostigmine in 60mg tablets (Mestinon). They are interchangeable, but most patients prefer pyridostigmine because its action is smoother and longer lasting. It is reasonable to commence with 60mg pyridostigmine three times a day, taken with meals, and patients may feel able to tailor the dosage to suit their particular needs. These drugs rarely produce complete relief of symptoms and some patients may take up to 15 tablets a day. Over-dosage itself may exacerbate weakness by producing a depolarising block at the neuromuscular junction.

The side-effects of anticholinesterase include nausea and vomiting, increased salivation, diarrhoea and abdominal cramps. Pyridostigmine produces fewer of these unwanted effects than neostigmine and propantheline bromide or atropine may give relief if they are particularly troublesome.

Anticholinesterase drugs may be all that is required in patients with mild disability, particularly when ocular symptoms predominate. These drugs control symptoms, but therapy aimed at inducing remission of the disease itself is now frequently attempted at an early stage (Rowland, 1980). The therapeutic choices include thymectomy, immunosuppression with prednisolone alone or in combination with azathioprine and, where available, plasmapheresis. Control trials on the relative efficacy of these various measures are needed but the consensus seems to favour early thymectomy, especially in young patients with generalised symptoms, following which about two-thirds of the patients will show improvement. In patients with a thymoma, the results are less encouraging but thymectomy is indicated because the tumour may infiltrate locally. In patients with severe and persistent disability, alternate-day prednisolone is frequently used though doubts still persist about the dosage and duration of treatment. When used in combination with azathioprine, prednisolone dosage can be reduced, thus lowering the incidence of long-term side-effects. Plasmapheresis may provide a dramatic short-term improvement which can be useful during a

severe exacerbation, and its role in the long-term management of patients with myasthenia is currently being evaluated.

The natural history of myasthenia is variable and in some patients weakness will remain restricted to the ocular muscles for many years and represent no threat to life. At the other end of the spectrum, however, there are patients with generalised disease who may require repeated admissions to hospital during acute relapses. Any profound exacerbation, particularly when the respiratory muscles are involved, will require immediate hospital referral because it may necessitate a period of assisted ventilation.

Emotional stress can lead to an increase in weakness and patients with myasthenia often need considerable psychological support. They should be advised to rest when weakness is generalised. Infection may lead to a deterioration which may be compounded if the patient attempts to carry on working. The severity of symptoms can increase during pregnancy but pregnancy is not necessarily contra-indicated unless the disease is severe and poorly controlled. Forceps delivery or caesarean section may be required to avoid the muscular effort which attends a normal delivery, and neonatal myasthenia occurs in one in eight babies born to myasthenic mothers. Management of a baby with myasthenia sometimes involves the use of anticholinesterase drugs but the symptoms of this condition do not last for more than a month.

DEMENTIA

The onset of dementia is usually insidious and there is a slow decline in intellect and personality. Memory, particularly short term, becomes impaired and this is accompanied by loss of judgement and reasoning ability. Change in personality and behaviour often alerts relatives that something is wrong, particularly when the deterioration in higher functions is subtle and effectively concealed by the patient. Focal neurological signs such as hemiparesis, hemianopia or language disturbance are usually absent but this should not preclude further investigation (Lishman, 1978).

When the disease starts in patients under the age of 65 years it is referred to as pre-senile dementia and over 65 years as senile dementia. However, dementia itself does not constitute a diagnosis and investigation is important in all age groups to exclude an underlying condition which may be amenable to treatment. The causes of dementia include those conditions characterised by primary neuronal loss of unknown cause such as Alzheimer's disease, Pick's disease and Huntington's chorea, as well as the secondary dementias in which neuronal loss occurs as a result of an underlying abnormality. Cerebrovascular disease may present as a step-wise dementing process usually with some physical signs, both the result of small multiple cerebral infarctions. Secondary dementia can also occur as a result of an underlying metabolic abnormality such as vitamin B_{12} deficiency or hypothyroidism. Non-specific intellectual decline or personality change may be a dominant symptom in patients with intracranial space-occupying lesions especially in the frontal lobes or with communicating hydrocephalus. Toxins, the most notable of which is alcohol, are sometimes responsible and neurosyphilis is still occasionally encountered.

Investigation has been greatly simplified by the CT scan and some patients can be effectively assessed on an outpatient basis. The metabolic dementias such as hypothyroidism and hypercalcaemia are excluded by the appropriate blood tests and the serum B_{12} should also be estimated. A WR should be performed to rule out neurosyphilis. A CT scan may indicate the degree of cerebral atrophy as well as excluding hydrocephalus and a treatable space-occupying lesion such as meningioma or subdural haematoma. A formal psychometric assessment is seldom required but may help when the distinction between depression and dementia is uncertain, and it also provides a baseline against which subsequent progress can be assessed.

After establishing that no specific therapy is available, the patient will want to know about prognosis particularly if he has had to give up work. It is best to err on the side of optimism because a gloomy prognosis leads to profound depression and a more lengthy explanation will almost certainly be forgotten. However, the patient's relatives will need a full and detailed account in order that the necessary adjustments can be made at home. One of the first problems which may have to be faced, particularly in pre-senile dementia, is that of continued employment. Some patients with less demanding work may continue for a surprising length of time, and understanding employers will sometimes make the necessary allowances once the situation has been explained.

The burden of care falls upon the family and their patience may be repeatedly tried as the disease progresses. Patients with dementia undoubtedly do better in familiar surroundings and hospital admission is best avoided although it should not be withheld when family strains build up.

Relatives may need advice on how to talk to and maintain the interest of a demented patient. They should be encouraged to follow the conversational leads given by the patient rather than introducing new topics beyond the patient's grasp. With help they may learn how to manage episodes of disturbed and aggressive behaviour.

The drug treatment of patients with dementia has three objectives. First, the judicious use of psychotropic preparations may benefit mood and sleep disorders; secondly, specific therapy is indicated for incidental illness during which the patient's mental state can deteriorate markedly and thirdly, treatment aimed at halting or reversing the demental process itself may sometimes be possible.

Psychotropic drugs

All sedatives are prone to cause confusional states and barbiturates in particular should be avoided. Simple hypnotics, such as one of the shorter-acting benzodiazepines (temazepam, oxazepam, lorazepam and triazolam) may be helpful when sleep is disturbed. If periods of restless agitation or aggressive withdrawal are prominent then small doses of promazine or thioridazine are helpful. When depression is a prominent feature, a trial of amitriptyline or imipramine may be indicated but these drugs have side-effects which can be particularly distressing in the elderly. The newer tricyclic antidepressants (mianserin, nomifensine and maptroline) are tolerated better and offer a reasonable alternative. The involuntary movements of Huntington's chorea can usually be reduced by tetrabenazine (Nitoman) but it is liable to cause depression. Drug regimens should be kept simple and where possible administration should be supervised by responsible relatives.

Incidental illness

In elderly and demented patients incidental illness may present as a confusional state without specific symptoms. Thus, episodes of cardiac failure, respiratory or urinary infection, and anaemia can present as an acute deterioration in mental function. Prompt antibiotic treatment aimed at any underlying infection is therefore indicated. It is worth remembering that faecal impaction or urinary retention may also present in this way and particular attention should be paid to maintaining adequate fluid and vitamin requirements.

Specific drug therapy aimed at arresting the dementing process

Dementias associated with vitamin B_{12} deficiency and hypothyroidism respond favourably to specific therapy which will halt and, on occasion, reverse the intellectual decline. Vasodilator substances have been tried in arteriosclerotic and other types of dementia but the overall impression remains that they have little place in management despite occasional claims to the contrary. Cyclandelate (Cyclospasmol), co-dergocrine mesylate (Hydergine) and naftidrofuryl oxalate (Praxilene) have all been subject to limited trials in demented patients with conflicting results and there is no convincing evidence of their efficacy. Even in arteriosclerotic dementia there is little rationale for prescribing these preparations because the dementia is almost always secondary to multiple cerebral infarction rather than to a primary reduction in overall blood flow. Sustained hypertension should of course be treated since this predisposes to further infarction, and anticoagulants or antiplatelet drugs (such as aspirin) may have a role in preventing further thrombotic episodes. In patients with Alzheimer's disease, the recent finding of a specific reduction in choline acetyl transferase in the cerebral cortex has prompted trials of choline and lecithin therapy, but preliminary results are disappointing.

REFERENCES

Agid, Y., Bonnet, A. M., Pollak, P., Signoret, J. L., and Lhermitte, F. (1979). Bromocriptine associated with a peripheral dopamine blocking agent in treatment of Parkinson's disease. *Lancet*, **1**, 570–2.

Cahill, G. F. et al (1976). 'Control' and diabetes. *New England Journal of Medicine*, **294**, 1004.

Canadian Co-operative Study Group (1978). A randomised trial of aspirin and sulphinpyrazone in threatened stroke. *New England Journal of Medicine*, **299**, 53–9.

Carter, A. B. (1965). Prognosis of cerebral embolism. *Lancet*, **2**, 514–19.

Fisher, C. M. (1979). Capsular infarcts. *Archives of Neurology*, **36**, 65–73.

Hughes, R. C. and Foster, J. B. (1971). *Current Therapeutic Research*, **13**, 63.

Lancet 1980. The Australian therapeutic trial in mild hypertension. *Lancet*, **1**, 1261–7.

Lishman, W. A. (1978). *Senile dementia, pre-senile dementia and pseudodementia*, In Organic Psychiatry: the Psychological Consequences of Cerebral Disorder, pp. 527–95. Blackwell Scientific Publications Ltd, Oxford.

Marsden, C. D. and Parkes, J. D. (1977). Success and problems of long-term levodopa therapy in Parkinson's disease. *Lancet*, **1**, 345–9.

Matthews, W. B. (1975). Paroxysmal symptoms in multiple sclerosis. *Journal of Neurology, Neurosurgery and Psychiatry*, **38**, 619–23.

Read, D. J., Matthews, W. B. and Higson, R. H. (1980). The effect of spinal cord stimulation on function in patients with multiple sclerosis. *Brain*, **103**, 803–33.

Rowland, L. P. (1980). Controversies about the treatment of myasthenia gravis. *Journal of Neurology, Neurosurgery and Psychiatry*, **43**, 644–9.

Sullivan, J. M., Harken, D. E. and Gorlin, R. (1968). Pharmacological control of thromboembolic complications of cardiac valve replacement. *New England Journal of Medicine*, **279**, 576–80.

VA Co-operative Study (1973). Treatment of cerebrovascular disease with clofibrate. *Stroke*, **4**, 684–93.

Weber, R. B. and Reinmuth, O. N. (1972). The treatment of migraine with propranolol. *Neurology*, **22**, 366–9.

WHO Clofibrate Trial (1978). A co-operative trial in the primary prevention of ischaemic heart disease using clofibrate. *British Heart Journal*, **40**, 1069–118.

Chapter 8   Gastro-intestinal tract disease

D. R. TRIGER MA, BM, BCh, DPhil, FRCP

INTRODUCTION

Many of the chronic disorders of the gastro-intestinal tract may be regarded as symptom complexes, in which the symptoms bear a variable and imprecise relation to the degree of measurable pathological disturbance and in which drug therapy is directed towards symptomatic relief rather than towards cure of the disease itself.

While drug therapy plays an important role in the management of most of these disorders, it is important to recognise that this is rarely the only means of treatment and a number of other vital factors should be borne in mind when managing such patients.

HIATUS HERNIA

Symptoms referable to hiatus hernia are caused by reflux oesophagitis and in their absence there is no indication for treatment. This is important since marked radiological, endoscopic and even histological changes may be seen at or near the gastro-oesophageal junction in the asymptomatic patient.

Although drug therapy plays an important role in the management of symptoms it may have little or no effect in many patients compared with other measures. Thus the obese patient who is resistant to many therapeutic manoeuvres may lose all symptoms if significant weight loss can be achieved. Significant oesophagitis is usually related to posture so elevation of the head of the bed at night and avoidance of activities which include bending will do much to relieve symptoms. Both cigarette and alcohol consumption as well as the ingestion of spicy food stimulate acid secretion and these should be avoided as they not infrequently aggravate oesophagitis.

Since many factors contribute to the symptoms associated with hiatus hernia, a number of very different drug regimens are effective.

Antacids

This group of drugs can be considered as the first-line method of drug therapy for reflux oesophagitis since antacids are cheap, easily available and generally very effective. They should be administered after meals and before the patient retires to bed. Although many are available in solid form, antacids are usually more effective when given as liquids, usually in 10ml doses.

The choice of antacid is arbitrary, although aluminium hydroxide, magnesium hydroxide and magnesium trisilicate are the most commonly used. Disturbances in bowel action are common, magnesium salts tending to induce diarrhoea and aluminium salts constipation. Sodium bicarbonate and calcium carbonate may also be used. Whereas antacids – frequently in combination with milk – are excellent for the relief of occasional symptoms, their prolonged use in high dosage should not be encouraged. Cardiac failure, hypercalcaemia and the milk-alkali syndrome are all serious and avoidable side-effects of antacids, while aluminium preparations are contra-indicated in patients with renal failure.

Other agents

Increasing the viscosity of the gastric contents reduces reflux. This is the rationale behind the use of alginic acid which is usually combined with an antacid (e.g. Gaviscon) and is undoubtedly effective in treating symptoms of hiatus hernia.

Another approach to symptomatic relief is the use of agents which act locally on the lower oesophageal mucosa. Local anaesthetic agents such as oxethazaine (Mucaine) are sometimes used but a more popular drug is dimethicone (Asilone). This is a synthetic coating agent which coats the lining of the lower oesophageal mucosa, thereby preventing acid from reaching the sensitive inflamed tissue. Both of these agents are marketed in combination with an antacid.

The H_2-receptor antagonist cimetidine (see below) may also be used, since effective blockage of acid secretion from the stomach may help to reduce continued inflammation of the oesophagus and the symptoms which this produces. Metoclopramide (Maxolon) may also be used, symptomatic relief being achieved through its ability to facilitate gastric emptying.

Drug therapy in practice

Although the drugs available for treating reflux oesophagitis vary widely in their mode of action we are unable to define any clinical features which enable us to predict with certainty which type of therapy is likely to be most effective.

Most patients with symptoms related to hiatus hernia only experience minor episodes of reflux oesophagitis from time to time and for such individuals an occasional dose of antacid coupled with attention to their diet and posture is all that is required. Where the symptoms are more severe or persistent, alternative drugs may be required. There is no evidence to suggest that any one group of agents is superior to the others although some patients may find one more effective or acceptable than another.

Usually a single drug taken regularly is sufficient to control symptoms within a week or two, but in cases of severe reflux oesophagitis it may be necessary to use two or even three drugs. A regimen which I find very effective in such severe cases is the combination of an alginate, an agent which coats the oesophageal mucosa and metoclopramide, each prescribed in full dosage. Control of symptoms is usually achieved within two weeks, when one of the drugs can be omitted and, subsequently, the other drugs slowly reduced.

Attention to the time and method of drug administration is particularly important since this varies widely according to the agent used. Many patients experience their major symptoms of gastro-oesophageal reflux at night, so most drug regimens should include a dose to be taken on retiring to bed. In addition, antacids are best prescribed on a thrice-daily basis between meals whereas dimethicone, which coats the mucosa in preparation for the acid secretion induced by food, should be taken half an hour before meals. Alginates, on the other hand, should be taken after the ingestion of food, since they rely upon increasing viscosity of the gastric contents for their action. Patients with upper gastro-intestinal tract symptoms commonly experience difficulty in swallowing medicines and most of the drugs for treating these disorders are available in either tablet or suspension form. There is little to choose between the two either in efficacy or in cost, but in most cases the tablets should be chewed or sucked rather than swallowed. Failure of the patient to appreciate this is likely to lead to the drug being labelled as ineffective.

Reflux oesophagitis is occasionally complicated by the formation of oesophageal ulcers. Ulcer-healing agents such as carbenoxolone or cimetidine have been recommended but it is doubtful whether they are significantly superior to the other drugs used.

Once the symptoms of reflux oesophagitis have been brought under control it is usually possible to reduce or even discontinue the drugs, especially if the other measures referred to earlier have been effectively enforced. The patient should be advised to reduce the dose of drugs gradually to the minimum necessary to control symptoms and from experience many are able to predict the circumstances which will induce symptoms and can take a dose of the appropriate drug to counter them.

Many patients can be well controlled on such regimens for years but periodic exacerbations of symptoms sometimes occur which necessitate re-introduction of larger doses of drugs. Failure to control symptoms of oesophagitis despite a combination of drugs (together with the non-drug measures) is one of the indications for hiatus hernia surgery, a situation which is relatively uncommon with the present range of therapy available.

PEPTIC ULCER

The development and widespread use of fibre-optic endoscopy, together with the extensive clinical trials which have taken place to evaluate cimetidine, have taught us a great deal about the natural history of peptic ulcer disease, especially duodenal ulcer. The main points to emerge from such studies are:

1. Peptic ulcer disease is extremely common, with many ulcers appearing and spontaneously healing over a course of a few weeks.
2. Patients may lose the symptoms of peptic ulceration without macroscopic healing of the ulcers.
3. The natural history of peptic ulcer disease in most patients is one of intermittent remission and relapse over many years, if not for most of their life.

While mental stress, cigarette and alcohol abuse are related to peptic ulcer disease the exact relation is obscure and at present we have no evidence that any non-surgical measures can significantly affect the natural history. It is against this background that the drug management of peptic ulcer disease should be considered.

Duodenal ulcer

ANTACIDS

As with reflux oesophagitis, antacids remain the corner-stone of drug therapy for duodenal ulcer symptoms, particularly in the patient with mild 'indigestion' where, in combination with milk, they are highly effective in the relief of pain. When taken in doses of 10ml three or four times a day it is doubtful whether they can induce or promote healing although this can be achieved if sufficient alkali is given to neutralise the gastric acid output. This necessitates two-hourly administration of 20ml antacid throughout the day and night, a regimen which is unacceptable to most people, in Great Britain at least.

In practice most patients with chronic duodenal ulcer disease have mild intermittent symptoms which are easily controlled by occasional small doses of antacids, and the majority treat themselves without seeking any medical advice. Severe symptoms which require large amounts of antacids, or which are resistant to them, should be considered an indication for alternative therapy.

CIMETIDINE

This drug is, without question, highly effective in healing duodenal ulcers. The recommended dose of 1g daily (200mg three times a day and 400mg at night) will heal 70 to 80 per cent of ulcers within six weeks. Higher dosage regimens are unlikely to be more effective in uncomplicated ulcer diseases. Most patients lose their symptoms of dyspepsia within a few days of starting therapy, but they should be encouraged to complete the full six-week course since symptomatic relief is obtained long before ulcer healing occurs.

At the end of six weeks it is advisable to stop cimetidine and await symptoms. A minority of patients (10 to 20 per cent) will relapse almost immediately and, if their symptoms are sufficiently severe and there are no obvious contra-indications, such patients should be recommended for surgery. A further minority (about 20 per cent) will remain asymptomatic for a prolonged period while the remainder will relapse at varying intervals during the next year or so. They are likely to respond to a further course of cimetidine but their remission will once again be no more than temporary and consistent with the natural history of duodenal ulcer disease.

The position regarding long-term use of cimetidine in such patients is at present uncertain. Experience has shown that in many patients symptomatic relief can be obtained by continuing a nightly maintenance dose of 400mg, although on this regimen many patients relapse and the proportion appears to increase steadily with time. Most patients can be kept symptom-free for long periods of time on cimetidine when prescribed in full dosage, but this is expensive and the long-term effects of gastric acid suppression are as yet unknown. At present it seems advisable to reserve such a regimen for patients with severe peptic ulcer symptoms in whom surgery is contra-indicated for medical reasons such as

debility, cardiovascular disease or respiratory failure. Elderly patients with severe inflammatory joint disease who develop peptic ulcer symptoms on analgesic drugs are another suitable category for long-term therapy.

There is no convincing evidence that cimetidine stops bleeding or prevents re-bleeding from peptic ulcers. Thus patients with recurrent haemorrhage from ulcers should be considered for surgery rather than be treated medically in the hope that further bleeding can be prevented.

Side-effects from cimetidine to date are few and minor. Gastro-intestinal upset and skin rashes occur in some patients, while gynaecomastia and impotence are more spectacular but rarer complications. Metabolism of the drug may be impaired in the elderly as well as in hepatic or renal failure, when the dose should be reduced since toxic levels can induce confusion or coma. In such patients it is advisable to reduce the daily dose to 600–800mg.

A further H_2-receptor antagonist (Ranitidine) has recently come on the market. It is at least as effective as cimetidine but somewhat more expensive. Theoretically it should not cause cerebral confusion as it does not cross the blood-brain barrier, but there is as yet insufficient experience to be sure that it does not have other side-effects.

OTHER DRUGS

A number of other drugs have been shown to be effective in treating gastric ulcers (see below) but their value in the management of duodenal ulcer is questionable. Nevertheless, several drugs, notably bismuth preparations (Denol) and slow-release carbenoxolone (Duogastrone) have their advocates and may be useful in patients in whom cimetidine is contra-indicated.

CONCLUSION

The wide choice of drugs currently available for treating duodenal ulcer disease means that symptoms can almost invariably be controlled, but we have made no significant progress in curing the disorder medically. Chronic mild symptoms can be effectively suppressed by antacids while cimetidine can control more severe acute exacerbations. Long-term suppression of duodenal ulcer symptoms with antacids in large dosage may produce a number of undesirable effects, while the risks of cimetidine are as yet unknown. There is no evidence to suggest that medical therapy has appreciably reduced the place of surgery for duodenal ulcer disease, although it may relieve the symptoms which patients need to tolerate prior to operation.

Gastric ulcer

The time-honoured treatment of gastric ulcer by bed rest, abstention from cigarettes and alcohol, and a strict milk diet is clearly an effective regimen but this is no longer essential and many drugs are now available.

Antacids and cimetidine have comparable therapeutic effect in gastric ulcer as in duodenal ulcer. The former are useful in obtaining symptomatic relief without promoting healing, while a six-week course of cimetidine will heal three-quarters of all gastric ulcers but with a significant relapse rate after treatment.

Alternative drugs which are appreciably cheaper than cimetidine are also available. Sodium carbenoxolone, a derivative of liquorice, promotes gastric ulcer healing and this can be achieved in four to six weeks using a dose of 100mg three times a day. Unfortunately the drug has significant sodium-retaining properties so cardiac failure complicated by hypokalaemic alkalosis can easily be precipitated, especially in the elderly. This is preventable by simultaneous prescription of a diuretic, but thiazide diuretics tend to aggravate the hypokalaemia and the logical alternative, an aldosterone antagonist such as spironolactone, effectively blocks the ulcer-healing properties. For this reason carbenoxolone has largely disappeared from clinical use and has been supplanted by a preparation in which the glycyrrhizinic acid has been removed (Caved-S). This product lacks the sodium-retaining properties but is of comparable cost and effectiveness in healing ulcers.

A number of medications containing bismuth are available (e.g. Denol). These are definitely effective in promoting gastric ulcer healing but, like many of the other drugs, must be given for at least four weeks even if symptoms are relieved within a few days.

PYLORIC ULCER

Ulcers at the pylorus respond to drug therapy in much the same way as gastric ulcers but because of their anatomical position there is a major risk of obstruction due to stenosis. Ulcer healing tends to cause fibrosis which is likely to aggravate any narrowing of the pyloric canal. For this reason patients with an ulcer and symptoms suggesting significant pyloric stenosis should be referred for surgery and long-term drug therapy is not to be recommended.

The principles governing drug therapy of gastric ulcer differ somewhat from that of duodenal ulcer in that there is a definite association between gastric ulcer and gastric carcinoma. Thus drug treatment of gastric ulcers should not be embarked upon without excluding the possibility of malignant change, and even initial symptomatic response to appropriate drug therapy does not exclude the possibility of carcinoma. Similarly, long-term management of chronic or recurrent gastric ulcerations using drugs is to be discouraged, and such subjects should be referred for surgery unless there are pressing medical contra-indications.

GALLSTONES

During the last few years the possibility of gallstone dissolution by non-surgical means has aroused much interest with the development of chenodeoxycholic acid. There is now good evidence to show that many stones can be dissolved, but a number of factors limit the use of this drug. The patient must have a functioning gall bladder as judged by the ability to opacify during cholecystography. In addition the gallstones must be radiolucent, as calcified stones cannot be dissolved. The larger the stones, the longer it requires for dissolution to occur, and experience has shown that it is difficult to dissolve stones greater than 15mm diameter. Chenodeoxycholic acid has no major side-effects, but abnormalities in liver function have been reported in patients receiving it and it should be used with caution in patients with hepatic dysfunction.

The recommended dose is calculated according to body-weight, the average being 10–15mg/kg/day. Stone dissolution is slow, most calculi requiring at least 6 to 12 months to disappear and the drug must be continued indefinitely since recurrence can often be detected within three months or so of stopping the medication. The drug is expensive, the average daily dose costing about £1 so the economics of long-term medical management compare unfavourably with cholecystectomy.

In practice there are few situations in which chenodeoxycholic acid is clinically indicated. The large majority of patients with symptomatic gallstones do not satisfy the criteria for treatment, and therapy for pre-symptomatic subjects is questionable on economic and ethical grounds as we must assume that such patients will remain on the drug for life and possible long-term effects of the agent are unknown. The patient with symptomatic gallstones who is otherwise fit should be referred for surgery without consideration for medical therapy. There remains a small group of symptomatic people with stones suitable for dissolution who have major medical contra-indications to surgery such as severe cardiovascular disease. For such individuals alone chenodeoxycholic acid may be life-saving.

Ursodeoxycholic acid is another derivative of cholic acid which is now being marketed. It is of similar efficacy in dissolving gallstones to chenodeoxycholic acid but is believed to be less likely to induce diarrhoea.

CHRONIC PANCREATITIS

Drugs play a comparatively small role in the management of this chronic disorder. Pancreatic extracts can be given by mouth to replace deficiencies in secretion and these are indicated in patients suffering malabsorption due to pancreatic steatorrhoea. A number of such extracts are commercially available and while there is little to choose between them in content some patients appear to express a distinct preference for one or another. The optimum dose varies from patient to patient and is derived by titration against the clinical response.

Diabetes mellitus is a further complication of chronic pancreatic disease which, if uncontrolled, will increase the problem of malnutrition. This must be treated with insulin since there are usually insufficient functioning islet cells for oral hypoglycaemic agents to be effective. Comparatively small amounts of insulin are required and good control of the diabetes is usually easy to achieve.

Pain is a major symptom of chronic pancreatitis in some cases. This may be either chronic and persistent or acute and intermittent due to recurrent attacks of acute pancreatic inflammation on a background of chronic disease. The pain may be extremely severe and require analgesic relief comparable with that given for malignant disease. Unless there are other contra-indications, however, such patients should be referred for surgical pancreatectomy which is usually highly effective in the treatment of severe pain.

In managing chronic pancreatitis it is important to bear in mind that this condition usually occurs in association with either alcohol abuse or gallstones. Ability to treat these precipitating factors is likely to facilitate the management of the pancreatic problem.

CHRONIC LIVER DISEASE

Drug therapy in chronic liver disease can be considered in two distinct parts – the treatment of chronic liver disorders *per se* in an attempt to halt or slow down their rate of progression, and the management of the complications which arise secondary to hepatic dysfunction.

Treatment of liver disease

Unfortunately our present knowledge of chronic liver disorders is such that few types of liver disease can be treated by any form of drug therapy. The most out-standing exception is Wilson's disease, the rare genetic disorder of copper metabolism in which spectacular improvement can be achieved by the use of the chelating agent D-penicillamine. The rarity and complexity of this disorder is such that it should not be managed without the advice of a specialist unit and detailed consideration is outside the scope of this book.

The only other chronic liver disease in which drugs have an established role in primary treatment of the disorder is chronic active or auto-immune hepatitis. This is the chronic liver disease characterised by a histological appearance of chronic aggressive hepatitis accompanied by serum auto-antibodies, high serum immunoglobulins and other auto-immune disorders which predominate in young and middle-aged females. There is now good evidence that the use of corticosteroids significantly prolongs survival. The diagnosis should always be clearly established by liver biopsy and treatment is indicated according to the degree of liver cell inflammation which is most simply assessed by serum transaminase measurement. Where there is evidence of marked inflammation, high-dose steroids (40–60mg daily prednisolone) should be instituted. At this level biochemical improvement is usually detectable within a few days, whereupon the dose can be slowly reduced. The rate and extent of steroid reduction is dependent largely upon the clinical and biochemical response but even in uncomplicated cases it is usually necessary to prescribe steroids for a minimum of a year. In such patients one may be able to discontinue the steroids completely but continued observation for clinical and biochemical evidence of relapse is essential, when re-introduction of the drug may be necessary. Many patients are unable to tolerate withdrawal of steroids without a relapse, in which case long-term administration may be necessary. Here azathioprine is a useful additional drug. Although relatively ineffective when used alone, its combined administration with prednisolone will enable adequate control of liver inflammation to be achieved with a lower dose of the latter, and a consequent reduction in side-effects. The dose of azathioprine required is comparatively low (50–75mg daily) so the marrow depressant effects are unlikely to be significant. Periodic monitoring of the blood count is nevertheless advisable. Whereas steroids usually have a demonstrable action within days, the effect of azathioprine is not seen for several weeks after introduction so the drug should only be introduced if its long-term use is planned.

It should be stressed that corticosteroids and azathioprine are only indicated when there is evidence of significant active liver inflammation and the histological diagnosis of chronic aggressive hepatitis with little or no elevation in transaminases is insufficient grounds for treatment. In such cases inflammation is unlikely to be suppressed by these drugs and the possible benefits of drug therapy are likely to be outweighed by their side-effects. Similarly, once inflammation has been brought under control it is advisable to maintain patients on as low a dose of drugs as possible.

The role of drug therapy in chronic active hepatitis of viral aetiology is controversial. Not only is the prognosis of chronic viral hepatitis extremely variable, but the clinical and biochemical pattern of inflammation may fluctuate and be unpredictable. Nevertheless in patients with good evidence of *persistent* liver inflammatory activity (e.g. for a minimum of four months) it is reasonable to consider drug treatment. Corticosteroids should be used in the first instance, but unless there is a significant biochemical response within the defined period (three to six months) they should be discontinued as their side-effects are likely to outweigh any benefits.

It should be emphasised that long-term drug therapy should not be embarked upon without adequate investigation and preferably in consultation with a hospital unit.

The role of drugs in other forms of chronic liver disease is unproven. The iron overload which accompanies haemochromatosis can be treated with the chelating agent desferrioxamine but regular venesection is a safer and more effective means of treatment.

Treatment of complications of liver disease

Pruritus, encephalopathy and ascites are the three major complications of chronic liver disease which are amenable to drug therapy.

PRURITUS

Cholestyramine is undoubtedly the most effective drug available for treating this distressing complaint of chronic liver disease. It is an anion-exchange resin which is marketed in sachets each containing 4g of anhydrous powder. It should not be taken in its dry form and is best mixed with a flavoured liquid such as orange juice since many patients find it unpalatable. It acts by binding with bile salts in the gastro-intestinal tract and preventing their re-absorption. It is therefore only effective in patients with partial biliary obstruction, so it is unlikely to be helpful in individuals with high grade malignant obstructive jaundice.

Cholestatic disorders such as biliary cirrhosis or drug cholestasis are the major hepatic conditions producing pruritus. The itching is often variable and unpredictable, but most patients suffer their major symptoms at

night, possibly because at this time there is usually little to distract their attention. One sachet of cholestyramine taken in the early evening is often sufficient to control their symptoms, but in more intractable cases it may be necessary to take several sachets throughout the day. A dose of one sachet daily rarely produces diarrhoea, but larger doses commonly do so and this is frequently the dose-limiting factor. As well as diarrhoea cholestyramine may also induce steatorrhoea which, when gross, quickly leads to troublesome symptoms. Lesser degrees of steatorrhoea, however, may not give rise to any complaints but may lead to malabsorption over a period of time, producing osteomalacia due to vitamin D deficiency as well as coagulation abnormalities from vitamin K malabsorption. For this reason it is particularly important to restrict the long-term use of cholestyramine to a minimum and since pruritus in chronic liver disease may fluctuate considerably from month to month patients should be encouraged to titrate the dose against their symptoms. In practice the unpalatability of the drug is often an advantage since many patients are reluctant to take it unless they have to and a few will even prefer to put up with pruritus. The binding properties of cholestyramine are such that it may interfere with the absorption of other drugs; care should be taken to avoid giving oral medications at the same time as the cholestyramine.

Alternative drugs to control pruritus are of less value, but may be useful in patients with minor symptoms and in those who cannot tolerate cholestyramine. By analogy with allergic pruritus, antihistamines are prescribed in an attempt to control the itching of cholestasis. It is doubtful whether this group of drugs achieves any symptomatic relief beyond making the patient so sleepy that they are able to ignore the irritation! A similar argument probably applies to the barbiturates (phenobarbitone being the most popular) although this group of drugs is also able to induce hepatic microsomal enzymes and affect bilirubin metabolism. Both antihistamines and barbiturates may occasionally play a small but useful role but caution should be exercised in prescribing them in patients with hepatic dysfunction. The altered effects of drug metabolism in liver disease may lead to excess serum or tissue levels which can produce undue sedation.

Extra-hepatic obstruction of the biliary tree is a major cause of pruritus associated with liver abnormalities and is particularly important since surgery may dramatically alter its prognosis. It is essential to exclude any surgically remediable lesions before embarking upon the long-term medical management of pruritus.

ASCITES

The onset of ascites in a patient with non-malignant chronic liver disease is usually a sign of marked hepatic functional impairment and of quite significant portal hypertension. The introduction of powerful diuretics during the past decade or so has greatly simplified the management of these patients, such that all but the most severe and resistant cases can be adequately managed on an outpatient ambulatory basis. Nevertheless, the time-honoured means of treatment, namely bed rest and salt restriction, should not be totally ignored. Bed rest almost certainly has a beneficial effect on liver function since hepatic blood flow is significantly increased in the recumbent position. Furthermore alcohol is the major aetiology of cirrhosis in this country so the act of confining such a patient to bed usually has a significant impact on its continued consumption! Modern diuretics are sufficiently effective that sodium restriction is usually unnecessary, but it should be considered in patients who require very large doses of diuretics and in those who develop renal problems on increasing the dosage of such drugs.

Aldosterone antagonists (e.g. spironolactone) are the first choice of diuretics in the management of ascites. As mentioned earlier, alcohol abuse is the commonest cause of cirrhosis and such patients are particularly prone to hypokalaemia since ethanol has a significant kaliuretic effect. Spironolactone not only induces urinary excretion of sodium and water but it also conserves potassium, in contrast to the thiazide diuretics, whose action is likely to induce or aggravate potassium depletion. The rate of action of spironolactone is very slow compared with other diuretics, four or five days elapsing before any significant effect is detectable. Whereas at first sight this would appear to be a major drawback, the slow rate of action is actually beneficial since patients with severe liver disease do not tolerate large and rapid shifts of fluid and electrolytes. It should be remembered however that it may take as long as 10 to 14 days for the effects of aldosterone antagonism to wear off once the drug is stopped.

Patients with ascites should be started on a relatively small dose of spironolactone (e.g. 50–100mg daily). If no significant effect is detectable after a week the dose can be increased gradually up to a maximum of 400mg daily. Higher doses are occasionally used but these should be prescribed with great care since at this level side-effects (see below) may be quite considerable. Because of its slow action spironolactone need only be given on a once-daily basis. Alternatively, once aldosterone blocking has been achieved and the serum potassium level is satisfactory, a further diuretic such as frusemide can be added. The combination usually produces a synergistic action. A small dose of frusemide (40–80mg daily) is usually sufficient in this context since the aim should be to produce a slow but sustained diuresis. Milder thiazide diuretics (e.g. cyclopenthiazide) are of little value in the treatment of ascites, but recently amiloride has been used as an alternative to spironolactone. Relatively large doses (20–30mg daily) are required and at this dosage much greater care must be taken to avoid hyperkalaemia than with spironolactone.

Patients with advanced liver disease tend to lose the ability to regulate fluid and electrolyte balance. The problems of diuretic-induced hypo- and hyperkalaemia have already been alluded to, but these are most likely to occur within the first few weeks of introducing the diuretics. Large doses of such drugs may also induce renal failure. This may result from excessive diuresis, when the patients become dehydrated and hypovolaemic, but renal failure may appear in their absence. This is marked by oliguria and a rising blood urea, which is reversible if the drugs are withdrawn early but may otherwise prove progressive and fatal. Hyponatraemia is another complication of diuretic therapy in this setting, although it tends to occur when there is incipient or overt renal failure. A low serum sodium (< 125 mmol/litre) should be considered a contra-indication to diuretic therapy. Diuretics may also precipitate encephalopathy as a result of the fluid and electrolyte shift they can induce. They should be used only with great caution if encephalopathy is already present.

Other side-effects of diuretics in chronic liver disease are trivial by comparison. Gynaecomastia is a well-recognised complication of spironolactone, which may sometimes be quite painful. This usually improves on withdrawal of the drug but it should be remembered that it is also a recognised complication of cirrhosis, particularly that secondary to alcohol abuse. Skin rashes and nausea are occasional side-effects of all diuretics.

ENCEPHALOPATHY

Chronic hepatic encephalopathy, like ascites, is a sign of severe liver dysfunction. It may either arise spontaneously in chronic progressive liver damage or it may be precipitated by some factor complicating an otherwise well-compensated case of cirrhosis. Recognition of the latter is particularly important since attention to the precipitating factor or factors may result in rapid clinical improvement. Surgery and infection are well-recognised aggravating insults but drugs, especially sedatives and diuretics, are other important causes.

Current management of hepatic encephalopathy is

based upon two drugs which act in very different ways. It is generally believed that this clinical disorder is at least partly due to toxic metabolites produced by urea-splitting organisms in the colon which by-pass the liver via the collateral circulation that arises in cirrhosis and portal hypertension. Neomycin is a broad-spectrum antibiotic which is poorly absorbed from the gastro-intestinal tract and thus acts by killing the bacterial flora of the colon. It is given by mouth (although in exceptional circumstances may be used in a retention enema) in divided doses of 2–3g per day. Recently it has fallen somewhat into disfavour as a long-term therapeutic agent since it is not as poorly absorbed as was originally thought and cases of nephrotoxicity and deafness have been recorded in association with its use. Nevertheless in such patients it is of undoubted therapeutic value and its safety can be improved by paying close attention to the dose prescribed.

Lactulose has emerged in recent years as an alternative treatment of encephalopathy and is probably the first drug of choice today. It has two distinct modes of action. It acidifies the bowel contents, and since most of the urea-splitting bacteria require an alkaline medium for survival this effectively destroys the organisms. In addition the hypertonic nature of lactulose makes it an effective laxative, a property which is most useful in the treatment of encephalopathy since constipation is a potent cause of precipitating confusion or even coma in patients with chronic liver disease. The amount of lactulose required is rather variable, ranging from 10ml to 40ml daily in divided doses. In theory lactulose should be given until the stool pH is acid, but in clinical practice it is rarely possible to monitor stool acidity so the correct dose is derived somewhat empirically by giving sufficient lactulose to produce symptomatic improvement without excessive diarrhoea. Once this has been achieved lactulose can be used with no apparent ill-effect over a prolonged period of time. Diarrhoea is the only major complication which may be critical in patients whose fluid and electrolyte balance is somewhat tenuous.

The role played by the liver in drug handling is so important that metabolism of many, if not most, therapeutic agents is likely to be altered in chronic liver disease. The factors involved are varied and complex, but in general terms caution should always be exercised when prescribing any drug for a patient with hepatic dysfunction. Hypnotics, anticoagulants, anticonvulsants and hypoglycaemic agents are particularly important groups of drugs in this respect.

INFLAMMATORY BOWEL DISEASE

Both ulcerative colitis and Crohn's disease should be viewed as chronic disorders which tend to relapse and remit over many years. As in the case of chronic liver disease, therapy should be considered in two parts; (a) the control of acute exacerbations and the induction of maintenance of remission and (b) treatment of the complications of the diseases.

Ulcerative colitis

Acute relapses of ulcerative colitis vary in severity from episodes of minor bloody diarrhoea to fulminant life-threating colitis. Severe episodes should be managed in hospital since many manoeuvres in addition to drug therapy, such as intravenous fluids, blood transfusion and surgery may be required.

Corticosteroids are undoubtedly the most effective drugs for inducing remission in both mild and severe inflammation. In mild attacks they can be given rectally, either in the form of a prednisolone-containing suppository or as a retention enema containing prednisolone-21-phosphate (Predsol). These contain 5mg and 20mg prednisolone respectively. More recently an enema containing hydrocortisone acetate as a foam preparation (Colifoam) has been introduced and this is favoured by many patients as it is less uncomfortable to insert and easier to retain. These preparations are in many respects preferable to systemic steroids since they are particularly effective locally at or near the site of inflammation and they are less likely to result in steroid side-effects. Nevertheless, an appreciable proportion of each drug is absorbed. Despite their local application, it has been shown that steroid enemata are absorbed as far as the transverse colon so they can be used in colitis which is not confined to the rectum alone. In relatively mild cases prompt remission can be induced by twice-daily application of enemata and once this has been achieved these can be gradually reduced to once daily, alternate days and finally discontinued. Patients may need to be shown initially how to insert them and they should be encouraged to retain them for at least half an hour. This involves lying down for at least this length of time, which is very easy in the evening but often difficult to manage in the morning if the patient is working.

Local steroid application is often limited by the severity of the colitis, as patients with profuse diarrhoea or active ano-rectal disease are unable to retain the preparations for long enough. In such cases systemic steroids may be indicated and while, ideally, many such patients should be admitted to hospital this is often impractical and more and more severe attacks are being treated on an outpatient basis. Prednisolone is the drug of choice, and it should be given in comparatively high doses starting with 30 or 40mg daily. Such a high dose should only be necessary for a few days, after which the dose can be tailed off as maintenance therapy is introduced (see below). Failure to respond after a few days, or continuing systemic features such as pyrexia and weight loss, are indications for hospital admission and treatment with parenteral steroids – either hydrocortisone or prednisolone-21-phosphate. There is little objective evidence to suggest that ACTH is superior to prednisolone.

Mild attacks of ulcerative colitis can be controlled with sulphasalazine (Salazopyrin) which is the treatment of choice for the prevention of relapse. It has been shown repeatedly that once remission has been conducted, daily sulphasalazine will keep most patients relatively or completely free of symptoms for many years. The sulphasalazine should be continued indefinitely as experience has shown that if it is stopped, even in patients with total remission for as long as ten years, there is a high rate of relapse. The recommended daily dose is 2g for maintaining remission, but a higher dose (3–4g daily) is usually required to treat mild acute attacks. Some patients prefer to try and lower their own maintenance dose which is often, though not always, effective. Side-effects are, unfortunately, quite common. Nausea, anorexia and other gastro-intestinal disturbances are particularly frequent, but these can be minimised by taking the tablets with meals and also by the use of an enteric-coated preparation. More recently sulphasalazine has become available in an enema preparation. While undoubtedly useful as an alternative to the oral form the full role of sulphasalazine enemata in long-term management remains to be assessed. Allergic skin rashes are a troublesome complication of the drug, but such is its importance in the long-term management of ulcerative colitis that it is worth desensitising such patients to the drug by slowly increasing oral doses, starting with as little as 5mg daily and building up to the full dose over several weeks. Blood dyscrasias and photosensitivity are more serious though rare complications of the drug. Most side-effects occur within the first two weeks of introducing sulphasalazine. Later complications are rare and many patients with ulcerative colitis have been taking the drug regularly for over 15 years without any apparent ill-effects. Recently, subfertility among males due to reduction in sperm count and an increase in abnormal sperm forms has been reported, but this is probably only an occasional problem and there is no evidence of any teratogenic effects.

While most remissions can be induced by either steroids and sulphasalazine and maintained on the latter alone, there remain a small group of patients who are unresponsive to this regimen. Corticosteroids may be required on a long-term basis to control symptoms but, in view of their serious potential side-effects, the dose should be kept as low as possible and it may be preferable to allow some bowel inflammation as the price for keeping the steroid dosage low. The additional small dose of azathioprine (50–75mg daily) will often enable good control of the colitis to be achieved with a much smaller dose of steroids. Sodium cromoglycate (Intal) has recently been advocated as an alternative drug for ulcerative colitis. Despite some initially promising reports, controlled trials have not shown it to be particularly effective but it may have a role in the management of patients who are unresponsive or sensitive to sulphasalazine.

Patients whose inflammatory bowel disease is poorly controlled on the above regimen or who require large doses of steroids over a period of time should be considered for surgery, especially if the inflammation involves most or all of their large bowel. With the exception of this situation, the site or extent of colonic inflammation does not significantly effect the choice of drugs used, although distal colitis is more likely to be responsive to local agents.

Non-specific diarrhoea and iron deficiency are the major complications of ulcerative colitis requiring drug therapy. Codeine phosphate, loperamide (Imodium) and diphenoxylate (Lomotil) are useful drugs in controlling the former and there is probably little to choose between any of them although diphenoxylate is probably less powerful. Many patients, however, are unable to tolerate one or other and the most appropriate agent for each individual is arrived at by a process of trial and error. The therapeutic dose is very much dependent upon the individual's response. In the case of loperamide, patients are advised to take one capsule after each bowel action, while the daily dose of codeine phosphate necessary to control symptoms may vary from 30mg to 180mg. Patients should be advised to experiment with the tablet dose themselves, but in either case they should be given a maximum daily dose which is not to be exceeded. If symptomatic relief is not achieved with a daily dose of eight × 30mg codeine phosphate tablets, eight diphenoxylate tablets, or eight loperamide tablets an alternative therapy should be tried. Patients should be warned against developing constipation as a result of taking anti-diarrhoeal agents as this may cause them considerable abdominal discomfort, so the above dose needs to be carefully adjusted. In practice, the patient alone is capable of finding the correct dose and if trouble is taken to explain the principles, most individuals quickly acquire the ability and are able to adjust their own dose from day to day.

Iron deficiency anaemia is an occasional long-term problem in patients with ulcerative colitis, particularly in those whose inflammation is never totally quiescent. Most patients tolerate oral iron preparation without any difficulty although in some cases parenteral iron may be necessary. Patients should not be given iron supplements unless there is good evidence of deficiency and they need not be continued once the colitis is controlled adequately and there is no rectal bleeding. B_{12} and folate deficiency are not features of ulcerative colitis; if either is present small bowel involvement with Crohn's disease should be suspected (see below).

Crohn's disease

Treatment of all aspects of this disease is much less satisfactory than that for ulcerative colitis, since the clinical course, anatomical involvement and complications tend to be much more variable and protracted. Whereas mild uncomplicated cases of ulcerative colitis can be satisfactorily managed in general practice, the long-term treatment of Crohn's disease is best directed from a specialist hospital clinic. As with ulcerative colitis, corticosteroids, sulphasalazine and immuno-suppressives provide the basis of treatment of Crohn's disease, although their effectiveness is less certain and indications for their use are somewhat different.

CORTICOSTEROIDS

Steroids are undoubtedly effective in suppressing inflammation in most patients with active Crohn's disease although quite large doses (40–60mg daily) may be necessary. Because of the nature of the disease the place of local steroids is limited although enemata and suppositories may be highly effective when symptoms are confined to the ano-rectal area. Once control of inflammation is achieved, the prednisolone dose should be reduced steadily and discontinued if possible. While many patients require long-term steroids because the drug cannot be stopped without a relapse, others may remain in remission and there is no evidence that in such patients long-term steroid therapy effectively prevents relapse.

SULPHASALAZINE

Sulphasalazine may be of value in inducing remission in patients with mild attacks, but in general the drug is much less effective than corticosteroids. Unlike in ulcerative colitis, sulphasalazine has not been shown to be useful as a means of maintaining patients with Crohn's disease in remission.

IMMUNOSUPPRESSIVES

Azathioprine alone is of little or no value in the treatment of acute exacerbations of Crohn's disease, but some studies have shown that it may reduce the relapse rate in patients whose remission has been induced by steroids. It is particularly useful in patients who relapse quickly on withdrawing prednisolone and also in those who require long-term steroids in substantial dosage in order to suppress symptoms, where it usually enables a smaller dose to be used with consequent reduction in side-effects. Early anecdotal reports of the value of azathioprine in healing fistulae and fissures in Crohn's disease have not been substantiated by subsequent prospective studies. As a daily dose of 100–150mg is usually required marrow suppression is the commonest side-effect so regular monitoring of the peripheral blood count is essential. As has been mentioned earlier the effect of azathioprine is usually quite slow so the drug must be given for weeks if not months before any benefit can be seen.

While azathioprine has been the most extensively used cytotoxic agent its metabolite, 6-mercaptopurine, has also been shown to be effective in ameliorating the signs and symptoms of Crohn's disease and permitting reduction in steroid dosage. When given in a dose of 1.5mg/kg, 10 per cent of patients develop toxic reactions necessitating withdrawal (usually haematological complications). As with azathioprine, 6-mercaptopurine has to be given for a period of several months before significant effects can be seen.

OTHERS

Other drugs, notably metronidazole and dapsone have been reported to have beneficial effects on patients with Crohn's disease both in suppressing activity and in healing fistulae. While such claims should be treated with caution there is no doubt that bacterial overgrowth (see below) may complicate the disease and appropriate chemotherapy can greatly improve symptoms.

There is no evidence to justify initiating maintenance therapy in patients who are asymptomatic or who have recently undergone surgical resection in an attempt to delay or prevent future recurrence of Crohn's disease.

Complications of Crohn's disease

Due to the nature of the disease its potential complications are much more varied and extensive than those encountered in ulcerative colitis. Many of these complications occur as a result of chronic damage and may not bear any direct relation to disease activity.

DIARRHOEA

This is a common complaint in Crohn's disease and may occur for many reasons. Identification of the cause is important as this may radically alter management. Frequent bowel actions may reflect active inflammation, in which case this should be treated according to the regimens mentioned above. In addition symptomatic relief may be obtained by the use of the anti-diarrhoeal agents described under ulcerative colitis. Disordered bowel motility is a mechanism frequently invoked to explain intermittent diarrhoea in Crohn's disease. This condition is poorly understood, but its symptoms frequently respond to dietary fibre (this is considered in detail later in the chapter). Diarrhoea is not infrequently a manifestation of steatorrhoea which in Crohn's disease is a sign of small bowel involvement (or resection) and failure to absorb dietary fat. The treatment of this is described below as part of the management of malabsorption.

Less common causes of diarrhoea in Crohn's disease include bacterial overgrowth and bile salt diarrhoea. Patients with extensive small bowel disease – with or without surgical resection – may acquire regions of stasis in which overgrowth with one or more species of bacteria may occur. Four to six weeks of antibiotic therapy is required to treat this; tetracycline or lincomycin are the traditionally favoured drugs but others such as metronidazole are probably equally effective.

Diarrhoea due to bile salt deficiency is a complication which is particulary likely to occur in patients who have undergone ileal resection. It usually responds dramatically to regular cholestyramine (one sachet daily) and such therapy is worth trying empirically in such patients with diarrhoea. It should, however, be used with considerable caution in patients who have steatorrhoea, where the bile salt chelating agent may potentiate the faecal fat excretion.

While diarrhoea is a troublesome complaint the opposite may also produce undesirable symptoms in patients with Crohn's disease. Abdominal pain and even intestinal obstruction are well-recognised complications of constipation in such patients. Anti-diarrhoeal agents should therefore be used with caution.

PAIN

Abdominal pain is a much commoner problem in Crohn's disease than in ulcerative colitis, and it may signify bowel inflammation or some element of obstruction. Care should be taken in prescribing analgesics for such patients, since most analgesic drugs tend to constipate and may aggravate or complicate the clinical picture.

MALABSORPTION

Attention to, and correction of, deficiencies due to malabsorption form an important part of the long-term management of Crohn's disease. Vitamin B_{12} deficiency will inevitably develop in patients who undergo resection of the terminal ileum although it may be several years before it is clinically apparent. It is advisable to forestall this complication by instituting regular intramuscular vitamin B_{12} shortly after surgery. 1000 micrograms is usually given at monthly intervals, but two-monthly injections are perfectly sufficient. Less commonly, vitamin B_{12} deficiency may complicate Crohn's disease involving the small bowel in the absence of surgery.

Folic acid deficiency is a much more common cause of macrocytic anaemia which can be effectively treated with oral supplements in even the most severe cases of small bowel damage. One 5mg tablet taken three times daily is advised for patients with folic acid deficiency but once, or at most, twice-daily dosage is more than adequate as a maintenance dose.

Iron deficiency may occasionally be due to failure to absorb the element from the intestinal tract, but is more commonly caused by blood loss. Despite the anorexia and nausea which often accompanies Crohn's disease, most patients are able to tolerate ferrous sulphate tablets although occasionally other more expensive iron preparations may be necessary. Parenteral iron is rarely required and should be avoided if possible. The dose of iron should be reviewed from time to time according to the patient's clinical condition. Long-term iron therapy is often unnecessary and may lead to haemosiderosis.

Deficiency of the fat soluble vitamins A, D and K may also develop as a complication of malabsorption, although these are only rarely of clinical importance even in patients with extensive surgical resection. Vitamin K deficiency can result in prolongation of the prothrombin time to the extent of producing undue bruising. Monthly intramuscular injections of the vitamin will suffice to correct this. Clinical osteomalacia or hypocalcaemic tetany are very unusual complications of vitamin D deficiency in Crohn's disease and, when present, require oral calcium supplements together with monthly intramuscular vitamin D (100 000–300 000 units). Sub-clinical forms of vitamin D deficiency occur much more commonly, osteomalacia being detectable by invasive techniques such as bone biopsy. In patients with extensive small bowel involvement due to Crohn's disease it may be advisable to prescribe regular calcium and vitamin D prophylactically as an oral preparation (one tablet contains 500 units vitamin D, 450mg calcium sodium lactate and 150mg calcium phosphate). Care should be taken in prescribing vitamin D supplements on a long-term basis since overdosage may lead to hypercalcaemia and renal failure. The fact that vitamin D is available in widely differing dosage may lead to confusion and the high dose required for osteomalacia should not be given under any circumstances for prophylaxis. All patients receiving vitamin D supplements should have periodic estimations of serum calcium.

Weight loss and malnutrition may result from either steatorrhoea and/or protein-losing enteropathy, both of which are difficult to treat. Excessive fat loss may be irksome to the patient who produces bulky offensive motions as a result. This can often be minimised by reducing dietary fat intake, but it is important to remember that fat accounts for a major part of the calorie intake and loss of this may aggravate the problem of malnutrition. Substitution of fat with medium chain triglycerides (e.g. Portagen) is a method of providing easily absorbable fatty acids to such patients. There is no single satisfactory way of overcoming chronic protein-losing enteropathy other than by increasing the dietary intake of protein. This, however, is frequently impossible for chronically ill patients who may find it difficult to eat sufficient protein, quite apart from the added expense of providing such a diet.

Dietary supplementation with preparations such as Complan (a mixture of dried skimmed milk, vegetable oils, sucrose and minerals) may be of value in providing additional calories for the chronically malnourished patient. A number of similar preparations of different composition are currently on the market, but from a practical point of view there is little to distinguish between them. They are, however, appreciably more expensive than an ordinary diet and their use should be limited to patients who are physically unable to take in sufficient calories in the form of normal food.

Elemental diets (Vivonex, Flexical), in which there is little or no residual volume have a limited place in the management of chronic gastro-intestinal disease. It is claimed that their use in patients with chronic inflammation may allow resting of the bowel, and complications such as intestinal fistulae may heal under such circumstances. While of definite value in the acute situation, the place of elemental diets in the management of chronic disease is less certain and such costly treatment should only be embarked upon under expert guidance.

Patients whose bowel disease is so extensive that they are unable to maintain an adequate long-term nutritional balance despite these manoeuvres should be considered for parenteral nutrition. This technique, which involves the insertion of an intravenous central line, is now practised by an increasing number of centres and patients may be maintained for years on this alone. The details are beyond the scope of this book since such procedures should only be embarked upon and managed by specialist centres.

Bowel motility syndromes

This term is used here to describe a variety of conditions whose aetiology is poorly understood, but which are currently thought to involve disturbances in bowel motility. These include such conditions as irritable bowel syndrome, spastic colon and diverticular disease of the colon, terms which are often used without any clear definition and whose major symptoms include abdominal pain, constipation and diarrhoea. In most cases the diagnosis is an imprecise one which is derived by exclusion of other pathology. Apart from organic disorders such as carcinoma or inflammatory bowel disease, it is important to exclude medications as a cause of either diarrhoea or constipation. Obvious causes of the latter include analgesics such as codeine phosphate while long-term antibiotics have a tendency to produce frequent loose bowel actions. Unconscious or surreptitious use of laxatives is an important cause of chronic diarrhoea.

Current opinion favours the idea that in many cases the symptoms are related to the lack of bulk in the diet arising from a deficiency of fibre. As a consequence the prescription of a high-fibre diet, notably cereal products such as wholemeal and brown bread, wholewheat or bran-containing breakfast cereals, or bran itself is often highly effective in ameliorating symptoms. These are the most obvious bulking agents but other constituents in the diet such as vegetables are also rich in fibre and it is often useful to hand the patient a diet sheet outlining the various high-fibre foodstuffs. Alteration of fibre intake by dietary means is unquestionably the most satisfactory approach but some patients find bran and wholemeal unacceptable, in which case preparations of ispaghula (e.g. Isogel) or sterculia (e.g. Normacol) are often useful. The recommended dose is usually one to two teaspoons twice daily, mixed with water and allowed to swell before ingestion. Individual tolerance varies from patient to patient, many finding a much smaller dose perfectly adequate.

In recent years the treatment of diverticular disease of the colon has swung diametrically away from a low residue diet to one favouring fibre, so the drug management of the condition is now similar to that advocated for the irritable bowel syndrome.

While a high-fibre diet often produces dramatic improvement in patients with constipation and abdominal pain, the response is less satisfactory in those in whom diarrhoea is a major symptom. The anti-diarrhoeal agents recommended for inflammatory bowel disease (codeine phosphate, loperamide and diphenoxylate) may be tried, but these drugs may reduce the number of bowel actions at the risk of aggravating the abdominal pain. Antispasmodic drugs are sometimes of value in this situation, although their effectiveness is variable and unpredictable. The belladonna alkaloids (often combined with a barbiturate) are little used today, having been replaced by the synthetic atropine-like drugs such as hyoscine derivatives or propantheline, and more recently related antispasmodics like dicyclomine (Merbentyl) or mebeverine (Colofac) which act directly on intestinal smooth muscle. There are no clinical signs or symptoms to indicate that one drug is preferable to another and one or more is worth trying in an effort to control symptoms. Because of the atropine-like effect they should be avoided in patients with glaucoma and prostatism.

Many patients with irritable bowel syndrome often display symptoms of anxiety, depression or other known nervous disorders. Psychotropic drugs such as diazepam may be effective in controlling the nervous symptoms and consequently may result in improvement of the bowel complaints.

Constipation

This merits special mention as it is such a common complaint. Many people have been brought up to consider that a daily bowel movement (usually shortly before or after breakfast) was an essential prerequisite to healthy life and any deviation had to be corrected at all costs. In recent years both doctors and patients have become less concerned about bowel regularity but there remain a large portion of the population (mainly middle-aged and elderly females) who habitually take regular laxatives including senna, phenolphthalein magnesium sulphate, liquid paraffin, methyl cellulose

and cascara. When pushed to extreme such preparations may lead to electrolyte imbalance, diarrhoea and melanosis coli. Constipation may be a side-effect of medication such as analgesics or it may form part of the irritable bowel syndrome, but in many patients the habit of opening bowels once every two or three days is quite normal and does not require any manoeuvres to alter this in the absence of any symptoms. The sudden development of constipation in a patient with previously normal bowel habit should be treated seriously, particularly if the patient is elderly. Such symptoms should be investigated to exclude organic pathology.

BIBLIOGRAPHY

Much of this chapter is concerned with current and controversial topics. For more detailed information the reader is referred to the following references.

Greenberger, N. J., Arvanitakis, C. and Hurwitz, A. (1978). *Drug treatment of gastrointestinal disorders.* Churchill Livingstone, Edinburgh.

Misiewicz, J. J. (1979). *Medical treatment of gastric and duodenal ulcer.* In *Advanced Medicine*, 15, pp. 219–27. (eds Harper, P. S. and Muir, J. R.) Pitman Medical Books, London.

Myren, J. and Schrumpf, E. (eds) (1980). Symposium on pathophysiology and drug therapy of peptic ulcer. *Scandinavian Journal of Gastroenterology*, Supp. **58**, 7–97.

Sleisenger, M. H. (1980). How should we treat Crohn's Disease? *New England Journal of Medicine*, **302**, 1024–26.

Triger, D. R. (1981). *Practical management of liver disease.* Blackwell Scientific Publications Limited, Oxford.

Truelove, S. C. and Heyworth, M. F. (eds) (1978). *Dietary fibre.* In *Topics in Gastroenterology: 6*, pp. 3–113. Blackwell Scientific Publications Limited, Oxford.

See Appendix overleaf: Average daily cost of some drugs commonly prescribed for chronic gastro-intestinal disorders

APPENDIX

Average daily cost of some drugs commonly prescribed for chronic gastro-intestinal disorders

Drug costs assume particular importance when long-term prescription is contemplated. This list illustrates the comparative cost of the major drugs mentioned in this chapter. There is no implication of cost-effectiveness, but in some instances cited in the text the initial choice of drug may be arbitrary, so cost may be a relevant factor.

Prices are based on the monthly index of Medical Specialities, November 1981, except for the calorie supplements which are obtained from the Chemist and Druggist price list January 1982.

	Drug	Dosage	Cost
Hiatus hernia peptic ulcer	simple antacids	5ml q.d.s.	5–15p
	antacid plus dimethicone	5ml q.d.s.	14–20p
	antacid plus alginic acid	5ml q.d.s.	17–30p
	bismuth colloid	5ml q.d.s.	10–37p
	carbenoxolone	50mg t.d.s.	31p
	deglycyrrhizinised liquorice	2 t.d.s.	25p
	cimetidine	1g	66p
Gallstones	chenodeoxycholic acid	750mg	£1.08
Chronic pancreatitis	pancreatic extracts	t.d.s.	6–45p
Chronic liver disease	frusemide	40mg	6p
	spironolactone	100mg	25p
	lactulose	30ml	22p
	neomycin	2g	38p
	cholestyramine	1 sachet	39p
Inflammatory bowel disease	sulphasalazine tablets	2 b.d.	23–30p*
	sulphasalazine suppositories	1	23p
	sulphasalazine enemata	1	£1.40
	hydrocortisone/prednisolone enemata	1	50–80p
	prednisolone	10mg	2–10p*
	azathioprine	50mg	32p
	codeine phosphate	30mg q.d.s.	15p
	diphenoxylate	q.d.s.	8–18p
	loperamide	q.d.s.	45p
Calorie supplements	Vivonex	1000 kilo calories	£3.71
	Flexical	1000 kilo calories	£4.68
	Portagen	1000 kilo calories	£2.63
	Caloreen	1000 kilo calories	86p
	Complan	1000 kilo calories	59p
Bowel motility disorders	dicyclomine	1 t.d.s.	6p
	probanthine	1 t.d.s.	6p
	sterculia/ispaghula	10ml	10p

* The more expensive preparations are enteric-coated

Chapter 9   Urinary tract disease

ANTHONY J. NICHOLLS MB, MRCP

and COLIN B. BROWN BSc, MB, MRCP

In general terms, there are two major categories of renal disease which may involve long-term chemo-therapy. First, there are serious diseases such as glomerulonephritis and chronic pyelonephritis which can lead to progressive impairment of renal function and, secondly, there are the far more common diseases such as urinary tract infection and stone which lead to considerable morbidity but only rarely cause renal failure.

Unfortunately, drug treatment of diseases in the first category may fail to avert renal destruction, but it may prevent major non-renal complications. The overall management of these patients is best co-ordinated by a nephrological unit for two reasons. First, the development of end-stage renal failure is a relatively uncommon event, with around 60 new patients per million population requiring renal replacement therapy annually. The survival of such patients is good, with an annual mortality of 8 to 10 per cent and the total number of patients in the community alive on dialysis or with a functioning renal transplant will eventually reach at least 600 per million population (or higher if patients over 60 years old are treated). Nonetheless, the average general practitioner may expect to have on his books only one or two patients on renal replacement therapy, and a few others with varying degrees of renal impairment. The second main reason for the involvement of a nephrologist in the care of patients with destructive renal diseases is the need for early preparation for dialysis, and careful judgement of the time to introduce it.

Diseases in the second category mentioned above – those conditions with high morbidity but little serious import – are clearly far too common for all patients to be seen in a specialist unit. However, misconceptions about both prognosis and the rationale for long-term treatment often exist. The guidelines which follow may clarify some of these issues and help in the management of problem patients.

The above classification of urinary tract diseases of course ignores the possibility of overlap between the groups; for example, patients with stones may develop obstructive uropathy and renal failure, and only some glomerular diseases lead to uraemia. Nonetheless, the broad differentiation between serious, but unusual diseases, and common, but often trivial disorders offers practical advantages, particularly in terms of the overall strategies of chronic drug treatment. It is thus proposed in this review to concentrate on the commoner renal diseases requiring long-term medication, and to outline the principles of therapy in some of the more serious disorders.

URINARY TRACT INFECTION

The widespread availability of quantitative urine bacteriology, and the screening of vulnerable groups of patients for urinary infection have led to enormous advances in the concepts of urinary tract infection (UTI) in the past 20 years. It has become clear that the syndromes of asymptomatic bacteriuria, symptomatic urinary infection, and chronic pyelonephritis (CPN) are separate entities; and that the outcome of UTI is crucially dependent on the presence or absence of anatomical abnormalities. The relationships between asymptomatic bacteriuria, symptomatic infection and CPN have been recently reviewed in detail by Sussman and Asscher (1979); in essence, it has been shown that symptomatic infections commonly follow asymptomatic bacteriuria in pregnancy, but in other situations the relationship is much less clear. Furthermore, although in early childhood bacteriuria is clearly associated with the development of pyelonephritic scarring when there is vesico-ureteric reflux, it is much less certain if infection of a non-obstructed urinary tract in adolescence or adult life leads to progressive renal damage even in the presence of previously acquired cortical scars.

The enigma of CPN as a cause of renal failure in adult life is the lack of our ability to identify factors responsible for loss of renal tissue; both recurrent infection and hypertension have been proposed as causes of progression of CPN, but they do not provide the whole answer. Nonetheless, treatment of both these complications is still to be advocated, but perhaps with more hope than belief that renal function will be preserved.

It should also be made clear that a large number of patients with radiological evidence of CPN have had no identifiable episodes of UTI. Some of these patients will have recognisable aetiologies such as analgesic abuse, but in many no predisposing cause can be found. Some authors would prefer the term chronic interstitial nephritis for those cases where infection is unproven. It is not proposed to discuss these noso-logical issues further; instead a guide to the therapy of chronic or recurrent UTI in various clinical settings will be outlined.

UTI in childhood
In children there are grounds for investigating even the first attack of UTI by intravenous urography (IVU) and micturating cystourethrography (MCU), as the likelihood of anatomical abnormality is high, and the possible consequences of recurrent infection are serious. Clearly obstruction will need surgical inter-vention, but more commonly vesico-ureteric reflux will be found. The work of Hodson and others (Editor-ial, 1974) has shown that the characteristic renal scar-ring of CPN is due to intra-renal reflux of infected urine. Hence the prevention of progressive renal scar-ring in childhood has concentrated on eliminating infection, or reflux, or both. However, although surg-ical correction is probably indicated when gross bilat-eral reflux is present, most children with less severe degrees of reflux can be managed with chronic low-dose antibiotic therapy (Smellie and Normand, 1968; Grüneberg et al, 1973). There are clear differences in the response to different antibiotics, and Table 1 lists in order of efficacy several common antibiotics for UTI prophylaxis in children. Prophylactic drug therapy will not prevent occasional symptomatic relapses, and these should be treated conventionally with normal doses of an antibiotic chosen according to sensitivities.

Table 1 Suggested prophylactic antibiotic regimens for children with recurrent UTI ($\pm$ reflux)

Nitrofurantoin	1.25mg/kg/day: nocte
Nalidixic acid	30mg/kg/day: 2–4 divided doses
Co-trimoxazole	12mg/kg/day: 1 or 2 doses
Trimethoprim	2.5mg/kg/day: 1 or 2 doses
Cephalexin	125mg nocte

The duration of long-term antibiotic prophylaxis of childhood UTI is determined by several factors. In general terms it should be continued if breakthrough infections occur or if MCU shows persisting reflux, but may be discontinued when reflux disappears (as it often does in adolescence) and the urine remains sterile.

UTI in women
The symptoms of cystitis in women of childbearing age – frequency, dysuria, haematuria – lead to an extremely large number of consultations in general practice. While many of these illnesses respond readily to a short course of antibiotics, there are some women who suffer repeated attacks of cystitis. Such women fall into two groups – those with recurrent bacterial urinary infection, and those with repeatedly sterile urine cul-tures.

Those women with proven infection are the easiest to manage, though there are several possible reasons for relapsing infection:

(1) an inappropriate drug may have been started before the antibiotic sensitivity of the pathogen was known;
(2) emergence of resistant organisms: this is highly unusual and can be disregarded;
(3) failure to take the prescribed course of therapy: this is probably unimportant if at least three days' treatment has been taken;
(4) inadequate concentration of antibiotic: when renal infection is patchy (either within both kidneys or in a unilaterally diseased kidney), the excretion of the drug by normal renal tissue may prevent a thera-peutic concentration within the diseased parts. This problem can be overcome either by high-dose bactericidal drugs such as gentamicin, or by nephrectomy when a unilaterally diseased kidney has little function (Editorial, 1976).
(5) renal calculi and anatomical abnormalities of the urinary tract: these will be considered as separate topics below;
(6) true re-infection: this accounts for the large major-ity of recurrent symptoms after antibiotic treat-ment of UTI, and a variety of measures are helpful in prophylaxis. As many infections can be shown to be related to sexual intercourse, strict perineal hygiene and voiding after intercourse may produce some benefit, but the most successful method of preventing recurrent infections is the long-term administration of low-dose antibiotics.

Several drugs have been clearly shown to be highly effective in this situation: nitrofurantoin 100mg, co-trimoxazole one tablet, or cephalexin 125mg should be given nightly and continued for a year or longer. Around 80 per cent of women with uncomplicated recurrent UTI will have their symptoms relieved by such therapy.

Unfortunately about a half of women who suffer recurrent attacks of cystitis have repeatedly sterile urine cultures, and the factors listed above are largely inapplicable. The management of these patients with the so-called 'urethral syndrome' is difficult, as the pathogenesis of the condition is obscure. While recent work suggests a possible role for fastidious micro-organisms which may be undetected by routine laboratory techniques, so far there are no promising therapeutic advances. Some women may be helped by perineal hygiene, voiding after intercourse, a high fluid intake, and urethral dilatation. Although long-term antibiotic prophylaxis is of no proven value, it is worth trying.

UTI, obstruction and stones

As has been emphasised above, one's approach to the problem of UTI hinges crucially on the presence or absence of obstruction. (Hence, of course, the need for investigation by IVU of even single episodes of UTI in infants and males of all ages, and of girls and women with recurrent UTI.) In particular, the aim of treatment of infection of the non-obstructed urinary tract – uncomplicated UTI – is the relief of symptoms alone. On the other hand, when there is obstruction, renal function is at risk and must be preserved as well.

The biggest problem is that of staghorn calculi, which rapidly form in the alkaline urine characteristic of the urease-producing organisms *Proteus sp.* and *Pseudomonas pyocyaneus*. Even after pyelolithotomy there is a persisting risk of re-infection and recurrent stone formation. Hence there are good reasons for long-term low-dose antibiotic therapy in these patients after removal of stones. Some patients who have had surgical correction of obstruction may be left with a minor degree of obstruction as demonstrated by postoperative IVU. Again, UTI is potentially damaging in this situation, and long-term low-dose antibiotic prophylaxis is indicated even for asymptomatic bacteriuria.

UTI in renal failure

The major problem here is that of eradicating infection owing to difficulty of obtaining therapeutic urinary antibiotic concentrations. Leaving this problem aside, the long-term use of nitrofurantoin is contra-indicated in severe renal failure as its accumulation may produce irreversible peripheral neuropathy; in milder degrees of renal failure (GFR 20–50ml/min) the chronic low-dose should be reduced to 50mg daily for adults.

UTI in diabetics and immunosuppressed patients

The spectrum of renal involvement in diabetes is very wide, encompassing glomerular disease, vascular disease and pyelonephritis. Diabetic patients have an increased susceptibility to infection, and asymptomatic bacteriuria is several times more common than in non-diabetic persons. Furthermore, the frequent co-existence of vascular and infectious processes may lead to necrosis of the renal papillae. Hence the eradication of UTI (even when asymptomatic) is important, and long-term low-dose antibiotics should be employed along the lines outlined previously.

The immunosuppressed patient is at risk of infection by unusual micro-organisms, but more commonly the standard urinary pathogens will be found. Hence antibiotic prophylaxis of recurrent UTI in these patients should not differ from that used in other patients.

The problem of recurrent UTI in patients with kidney transplants has come under close scrutiny. There is little evidence to suggest that renal function is in jeopardy from such infections, but when recurrent symptoms are a feature, again low-dose nightly antibiotics offer relief.

UTI in men

Enlargement of the prostate is clearly the most important predisposing feature here, but some men have recurrent UTI without obstruction. Rather than use long-term antibiotic therapy in this situation, one should first consider whether prostatitis is the source of recurrent infection. Ampicillin, sulphonamides, nitrofurantoin and some cephalosporins penetrate poorly or not at all into prostatic fluid, whereas trimethoprim, erythromycin and tetracycline are excreted in prostatic fluid and may eradicate prostatic infection.

RENAL STONES

Between one and five per cent of the population will develop a urinary tract stone in their lifetime. Few patients develop renal failure from stones, but morbidity is high and recurrent stones may plague the patient for many years. Although the production of dilute urine is fundamental to the prophylaxis of any stone disorder, the rational use of other specific measures depends on the diagnosis of the underlying problem predisposing to urolithiasis. Table 2 presents an aetiologic classification of stone disorders and is used as the framework for subsequent details of therapy.

Table 2 Causes of urinary tract stones

A. Metabolic Disorders

   (i) Hypercalcaemia
   (ii) Hypercalciuria (normocalcaemic)
   (iii) Urate stones
   (iv) Hyperoxaluria
   (v) Associated with gastro-intestinal disease
   (vi) Other idiopathic syndromes

B. Renal Tubular Syndromes

   (i) Cystinuria
   (ii) Renal tubular acidosis

C. Secondary Urolithiasis

   (i) Infection
   (ii) Obstruction
   (iii) Medullary sponge kidney
   (iv) Urinary diversion

Hypercalcaemia

Therapy for these patients is dictated by the cause of hypercalcaemia – most commonly primary hyperparathyroidism. This group of stone formers will not be discussed further.

'Idiopathic' hypercalciuria

Around 50 per cent of recurrent stone formers have hypercalciuria in the presence of a normal serum calcium and a low or low normal phosphate. Such patients are typically male and produce calcium oxalate and/or calcium phosphate stones. Most of them show increased calcium absorption from the gut in response to elevated circulating levels of the biologically active form of vitamin D, 1,25-dihydroxycholecalciferol: so-called 'absorptive hypercalciuria'. A smaller subgroup of patients with hypercalciuria appear to have a primary renal leak of calcium, with associated secondary hyperparathyroidism.

Apart from a high fluid intake and dietary restriction of calcium, two specific therapies for hypercalciuria can be considered. Phosphate salts have been used for many years to bind dietary calcium within the gut, and hence reduce its intestinal absorption. In addition the absorbed phosphate leads to increased urinary excretion of pyrophosphate which inhibits stone formation. In several series the use of oral orthophosphate 1.5–2.5g daily in three to four divided doses has been reported to reduce or prevent stone formation in up to 90 per cent of patients with hypercalciuria.

The major side-effect of orthophosphates is diarrhoea which usually subsides after the first few weeks; less frequently, dyspepsia is troublesome. Some patients treated with orthophosphates will pass a stone, possibly with colic, during the first six months of treatment. This does not imply treatment failure, but merely indicates a reduction in the size of stone so that it can be passed. Occasionally, ectopic calcification has been reported during long-term orthophosphate therapy, but this is probably only a risk in the presence of renal failure. Secondary hyperparathyroidism is also a potential theoretical complication of long-term therapy, but has not been demonstrated convincingly. Orthophosphates should not be given when the glomerular filtration rate (GFR) is less than 30ml/min, or when infection complicates stone formation. In these situations the phosphate load may itself encourage stone growth.

An alternative to orthophosphate as a calcium binder is cellulose phosphate, an ion-exchange substance with affinity for divalent cations. A dose of 12–15g daily with meals leads to increased faecal loss of calcium and a lowering of urinary calcium excretion. Experience with this agent has shown no major side-effects, and it is of value in those unable to tolerate orthophosphate therapy.

A further calcium-binding agent is sodium phytate, but it has no particular advantages over orthophosphates or cellulose phosphate.

An alternative approach to hypercalciuria, particularly when calcium absorption is normal and there is a primary renal leak of calcium, is the use of thiazide diuretics. Bendrofluazide 5mg daily or hydrochlorothiazide 50mg b.d. will reduce urinary calcium excretion by 40 to 50 per cent, and thus reduce stone formation, but this effect may be lost when there is sodium loading. Hence dietary sodium should be restricted before thiazide diuretics are considered ineffective.

Side-effects of long-term thiazide administration are predictable, but only lead to cessation of therapy in around 10 per cent of patients. The commonest side-effects are fatigue, mild hypokalaemia, hyperuricaemia (± gout) and impaired glucose tolerance; hence patients on long-term therapy need regular biochemical monitoring. Potassium supplements are unnecessary as a routine.

Urate stones

Uric acid calculi account for about 20 per cent of stones. Most patients are free from gout, have normal serum urate, normal or elevated urate excretion, and typically show persistently acid urine. About a quarter of urate stone formers have gout, and a small minority of patients have increased purine breakdown in association with myeloproliferative diseases.

Irrespective of the exact cause of urate stones, treatment is generally very satisfactory. Urine volume should be increased to three litres daily, urinary acidity corrected to pH 6.5 with sodium bicarbonate, and allopurinol given in a dose of 300mg daily. If stones no longer form, allopurinol can be discontinued in cases of idiopathic urate lithiasis, but should be continued indefinitely in gout and myeloproliferative disease.

Some normocalciuric idiopathic recurrent calcium stone formers exhibit hyperuricosuria. Despite the fact that urate stones *per se* are not passed, it has been suggested that urate crystals in urine may induce the precipitation of calcium oxalate stones. There may therefore be a place for allopurinol in the treatment of calcium oxalate stones when excess urate excretion can be demonstrated, but only as an adjunct to thiazide or phosphate therapy.

Hyperoxaluria

Hyperoxaluria can contribute to calcium oxalate stone formation in three conditions: in primary hyperoxaluria, a rare hereditary enzyme disorder; in association with gastro-intestinal disease (see below); and as a feature of some cases of normocalciuric stone formers without an enzyme defect.

Primary hyperoxaluria is disappointing to treat; at least 50 per cent of patients are dead or in renal failure by adulthood. Perhaps the most encouraging benefits have been produced by combined therapy with orthophosphate and pyridoxine (150mg/day). Pyridoxine reduces the oxalate pool and its excretion by enhancing the conversion of glyoxalate (the precursor of oxalate) into glycine.

In hyperoxaluria unassociated with a defect of glyoxalate metabolism, there is little evidence to support the routine use of pyridoxine; rather orthophosphate should be used.

Renal stones associated with gastro-intestinal disease

Several complications of gastro-intestinal (G–I) disease increase the risk of stone formation. Diarrhoea, with the consequent loss of water and bicarbonate from the gut, results in a low volume of acid urine; hence urate stones readily form. Furthermore, acquired or enteric hyperoxaluria is a feature of several conditions, including small bowel resection, blind-loop syndrome, bacterial overgrowth, coeliac disease, small bowel Crohn's disease, chronic pancreatitis and primary biliary cirrhosis. In these conditions the excess fat present in the colon precipitates with dietary calcium, and there is

consequent increased absorption of dietary oxalate by the colon. Hence hyperoxaluria is not present after total colectomy.

Treatment of stones associated with G–I disease is difficult owing to the problem in many patients of coping with a high fluid intake. Urate lithiasis, even when urate excretion is normal, should be treated with allopurinol in a dose of 300mg daily. The prime approach to enteric hyperoxaluria is the restriction of dietary oxalate. Additionally cholestyramine (4g three or four times daily) non-specifically chelates oxalate and reduces its absorption.

Cystinuria

Cystinuria comprises a defect in tubular handling of cystine, ornithine, lysine and arginine: clinically, the only problem relates to the formation of cystine stones and consequent renal damage. General therapeutic measures involve increasing urine volume to four litres daily, alkalinising the urine to pH 7.5–7.8 by the use of citrate 15mmol four times daily and reducing cystine excretion by limiting protein intake (in particular methionine). Specific treatment with D-penicillamine has been used successfully in some patients: the disulphide cysteine-penicillamine is much more soluble than cystine and stones can not only be prevented, but may also dissolve with its use. However, major side-effects including agranulocytosis, nephrotic syndrome, skin rashes, arthralgia and lymphadenopathy complicate the use of D-penicillamine and may lead to its withdrawal. It should only be used in those patients with extreme cystinuria in whom supersaturation cannot be controlled by fluids and alkalis.

Renal tubular acidosis

Type I, or distal, renal tubular acidosis (RTA) is characterised by the inability to excrete a urine of pH<5.8, systemic acidosis, hyperchloraemia, hypokalaemia, and excessive urinary loss of sodium, potassium, calcium and phosphate. Renal stones and nephrocalcinosis are typically found in this variety of RTA unlike the proximal tubular disorder (Type II RTA) where they do not occur.

The primary treatment of Type I RTA involves correction of the metabolic acidosis with 60–120mmol bicarbonate or citrate daily, and replacement of sodium and potassium as needed. Shohl's solution (citric acid 140g, sodium citrate 98g in water one litre) given in a dose of 50–100ml eight-hourly is a convenient way of giving this alkali, and should be continued indefinitely. Urinary calcium excretion will decrease with correction of the acidosis, but the increased urinary pH favours precipitation of calcium-containing stones.

Thus there will be some patients in whom stone formation and nephrocalcinosis progress despite adequate correction of acidosis. These patients should be given orthophosphate or cellulose phosphate as described under hypercalciuria.

Stones in association with infection and obstruction

This has been largely considered in the section on urinary tract infection above. It is important to appreciate that so-called 'secondary urolithiasis' may complicate an underlying metabolic disorder. Hence, a comprehensive evaluation of all possible predisposing factors is necessary even when dealing with apparently typical infective staghorn calculi.

Urinary diversion procedures

After uretero-sigmoidostomy, calculi are common owing to the co-existence of infection, acidosis and hypercalciuria. Better results are obtained with ileal loop ureterostomy, but large upper tract calculi may still form. Long-term antibiotic therapy is not indicated, but correction of any metabolic disorder is essential.

Idiopathic recurrent stone formers not otherwise classified

A substantial proportion of patients have no demonstrable predisposing cause for stone formation, yet continue to form stones in the face of dietary restriction of calcium and oxalate and increased fluid intake. Treatment with calcium-binding agents should be tried in these patients initially, with thiazides or allopurinol for non-responders. Such therapy is entirely empirical, but occasionally helpful.

RENAL HYPERTENSION

The management of hypertension has been considered in Chapter 2. So far as hypertension in the presence of severe renal failure is concerned, it is worth making three points specifically.

1. Very large (500–2000mg/day) doses of frusemide will sometimes lower blood pressure when other drugs have failed.
2. When blood pressure fails to respond to conventional drugs, minoxidil and captopril are strikingly effective, and are needed far more often than when renal function is normal.
3. Failure to control blood pressure adequately should be a major factor in the decision to start dialysis in advanced renal failure.

PRIMARY GLOMERULAR DISEASE

The various morphological types of glomerular disease can present clinically in a range of overlapping syndromes; for a fuller discussion of the problems of classification one should consult the recent review of Cameron (1979). Rational therapy of glomerulonephritis depends on the histological type of disease present so renal biopsy is essential in all patients apart from most children with nephrotic syndrome. Unfortunately our ability to treat glomerulonephritis is limited, and useful drugs are few: therefore for many diseases no specific therapy can be offered. However, in these cases it is equally important not to give ineffective and potentially harmful therapy; treatment here should be limited to control of individual clinical manifestations of disease such as oedema and hypertension. The following resumé will deal with specific treatment of individual glomerular diseases and mention symptomatic therapy of the nephrotic syndrome. For treatment of secondary glomerular disease as found in the connective tissue diseases see page 113.

Minimal change disease

This is the characteristic lesion of childhood nephrotic syndrome, and also causes a substantial proportion of adult nephrosis. Patients are treated routinely with steroids (e.g. prednisolone 60mg/m²/day), and most will be in remission within six to eight weeks of starting treatment. The 10 per cent or so of patients who fail to respond to steroids can be expected to respond to cyclophosphamide (2–3mg/kg/day for six weeks).

Following the initial response to steroids, patients follow one of several courses. Thirty to 40 per cent of patients remain free of disease indefinitely, while a further 10 to 20 per cent relapse occasionally and respond to a second course of steroids. These patients need be considered no further here. Up to 50 per cent of patients suffer recurrent relapses; a response to steroids is usually retained, and repeated courses can be given. If relapses are frequent, long-term low-dose prednisolone (e.g. 10mg on alternate days) is often effective. Major side-effects of long-term steroid therapy will inevitably be encountered in some patients (Table 3); in these patients a prolonged remission may be obtained with a short course of cyclophosphamide in the same dose as above. The acute side-effects of cyclophosphamide are predominantly on the bone marrow and are dose-dependent; chronic side-effects such as azoospermia, haemorrhagic cystitis and increased carcinogenesis seem to relate to the total dose administered. In particular, azoospermia is likely with a total dose of greater than 11g in adults, though children may tolerate a higher dose.

Table 3 Common side-effects of long-term steroid therapy

1. Increased risk of infections – bacterial
                                            viral
                                            fungal
                                            protozoal
2. Retardation of growth
3. Osteoporosis and avascular necrosis of bone
4. Gastro-duodenal bleeding
5. Hypertension
6. Obesity
7. Glucose intolerance
8. Cataracts
9. Pancreatitis
10. Acne

NB Side-effects are probably less when steroids are given on alternate days.

Should further relapses occur after cyclophosphamide treatment, steroids can again be used, with chlorambucil being reserved for occasional problem patients.

An important sub-group of patients who initially respond to steroids but immediately relapse on their withdrawal (steroid-dependence) should probably not be given cyclophosphamide as the subsequent course is then worse. These patients will therefore need long term steroid therapy.

A flow chart summarising the above treatments is given in Figure 9/1.

Membranous nephropathy

There is little evidence that corticosteroids, azathioprine or cyclophosphamide, alone or in combination, induce remission of the nephrotic syndrome or prevent uraemia in most patients with membranous nephropathy. Recently it has been claimed that a single brief course of high-dose steroid therapy prevented deterioration of renal function, but this apparent benefit might have been due to the heterogeneous nature of membranous nephropathy. The disease is insidiously progressive in most patients, but a minority run a more aggressive course with early renal failure. Steroids may be indicated for this sub-group with rapidly declining renal function, but further trials are needed to clarify this issue.

Focal segmental glomerulosclerosis (FSGS)

The prognosis in this condition is almost universally poor, and unaffected by immunosuppressive therapy. Current therapeutic interest has focussed on platelet involvement in the pathogenesis of FSGS; treatment with aspirin 300mg daily and dipyridamole 100mg t.d.s. is worth trying in view of the gloomy outlook for this disease if untreated.

Membranoproliferative (mesangiocapillary) glomerulonephritis (MPGN)

MPGN can be characterised morphologically either by the type of immune deposits found – subendothelial (Type I), dense intramembranous (Type II) or subendothelial and subepithelial (Type III) – or by the glomerular architecture – focal, lobular or crescentic.

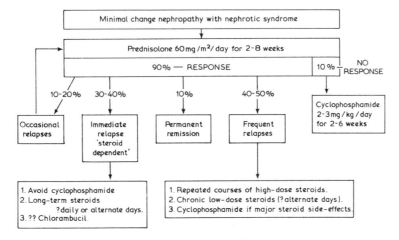

Fig. 9/1 Flow chart showing treatment of minimal change disease

Furthermore, the clinical course ranges from indolent progressive renal failure to a more rapid loss of renal function. In the past, clinical trials have tended to include all morphological types and clinical presentations of MPGN; the negative results of such studies led many nephrologists to adopt a nihilistic attitude to immunosuppressive therapy in the mid-1970s. However, it is now becoming apparent that selected patients with MPGN (particularly those with an aggressive tempo of disease clinically, Type I and II deposits, or very 'inflammatory' glomerular changes) may benefit from immunosuppression. In such patients treatment with prednisolone (initially 40–80mg daily) and azathioprine (1.5–3mg/kg/day) for several months is worth trying. If there is a response (assessed in terms of diminution of proteinuria and improvement or stabilisation of renal function), pred-nisolone 5–15mg/day and azathioprine 1–2mg/kg/ day should be continued indefinitely. The side-effects of azathioprine are given in Table 4.

Table 4 Side-effects of azathioprine

1. Marrow suppression: predominantly granulocytes and platelets
2. Increased risk of skin and lymphoid malignancy
3. Liver dysfunction

NB The effects of azathioprine are enhanced by allopurinol. When used concurrently, the dose of azathioprine should be cut to about $\frac{1}{4}$ to $\frac{1}{3}$ of the previous dose

Acute diffuse proliferative glomerulonephritis
Similar problems arise in this condition as in MPGN; again, studies in the past have included patients with widely differing aetiologies, clinical courses, and histo-logical patterns: immunosuppression has fallen into disrepute. However, in general terms, the more aggressive variants are well worth treating with steroids and azathioprine in doses similar to those suggested for MPGN.

Focal proliferative glomerulonephritis
Most patients in this category have glomerular disease secondary to systemic lupus erythematosus (SLE), polyarteritis or other systemic vascular disease. The primary condition is unusual, and should always alert one to the possibility of collagen-vascular disease. Selected patients with apparently primary focal pro-liferative glomerulonephritis respond to immunosup-pression, but it should not be routinely employed.

Mesangial proliferative glomerulonephritis
The prognosis is generally good, no specific therapy is available.

Mesangial IgA nephropathy
The long-term prognosis of this condition is uncertain, and renal failure undoubtedly occurs. A recent trial of phenytoin (which reduces serum IgA concentrations) has shown no benefit and no other therapy is of proven value.

Crescentic glomerulonephritis
This category is aetiologically heterogeneous, includ-ing idiopathic or primary renal disease, systemic vasculitis, and anti-glomerular basement membrane antibody disease (anti-GBM disease, or Goodpasture's syndrome). However, the presentation and clinical course of the renal disease is remarkably uniform. Rapidly progressive renal failure (often with oliguria or anuria) is characteristic, and the prognosis is deter-mined by the degree of glomerular involvement with crescents.

No controlled trials have been conducted in this condition, so the recommended treatment is empirical and open to criticism. It is customary to treat patients with steroids and immunosuppressive agents (azathioprine and/or cyclophosphamide), while some groups also use anticoagulants and antiplatelet agents. Recent interest has centred on the use of plasma exchange as an adjunct to drug therapy and encourag-ing results have been obtained especially in anti-GBM disease.

Irrespective of the initial agents used in crescentic nephritis, long-term drug therapy is indicated if renal function improves. In such cases treatment should con-tinue for several years at least, and possibly in-definitely.

Nephrotic syndrome
The underlying glomerular disease in adult nephrotics is not always amenable to specific therapy. Treatments directed towards the consequences of heavy pro-teinuria then have to be used.

Oedema should be treated in the first instance by restriction of dietary sodium to 20mmol/day, but most patients will also need diuretics as urinary sodium excretion is often as low as 10mmol/day. The aim of diuretic therapy in the nephrotic syndrome is not to render the patient totally free from oedema, but to increase sodium excretion and hence allow a palatable diet. Nephrotic patients have low plasma volumes by virtue of the hypo-albuminaemia, and over-aggressive diuretic therapy (often for cosmetic reasons) can lead to hypovolaemic shock and renal failure. If renal function is normal, 80–250mg of frusemide or 2–5mg bumetanide daily is sufficient; potassium supplements or an aldosterone antagonist can be added to prevent hypokalaemia. Patients refractory to diuretic therapy, or at particular risk of thrombosis, can be given weekly infusions of 2–4 units of salt-poor albumin. However, this product is in very short supply, and is not routinely recommended.

Nephrotic patients are prone to arterial and venous thrombosis; the platelets are hypersensitive and antithrombin III, the pivotal regulator of thrombin activation, is deficient. However, long-term anticoagulants or antiplatelet agents are not routinely recommended. Rather, they should be reserved for those with overt thrombotic disease.

Hyperlipidaemia is a characteristic feature of nephrotic syndrome, but clofibrate or other hypolipidaemic drugs are not recommended.

In the pre-antibiotic era, the leading cause of death in childhood nephrotic syndrome was infection. However, prophylactic antibiotic therapy is not indicated for either child or adult nephrotics.

SECONDARY GLOMERULAR DISEASE

Glomerulonephritis occurs as part of the clinical spectrum of several multisystem diseases which have a vascular basis. The following discussion will consider only the major variants of polyarteritis and also systemic lupus erythematosus.

Classical polyarteritis nodosa (PAN)
The renal manifestations of PAN commonly include microscopic haematuria and proteinuria, hypertension, acute nephritis and acute renal failure; pathologically the renal lesions range from frank renal infarction to necrotising glomerulonephritis, crescent formation and occasionally focal nephritis. High-dose steroids are always needed to control the disease, and recent evidence suggests that cyclophosphamide should also be used as initial treatment, rather than be added as a secondary measure when the disease is poorly suppressed by steroids alone. Life-long therapy with steroids, and possibly cyclophosphamide (or azathioprine) is necessary. Drug dosage should be the minimum necessary to control disease activity (assessed in terms of symptoms, renal function, urinary sediment and ESR). Crescentic nephritis in PAN has been discussed above.

Wegener's granulomatosis
The outlook in this condition was extremely gloomy until immunosuppressive therapy was employed. All patients should be treated with high-dose steroids, cyclophosphamide and possibly azathioprine. Should renal function be irretrievably lost, immunosuppressive therapy should be continued during chronic haemodialysis in order to control extrarenal disease. After kidney transplantation standard anti-rejection therapy is adequate.

Systemic lupus erythematosus (SLE)
Depending on the diagnostic criteria used, the incidence of renal disease in SLE varies from about 65 to 100 per cent. The striking improvement in five-year survival from 20 per cent to over 80 per cent in the past 25 years is attributable both to increased diagnosis and corticosteroid therapy, but the ideal treatment for renal SLE is not yet established. While diffuse proliferative glomerulonephritis undoubtedly carries a poor prognosis, focal lesions often resolve spontaneously, and membranous disease is also relatively benign. It is becoming increasingly apparent that a reduction in the incidence of renal failure using steroids is partly offset by an excess number of deaths due to sepsis and cardiovascular disease. Hence the exact place for steroids and immunosuppressive agents in renal SLE remains controversial. However, the available evidence suggests that the major hazards result from corticosteroids. Hence combined therapy with low-dose steroids and azathioprine may prove effective in controlling disease while minimising side-effects.

In general terms, patients with nephrotic syndrome, deteriorating renal function or diffuse glomerulonephritis on renal biopsy should receive steroids and azathioprine. When less severe renal disease is present, it is justifiable to withhold therapy initially provided adequate follow-up is undertaken. Special problems arise in pregnancy: a flare-up of disease activity is common in the puerperium, so increased steroid dosage should start some days before delivery.

CHRONIC RENAL FAILURE AND MAINTENANCE DIALYSIS

Chronic renal failure is accompanied by a broad spectrum of systemic upset. Many complications persist during maintenance haemodialysis and the principles of therapy are similar in both conservatively treated uraemic patients and dialysed patients.

Anaemia
The dominant reason for anaemia in uraemia is the lack of erythropoeitin; in addition red cell survival is often shortened, and the bleeding tendency of renal failure

may lead to menorrhagia and gastro-intestinal bleeding. During haemodialysis the problem is aggravated by dialyser blood trapping and loss of folate into the dialysate.

The assessment of iron status can be difficult as serum iron and iron binding capacity are unreliable guides owing to disordered iron utilisation. Furthermore, microcytic hypochromic red cells are not always found when true iron deficiency is present, as assessed by absent marrow iron stores. Currently, the assay of serum ferritin provides the best guide to iron balance in uraemia.

When iron deficiency is present, 100mg of elemental iron daily should be given orally in any of the many available preparations. Parenteral iron should never be given routinely as haemosiderosis will develop in a proportion of patients so treated.

Folate losses during dialysis are replaced by folic acid 5mg on dialysis days.

Androgen therapy undoubtedly improves the anaemia of renal failure, but the major side-effects – virilisation of women, hepatic dysfunction, acne and priapism – outweigh the benefits in almost all patients. Furthermore, in patients who have undergone nephrectomy, who often run the lowest haematocrits, androgens are ineffective.

Renal osteodystrophy

Renal osteodystrophy is a common, but not invariable, complication of uraemia; it encompasses to varying degree hyperparathyroidism, osteomalacia, osteopenia, osteosclerosis and ectopic calcification. The aetiology is not entirely clear, but two major factors are well recognised. First, phosphate retention secondary to nephron loss leads to mild hypocalcaemia and hence increased parathyroid activity. Calcium homeostasis is restored, at least temporarily, but only at the expense of the bones. The second major factor is deficiency of 1,25-dihydroxycholecalciferol (1,25DHCC), the biologically active metabolite of vitamin D. 1-α-hydroxylation occurs in the kidney, and this function is impaired even in early renal failure. The deficiency of 1,25DHCC leads to reduced intestinal calcium absorption and skeletal resistance to parathyroid hormone. It is probable that acidosis, and possible that heparin (in haemodialysis patients) play some additional part in bone disease.

The first step in the treatment of renal osteodystrophy is undoubtedly to control the serum phosphate. If the GFR is over 30ml/min, dietary restriction of phosphate is sufficient, but in more advanced renal failure, and in many dialysis patients, phosphate binders will be needed. Calcium carbonate effectively reduces phosphate absorption and also improves calcium balance, but its ability to control major hyperphosphataemia is limited as doses in excess of 20g daily are rarely tolerated. Therefore, many patients will also need aluminium hydroxide to bind phosphate in the gut and so prevent its absorption; this is most conveniently given in capsules (Alu-Cap), up to 18 (equivalent to 100ml aluminium hydroxide gel) being needed daily. Such therapy may enhance the risks of dialysis encephalopathy (due to aluminium toxicity), but if severe hyperphosphataemia is present no other therapy is available. It is important not to be over-zealous in the control of phosphate, as hypophosphataemia itself causes osteomalacia. A serum inorganic phosphate of 1.0–1.4mmol/litre is ideal.

Further treatment of renal osteodystrophy will involve vitamin D therapy in one form or another. Although cholecalciferol and dihydrotachysterol have been used in the past for this purpose, the response in renal bone disease is unpredictable. Furthermore, should hypercalcaemia be induced, it may last many months, whereas the newer vitamin D derivatives 1,25DHCC and 1-αHCC have a much shorter duration of action. These agents are now the drugs of choice as they combine relative safety with efficacy for most patients.

A dose of 1–2 micrograms/day of 1,25DHCC or 1-αHCC is needed for most patients, but regular and frequent measurement of the serum calcium is essential, especially during the start of therapy and also when the bones have healed. In dialysis patients it is safe to let the serum calcium run as high as 3.0mmol/litre before reducing the dose, but in the pre-dialysis phase of renal failure much stricter control of calcium is mandatory. Even small elevations of serum calcium have major adverse effects on the GFR, and end-stage renal failure may be precipitated by injudicious use of vitamin D analogues. However, provided the serum calcium remains properly controlled, there is no evidence that vitamin D or its derivatives jeopardise renal function.

Some patients become very hypercalcaemic on miniscule doses of 1,25DHCC or 1-αHCC without any healing of bone disease. Such patients typically have marked hyperparathyroidism and need parathyroidectomy. Alternative medical approaches are not yet available.

RENAL TRANSPLANTATION

Despite an enormous amount of clinical and laboratory research into organ transplantation in the past 25 years, it is remarkable that the vast majority of transplanted patients still receive only two immunosuppressive agents – a glucocorticoid and azathioprine. Furthermore, although there is considerable variation in the dosage of these drugs (particularly steroids) used in the early post-transplant period, there is remarkable uniformity in long-term management.

In brief, the doses used after the first six months are similar to those used in the long-term treatment of glomerulonephritis (see above); viz 10–20mg prednisolone daily (or double the dose on alternate days) and 1.5–3mg/kg/day azathioprine. Side-effects in transplanted patients do not differ from other patients, and are given in Table 3, p. 111 and Table 4, p. 112.

Other problems in transplanted patients – hypertension, anaemia, peptic ulceration, infections, etc – are, of course, common; treatment, however, is no different from that used in non-transplanted patients.

The recently introduced immunosuppressive agent, cyclosporin A, will not be discussed here as its use is still experimental.

DRUGS AND THE KIDNEY

Drugs in chronic renal failure

It is clear that drugs excreted in the urine accumulate in renal failure; what is less well known is that uraemia also affects drug absorption, volume distribution and protein binding. It is to be expected, therefore, that adverse drug reactions will be common in renal failure; a major problem arises with those patients with undiagnosed renal impairment who may unwittingly be exposed to the risk of a major side-effect of drug therapy. Most of these patients are elderly; hence, particular care should be taken when prescribing for them. Perhaps the biggest single hazard is the nephrotoxicity of tetracycline when used in renal impairment. The only safe guide to prescribing in renal failure is to consult the manufacturers data sheet, a pharmacist, or one of several exhaustive reviews on the topic (see Bibliography).

Drug-induced nephropathy

Many drugs can cause acute renal failure, but a discussion of this problem is outside the scope of this review. More relevant is chronic nephrotoxicity.

Analgesic nephropathy has been recognised as a global problem since 1953, and although the incidence has declined since the banning of phenacetin in many countries, many cases still occur. The toxicity of phenacetin is no longer in doubt, but the nephrotoxicity of other analgesics is more controversial: present evidence suggests that long-term administration of mixed preparations of analgesics should be avoided.

Several drugs have been implicated in causing a syndrome resembling SLE. The drug-induced syndrome may include renal involvement, and usually (but not always) the syndrome remits on withdrawal of the offending drug. The commonest drugs causing a lupus-like syndrome are hydralazine, isoniazid, procainamide, chlorpromazine, phenytoin, sulphonamides, penicillins, methyldopa and oral contraceptives. There are, as yet, no reliable methods for predicting susceptibility to drug-induced lupus.

The nephrotic syndrome occasionally complicates therapy with a variety of drugs, but the proteinuria commonly disappears with cessation of therapy. The drugs reported to have caused nephrotic syndrome include troxidone, tolbutamide, penicillamine, perchlorate, probenecid, gold and captopril.

REFERENCES

Urinary tract infection
Editorial (1974). V.U.R. + I.R.R. × C.P.N. *Lancet*, 2, 1120–21. (A discussion of the role of reflux in the pathogenesis of chronic pyelonephritis.)

Editorial (1976). Antibiotic treatment of kidneys of unequal function. *British Medical Journal*, 1, 4–5.

Editorial (1979). Bacteriuria – when does it matter? *Lancet*, 2, 1166–7.

Grüneberg, R. N., Smellie, J. M. and Leakey, A. (1973). *Changes in the antibiotic sensitivities of faecal organisms in response to treatment in children with urinary tract infection*. In Brumfitt, W. and Asscher, A. W. (eds). *Urinary Tract Infection*, pp 131–38. Oxford University Press, Oxford.

Smellie, J. M. and Normand, I. C. S. (1968). *Experience of follow-up of children with urinary tract infection*. In O'Grady, F. and Brumfitt, W. (eds). *Urinary Tract Infection*, pp 123–35. Oxford University Press, Oxford.

Sussman, M. and Asscher, A. W. (1979). *Urinary tract infection*. In Black, D. and Jones, N. F. (eds). *Renal Disease*, pp 400–36. Blackwell Scientific Publications Ltd, Oxford.

Primary glomerular disease
Cameron, J. S. (1979). *The natural history of glomerulonephritis*. In Black, D. and Jones, N. F. (eds). *Renal Disease*, pp 329–82. Blackwell Scientific Publications Ltd, Oxford.

BIBLIOGRAPHY

Renal stones
Coe, F. L. (1978). *Nephrolithiasis: pathogenesis and treatment*. Year Book Medical Publishers, Chicago.

Smith, L. H. (1979). *Urolithiasis*. In Earley, L. E. and Gottschalk, C. W. (eds). *Strauss and Welt's Diseases of the Kidney*, pp 893–931. Little, Brown and Co, Boston.

Thomas, W. C. (1976). *Renal Calculi: A Guide to Management*. Thomas, Springfield, Ill.

Yendt, E. R., Gagné, R. J. A. and Cohanim, M. (1966). The effects of thiazides in idiopathic hypercalciuria. *American Journal of the Medical Sciences*, **251**, 449–60.

Primary glomerular disease

Earley, L. E. and Forland, M. (1979). *Nephrotic syndrome*. In Earley, L. E. and Gottschalk, C. W. (eds). *Strauss and Welt's Diseases of the Kidney*, pp 765–813. Little, Brown and Co, Boston.

Glassock, R. J. (1979). *Clinical aspects of acute, rapidly progressive, and chronic glomerulonephritis*. ibid pp 691–764.

Kincaid-Smith, P., d'Apice, A. J. F. and Atkins, R. C. (1979). *Progress in Glomerulonephritis*. Wiley Medical, New York.

Secondary glomerular disease

Berlyne, G. M. (1979). *Renal involvement in the collagen diseases*. In Black, D. and Jones, N. F. (eds). *Renal Disease*, pp 653–86. Blackwell Scientific Publications Ltd, Oxford.

Cameron, J. S., Turner, D. R., Ogg, C. S., Williams, D. E., Lessof, M. H., Chantler, C. and Leibowitz, S. (1979). Systemic lupus with nephritis: a long-term study. *Quarterly Journal of Medicine*, **48**, 1–14.

Donadio, J. V., Burgess, J. H. and Holley, K. E. (1977). Membranous lupus nephropathy: a clinicopathologic study. *Medicine* (Baltimore), **56**, 527–36.

Fauci, A. S., Haynes, B. F. and Katz, P. (1978). The spectrum of vasculitis: clinical, pathologic, immunologic, and therapeutic considerations. *Annals of Internal Medicine*, **89**, 660–76.

Chronic renal failure and maintenance dialysis

Ledingham, J. G. E. (1979). *Chronic renal failure*. In Black, D. and Jones, N. F. (eds). *Renal Disease*, pp 523–48. Blackwell Scientific Publications Ltd, Oxford.

Kennedy, A. C. (1979). *Maintenance dialysis*. ibid pp 549–87.

DeLuca, H. F. and Avioli, L. V. (1979). *Renal osteodystrophy*. ibid pp 766–803.

Renal transplantation

Morris, P. J. (1979). *Renal Transplantation: Principles and Practice*. Academic Press, London.

Drugs and the kidney

Bennett, W. M., Porter, G. A., Bagby, S. P. and McDonald, W. J. (1978). *Drugs and Renal Disease*. Churchill Livingstone, Edinburgh.

Bennett, W. M., Muther, R. S., Parker, R. A., Feig, P., Morrison, G., Golper, T. A. and Singer, I. (1980). Drug therapy in renal failure: dosing guidelines for adults. *Annals of Internal Medicine*, **93**, 62–89 and 286–325.

Evans, D. B. (1980). Drugs and the kidney. *British Journal of Hospital Medicine*, **24**, 244–51.

Rubin, A. L., Stenzel, K. H. and Reidenberg, M. M. (1977). Symposium on drug action and metabolism in renal failure. *American Journal of Medicine*, **62**, 459–60.

Chapter 10 Skin disorders

I. B. SNEDDON CBE, MD, FRCP

ACNE VULGARIS

This common complaint of adolescents is often regarded as untreatable, a concept supported by a recent review which discovered that only one-third of patients had ever had adequate treatment (Cunliffe et al, 1980). Even when treated well the relapse rate is high and patients and their parents should be told that repeated treatment will be required over a number of years if permanent ugly scars are to be minimised.

There is a strong genetic factor in acne and treatment should be more vigorous in those with a bad family history. Rational treatment aims to reduce sebum production, unblock the sebaceous glands, and control infection and the resultant inflammatory response.

Patients with mild acne need only topical treatment. Retinoic acid (Retin A) either as a lotion or a gel removes blackheads (comedones); patients should be warned that erythema and soreness may occur but is not an indication to stop treatment.

Benzoyl peroxide also in lotion, cream or gel is an effective bactericidal agent but again it may produce some redness and scaling. This may be compared to moderate sunburn. It should be applied once daily and as the skin becomes accustomed to it, twice daily. Retinoic acid and benzoyl peroxide have an additive effect if one is used in the morning and the other at night.

More severe acne needs treatment with an antibiotic. Oxytetracycline B.P. is usually the first choice since it is cheap and safe. It must be given before food since its benefit will be negated by milk and iron. Patients are often worried by the need to take tetracycline often for years but the only contra-indications are renal disease and pregnancy. Young girls should be warned of the risk to the fetus if they are on tetracycline and, if contraceptive pills are being taken, a high oestrogen-containing one such as Minovlar would be indicated as it might help the acne. Oxytetracycline 250mg twice daily for three months is the usual course for moderate acne. There is no advantage in the use of more expensive tetracycline and a combination with nystatin is unnecessary. Erythromycin 500mg b.d. is equally suc-cessful and is tolerated by the occasional patient who develops nausea with oxytetracycline. If these antibiotics fail, co-trimoxazole (Septrin, Bactrim) one tablet b.d. can be substituted but it carries the risk of sulphonamide drug reactions.

Clindamycin (Dalacin C) is very effective in severe cases of acne vulgaris but has fallen into disuse as prolonged treatment may cause pseudomembranous colitis.

Attempts to control sebum production with local and systemic anti-androgens such as cyproterone acetate have not proved satisfactory. In really difficult acne which is producing mental depression it is justifiable to combine prednisolone 5mg daily for a month with the antibiotic.

One advance in therapy which may be adopted, though it is at present only at the trial stage, is oral 13-cis-retinoic acid. It is not yet available on prescription.

Acne should be treated with enthusiasm and the patient encouraged to control exacerbations until natural remission occurs. This may be often much later than the early twenties and long supportive interviews may be indicated from time to time.

ROSACEA

Though of unknown etiology and not associated with excessive sebum production, this unsightly and chronic complaint of middle-age often needs prolonged treatment.

In the past local treatment with sulphur preparations was used; this has now been abandoned and simple emollients are all that are necessary. The most effective remedy is oral oxytetracycline 250mg twice daily taken on an empty stomach. Improvement may take several months and there may be difficulty in persuading the patient to continue treatment after improvement has occurred. Relapses are also frequent but respond again to another course of oxytetracyline.

Strong topical steroid creams have often been tried before treatment starts and they should be stopped. A warning must be given to the patient that a rebound flare-up of the eruption is probable and must be suffered in order to achieve cure.

Oxytetracycline may not be tolerated and is, of course, not permitted in pregnancy, when rosacea is often troublesome. Metronidazole (Flagyl) 200mg given twice daily is an effective substitute and can be used in pregnant women. A few cases of mild but reversible peripheral neuropathy have been described after its prolonged use but the complication is not severe enough to prevent its use.

PSORIASIS

The introduction of topical steroid creams and ointments was hailed as a great step forward in the management of chronic adult type psoriasis. It has now been realised that only the most potent steroids such as betamethasone valerate (Betnovate), clobetasol propionate (Dermovate) and fluocinolone acetonide (Synalar) will reduce the increased epidermal mitoses on the patches of psoriasis, but on thickened plaques even those are ineffective unless forced through the skin by polythene occlusion. Thus, much of the steroid cream prescribed for psoriasis is wasted as it is no more effective than an inert cream.

Prolonged treatment with potent steroids under occlusion causes local skin atrophy and, more important, systemic steroid effects such as hypertension, adrenal suppression or Cushing's syndrome. It has been calculated that more than 50g of clobetasol propionate ointment applied weekly is dangerous and especially so if the patient has liver disease.

Other drawbacks to the prolonged use of topical steroids are the rosacea-like changes if it is applied to the face, and the rebound pustular reaction which occurs in simple chronic psoriasis if treatment is stopped suddenly.

The disenchantment with topical steroids has led to a fresh look at dithranol. There is no doubt that dithranol preparations are effective but they have the disadvantage of staining the skin and clothes. Modern preparations such as Dithrocream and in combination with salicylic acid or urea are much more acceptable. Dithranol ointment (Stie-Lasan) can also be used for psoriasis of the scalp. The only complication of dithranol application is that erythema and burning may follow the use of too concentrated a preparation. This reaction is not a true allergic response and dithranol can be used again in a lower concentration when the acute reaction has subsided.

The usual strength used to start treatment is 0.1% Dithrocream which can be increased up to 0.5% if erythema is minimal. If a reaction occurs at higher concentrations a return to 0.1% is indicated.

Conflicting opinions have been given about the combination of topical steroids and dithranol. Some workers believe that psoriasis clears more quickly but relapses equally quickly. The only indication for systemic steroids in the treatment of psoriasis is in the rare exfoliative psoriasis which behaves in the same way as any erythroderma. In all other patients with psoriasis systemic steroids should be avoided.

Ultra-violet light therapy

Over 50 years ago Goeckerman showed that daily ultra-violet light given to patients who had applied tar in the form of paint or ointment on the patches of psoriasis, would clear the condition in a high proportion of patients. Ingram modified this technique by substituting dithranol in Lassar's paste instead of tar. The Ingram treatment is widely used in Britain but though successful is time-consuming and requires staff trained in the technique. Remissions last from 6 to 12 months and repeated courses of treatment are less and less successful. Some workers have claimed that a simpler form of treatment with ultra-violet alone is satisfactory.

Photochemotherapy

In 1974 the giving of oral 8-methoxypsoralen (8MOP) followed by exposure of the whole patient to long wave ultra-violet light (UVA) was shown to improve 90 per cent of psoriatics in five weeks. Psoralens and UVA have now been used on many thousands of patients. Methoxalen (8-methoxypsoralen) is given in a dose of 0.6mg/kg two hours before irradiation. The UVA measured in Joules per cm^2 should be carefully monitored and the dosage assessed by the patient's skin colour. Treatment is given three times weekly, at first with clearing in 5 to 12 weeks. Maintenance treatment every week or possibly once every three weeks will control the psoriasis. Cessation of treatment is followed by relapse at much the same rate as after the Goeckerman treatment.

SIDE-EFFECTS

An overdose of UVA causes burning. There is occasionally nausea, and dizziness and pain in the skin can occur. The eyes should be protected by sunglasses during the day of treatment, as otherwise cataract can occur. The main risk is of carcinoma of the skin with prolonged treatment but it is too soon yet to estimate the danger.

Some 10 per cent of patients do not respond to PUVA and may become tired of attending a special centre for treatment, and discontinue. It should not be used in childhood or in pregnancy, in patients with light sensitivity, and in mild cases who could be managed with other measures.

The main indications, are those with severely incapacitating psoriasis (though it does not help psoriatic arthritis) and in those who cannot be accepted for methotrexate therapy because of liver damage.

Methotrexate

This folic acid antagonist has proved over the years to be an effective systemic treatment for severe and intractable psoriasis. It has the great advantage of enabling the patient to continue to control the disease without the need for complicated apparatus or messy local applications. It can be given intravenously, intramuscularly or by mouth. The technique favoured by the author is a once-weekly oral dose of 15mg divided into 5mg given every 12 hours.

Since its greatest danger is its hepatotoxicity it is vital to check before starting treatment that the liver is healthy. Liver function tests have not proved sufficiently reliable and it is usual to carry out a liver biopsy before considering treatment. It is also important that the patient should realise that other liver toxins, especially alcohol, should be avoided. If there is any doubt about the patient's ability to forego alcohol, treatment should not be started. Aspirin and sulphonamides also potentiate its effect and should be avoided if possible.

Renal and bone marrow function should also be checked and patients on treatment should be told that a monthly blood count will be essential throughout the period of treatment. Repeat liver biopsy biennially is necessary though there is a possibility that a liver scan may prove just as effective and less traumatic.

Toxic effects include mouth ulcers, nausea which can be controlled by prochlorperazine maleate (Stemetil) 5mg given with the methotrexate, and megaloblastic anaemia. The latter can be reversed by folic acid 5mg daily without interfering with the antipsoriatic effect. Modest thrombocytopenia and mild leukopenia occur but are not indications for cessation of treatment.

Methotrexate therapy should be reserved for patients whose psoriasis cannot be controlled by other methods. It should be avoided in children, and pregnancy and conception should not be allowed within three months of taking methotrexate. Personal experience over 15 years has given confidence that this is a valuable form of treatment especially in erythrodermic, generalised pustular and arthropathic psoriasis. A recent review of 45 patients treated in this

way has shown that, provided they are selected carefully, the treatment is safe. The only disaster was in an unrecognised alcoholic who succumbed from cirrhosis of the liver.

Other antimitotic drugs have not stood the test of time, either proving too toxic or ineffective.

No discussion of the management of psoriasis is complete without the mention of the aromatic retinoids derived from vitamin A. Early reports record that Ro-10 9359 is effective especially in pustular psoriasis but the side-effects of hypervitaminosis A preclude high dosage. In their present form the aromatic retinoids are not a safe form of treatment but later compounds may well be more successful.

ECZEMA

Of the eczematous eruptions the most difficult problem is that of the atopic state which includes asthma and hay fever. The condition often starts with an eczematous eruption in the infant, usually at three to four months old. Successful management depends on obtaining the confidence of the parents of the baby, since the whole family become involved in the anxiety about the excoriated, crusted and possibly sleepless infant.

Atopy is genetically determined, some 70 per cent with the disorder having a first degree relative with a similar condition. In those affected there is an increased susceptibility to form IgE and to show acquired anaphylactic reactions to substances such as milk, protein, egg albumin and house dust and animal hair. A lowered resistance to infection is ascribed to defective T-cell immunity.

The eczematous eruption in infants usually starts on the head and the face, and later extends to the bends of the arms, the backs of the knees and, in severe cases, involves the whole body. These patients will require treatment over a long period of time, often many years, and this must be explained at the onset to the parents.

However, a recent long-term follow-up has revealed that the prognosis is better than previous workers have thought in that some 87 per cent clear somewhere between the ages of five and twenty (Vickers, 1980). Adverse features shown in the recent study were a late onset of the eczema, particularly after adolescence, and a reversed distribution of the eruption, i.e. involvement of the extensor surfaces rather than the flexor surfaces.

In the management of infants born into families with the atopic tendency there is now evidence that avoidance of exposure to well-known exciting causes of allergic reaction may lower the incidence of eczema

(Matthew et al, 1977). Thus breast feeding should be encouraged, cow's milk avoided and a soya bean substitute used instead. There has long been a tradition that goat's milk is preferable to cow's milk but there is no adequate evidence for this. Feathers in bedding and contact with domestic furry pets should be avoided. Once the eczema has started, skin tests to discover supposed allergens and diets are of no value. Occasionally urticarial reactions may be induced by food such as fish or nuts but the eczema remains largely unchanged.

Treatment of eczematous areas

The mainstay of treatment is the topical application of emollients such as ung. aquosum and the avoidance of soap which degreases the skin. Ung. emulsificans mixed with water can be used as a soap substitute or oilatum bath emollient (Stieffel) is effective. Creams containing urea (which is hygroscopic) improve the hydration of the skin, are comforting and harmless. Calmurid or Aquadrate, simple urea creams, or urea in combination with hydrocortisone in Alphaderm are pleasant to use and will control irritation in mild cases.

Though the mechanism of itching is not understood in atopic eczema, topical steroid applications will control the symptoms and allow the patient and the parents to attain a restful night.

As a principle the weakest steroid preparation which will control symptoms should be used. 1% hydrocortisone in cream or ointment is sufficient for mild cases and there is no need to be frightened that skin atrophy or systemic absorption sufficient to suppress the adrenal glands will occur. Parents who have read alarmist stories in the media may shy away from steroids but can be reassured that hydrocortisone is safe. Should hydrocortisone not be powerful enough to relieve symptoms then a stronger steroid should be used. Clobetasone butyrate (Eumovate), hydrocortisone butyrate (Locoid) or a 1 in 4 dilution in paraffin moll. of a stronger steroid such as betamethasone valerate (Betnovate) ointment may have to be used. There is also some point in switching from one steroid to another since the skin does become accustomed to a preparation which then may cease to be effective, a phenomenon known as tachyphylaxis. In the worst cases it may be useful to provide the parents with a large supply of weak steroid and a small tube of a stronger steroid and suggest that the strong steroid should be used for a day or so and then as soon as the exacerbation is better, a return to the weaker preparation should be made.

The three significant complications of the overuse of topical steroids are: (1) local atrophy and striae forma-tion; (2) a Cushingoid change in which the child puts on weight and growth is suppressed and (3) adrenal suppression so that they may not respond to a stressful situation such as infection.

Systemic steroids should never be used for eczema before puberty and only in very exceptional circumstances in adults. Occasionally children with severe eczema are receiving systemic steroids for their asthma but eczema is not an indication.

The only drugs which are of assistance are the antihistamines. These do relieve some of the itching. Hydroxyzine (Atarax) is both an antihistamine and a sedative and of great value. Promethazine hydrochloride (Phenergan) and trimeprazine (Vallergan) are safe, and should be used in sufficient dose to produce a good night's sleep. Systemic antibiotics may be required if the eczema becomes infected with pyogenic organisms. Erythromycin is preferred because many atopic sufferers develop urticaria with penicillin and the tetracyclines must be avoided in young children as they stain the second dentition.

Intractable atopic eczema in young adults may need systemic steroids though the need for this lessens as better local treatments become available. Short courses are valueless and one must expect to give prednisolone 15mg daily for between 6 to 12 months. During that time most girls will gain 6 to 12kg and they should be warned of this possibility; there is also a greater risk of hypertension in young men. It is better to avoid this regimen if possible.

Obviously hypertension and a history of peptic ulcer will contra-indicate the use of steroids, but in the young and active on a normal diet one sees little or no side-effects. The risk of decalcification or the activation of tuberculosis in this country is negligible. The real hazard is the automatic continuation of prednisolone for up to 20 years when cataracts may form, thromboses occur and intracranial hypertension may develop.

There is a slightly increased risk to the fetus if pregnancy occurs once the patient is on prednisolone and this must be clearly explained to the patient. Incidentally, the contraceptive pill has a mild steroid effect and the dosage of prednisolone can be lowered if an oestrogen-containing pill is taken simultaneously.

Long-acting ACTH can be used rather than prednisolone but this means injections which are never popular as a long-term treatment.

Before resorting to steroids a short period in hospital on intensive local treatment is in most situations a better solution. The steroids can be kept for the treatment of severe recurrence which may follow discharge from hospital.

The only other variety of eczema which needs long-term treatment is discoid or nummular eczema. This is a disorder of adults unrelated to atopy. Though chronic and recurrent individual lesions will respond to topical tar preparations, often local occlusion with Coltapaste or powerful topical steroids such as Betnovate and Dermovate need to be used. Occasional resistant patches can be cleared by subcutaneous intra-lesional hydrocortisone injection 25mg/ml. Systemic drugs are of no value and the prognosis of this condition is poor. Many patients continue to have recurrent nummular eczema over a period of many years.

IMMUNOSUPPRESSIVES AND THE SKIN

Many patients with skin lesions are taking immuno-suppressive drugs either because they have diseases which require them, such as lymphomata, or they are transplant patients. The effect of these immunosuppressives is to make the patients vulnerable to skin infections which otherwise would be negligible. Thus, disorders such as herpes zoster, herpes simplex, molluscum contagiosum, candidiasis and other fungus infections may become invasive and atypically ferocious.

The treatment of these infections does not differ from the conventional methods but it is right to be aware that violent attacks of these infections may well occur. It may be necessary to reduce the immunosuppression in order to control the infection.

One other complication of immunosuppression is that skin neoplasms may be triggered off by the depression of immunity. It has been particularly recognised that renal patients on immunosuppression are more prone to develop skin carcinomata or solar keratoses.

REFERENCES

Cunliffe, W. J., Clayden, D., Gould, D. J. and Simpson, N. B. (1981). Acne vulgaris – its aetiology and treatment. *Clinical and Experimental Dermatology*, **6**, 461–9.

Matthew, D. J., Taylor, B., Norman, A. P., Turner, M. W. and Soothill, J. F. (1977). Prevention of eczema. *Lancet*, **1**, 321–4.

Vickers, C. F. H. (1980). The natural history of atopic eczema. *Acta Dermatovena*, **Supp 92**, 113–15.

Chapter 11 The rheumatic diseases

M. THOMPSON MD, FRCP

PRINCIPLES OF GENERAL MANAGEMENT

It is evident that drugs occupy a predominant role in the management of chronic rheumatic disorders and will continue to do so in the forseeable future. Although there are examples where drugs are virtually specific in their action and sufficient by themselves to control the disease, e.g. allopurinol in the treatment of gout and prednisolone in the control of polymyalgia rheumatica, there is general recognition that drugs must be used in combination with various additional methods of treatment. For each patient there must be an individually prepared programme of management according to their needs. Many patients, especially those with milder forms of rheumatic disease, can be treated adequately with drug therapy alone but others with major, crippling disorders such as severe rheumatoid arthritis, osteoarthritis and ankylosing spondylitis, will require a regimen in which drug therapy will play an important but not an exclusive role. Rest in bed, physiotherapy, splints and appliances, joint aspiration, intra-articular injections, diet, reconstructive surgery and rehabilitation procedures involving occupational therapy, aids and adaptations to facilitate daily living activities and re-training for work or domestic independence may be needed. It is imperative that the doctor should define what needs to be treated, as symptoms may arise from various causes some of which are amenable to treatment by drugs while others require physical or surgical measures, e.g. pain and stiffness due to destroyed joints will require physical measures such as splints or surgery for satisfactory relief of symptoms. Table 1 shows the principal causes of symptoms in rheumatoid arthritis with the various measures required for their control. Disappointment and mistakes in the therapy of the chronic rheumatic diseases are usually due to failure to identify the precise causes of the symptoms or to a neglect of the basic regimen of treatment and failure to keep in touch with a changing situation over a period of time when progression of the disease and complications may radically alter the needs for treatment.

Table 1 Indications for treatment: symptoms in inflammatory polyarthritis

1. Local pain in joints and associated tissues due to inflammation; treatment by analgesic/anti-inflammatory drugs.
2. Joints distended by effusions; treat by aspiration and possible corticosteroid injection.
3. Pain due to disorganised joints; splints and/or surgery.
4. Nerve entrapment or compression, e.g. carpal tunnel in rheumatoid; treat by local steroid injection or surgery.
5. Anxiety and depression; if primary, with anxiolytic and anti-depressants; if secondary, then reassurance and pain relief.
6. Insomnia; identify cause and treat appropriately, more likely to be due to pain and stiffness requiring analgesic/anti-inflammatory drugs in preference to sedatives.
7. Visceral and systemic complications, e.g. pleuritis, severe anaemia and vasculitis in rheumatoid; may need steroids or immune-suppressive drugs.
8. Complications of therapy, mainly side-effects of drugs, e.g. myopathy with steroids and D-penicillamine.

Disease classification

The rheumatic disorders can be broadly classified into those diseases characterised by (1) *inflammation* in the joints (e.g. rheumatoid arthritis, ankylosing spondylitis, psoriatic arthritis etc); (2) *degenerative* forms of arthritis of which osteoarthritis and intervertebral disc disease are the most common; (3) *metabolic* disorders, gout, and other forms of crystal deposition disease in the joints, e.g. pyrophosphate arthropathy (pseudogout or chondrocalcinosis); and (4) *non-articular* rheumatic disorders, mainly due to traumatic and degenerative changes in tendons and ligaments but which may be associated with major arthritis or connective tissue disorders in some cases.

All of these conditions cause pain and stiffness and

have some component of inflammation even those caused by trauma and conditioned by degeneration. During the past two decades there has been a tendency to use the terminology 'osteoarthrosis' rather than osteoarthritis, but a recent recognition of the inflammatory changes that accompany or complicate degenerative joint disease has led to a resurgence of popularity for osteoarthritis. These inflammatory changes appear to be associated in some cases with the presence of hydroxyapatite crystals and in others to the mechanical derangement of the joint by destruction of cartilage, osteophyte formation and by the presence of loose cartilaginous bodies causing intra-articular trauma, synovitis and occasional haemarthrosis. Recognition of the role of inflammation in all of these groups, whether their origin and nature may be primarily inflammatory, degenerative, traumatic, metabolic or a mixture, is important in their management. While simple analgesics such as paracetamol or codeine will confer some measure of pain relief, the use of drugs which combine analgesic and anti-inflammatory properties has been shown to be significantly more effective in the relief of pain and particularly stiffness with reduction of swelling and other signs of inflammation. This is exemplified by the use of analgesic/anti-inflammatory drugs in the treatment of acute and chronic sports injuries in the young, and non-articular forms of rheumatism in the middle-aged and elderly.

CHOICE OF DRUG

The less severe forms of arthritis and rheumatic disorders will only require symptomatic relief which can be provided with milder and generally safer non-steroidal analgesic/anti-inflammatory drugs (NSAID). The more severe presentations of major arthritis, e.g. rheumatoid and spondylitis, will call for a decision as to whether additional drug therapy is needed for control or to suppress the disease process, e.g. gold, penicillamine, chloroquine. Safety is always important and in some cases a paramount factor, e.g. in sports injuries and milder disabling degenerative disease, powerful drugs with potential major hazards should not be used as their risks are not justified.

The development of analgesic and anti-inflammatory drugs has represented one of the major advances in pharmaco-therapeutics during the past 30 years. So much so, that the doctor is faced with a large number of drugs, many of which are similar in their chemical composition and properties and to add to the confusion they may be manufactured under different names and in different presentations. The main groups of analgesic and anti-inflammatory drugs are listed in Table 2. In the treatment of the inflammatory rheumatic disorders, these preparations are referred to as *first-line* drugs (analgesics and non-steroidal analgesic/anti-inflammatory drugs); *second-line* drugs with a slower effect upon the disease, including gold preparations; D-penicillamine; anti-malarial drugs; sulphasalazone and dapsone. The *third-line* drugs include the cortico-steroid group given by mouth or by injection over a long term, and the immuno-suppressive drugs (azathioprine, chlorambucil and methotrexate), and cytotoxic drugs (cyclophosphamide). Generally speaking, the policy is to initiate treatment with the mildest and safest drug in the minimal dosage requisite to give satisfactory relief and to progress cautiously to stronger drugs and higher dosage in more severe cases. Certain diseases and certain defined presentations will call for stronger measures initially, e.g. polymyalgia rheumatica with severe proximal joint stiffness and a rapid ESR will

Table 2 Drugs used in the treatment of rheumatic disorders

1. *Plain analgesics*, e.g. aspirin and its derivatives in small dosage; paracetamol; codeine and dihydrocodeine; dextropropoxyphene and pentazocine.
2. *Mild anti-inflammatory/analgesic drugs* aspirin and derivatives in dosage of 2.4–4g daily; ibuprofen; azapropazone; sulindac; mefenamic acid; piroxicam.
3. *Moderate anti-inflammatory/analgesic drugs* ketoprofen; fenoprofen; indoprofen; flurbiprofen; naproxen; feprazone; flufenamic acid; fenclofenac; diclofenac; benorylate and aspirin derivatives in dosage of 4g or more aspirin daily; tolmetin; benoxaprofen; tiaprofenic acid.
4. *Powerful anti-inflammatory drugs with analgesic effects*, e.g. phenylbutazone and oxyphenbutazone; indomethacin.
5. *'Second-line drugs'*, slow-acting and with a more specific effect on rheumatoid arthritis; gold, penicillamine, anti-malarial compounds, sulphasalazine and dapsone.
6. Anti-inflammatory corticosteroids and corticotrophin.
7. *'Third-line drugs'* for rheumatoid arthritis, e.g. azathioprin; chlorambucil and methotrexate (immuno-suppressants) and cyclophosphamide (cytotoxic).
8. Drugs with a specific effect on joint diseases, e.g. antibiotics for joint sepsis, and colchine and allopurinol for gout.

require immediate steroid therapy to relieve symptoms and prevent hazardous complications; severe and active rheumatoid arthritis with visceral and systemic complications will require both first-line and second-line drugs at an early stage with the probable need for steroid and/or immuno-suppressive therapy if vasculitis is present. However, a cautionary attitude prevails in the prescription of second-line and particularly steroids and third-line drugs in rheumatoid arthritis. When life-threatening complications such as vasculitis or severe visceral disease are present, or when one is dealing with the rarer rheumatic disorders where there is an adverse prognosis, e.g. systemic lupus erythematosus and polyarteritis nodosa complicated by renal involvement, then the prescription of steroids and immuno-suppressant drugs is not only justified but may be urgently needed as a life-saving measure.

FIRST-LINE DRUGS

'Simple' or 'plain' analgesics

The major problem facing the doctor embarking on long-term therapy for a rheumatic patient is to select the best regimen from the many drugs available. The prescription of a plain analgesic alone may suffice in the management of mild cases of non-articular rheumatism and in the milder forms of osteoarthritis, especially when dyspepsia or other relative contra-indications limit or preclude the use of stronger anti-inflammatory compounds. These mild analgesics are also frequently prescribed or self-administered by patients to supplement other therapy in the more severe forms of arthritis. One of the dangers of such self-medication is that patients may unwittingly take preparations containing phenacetin which has now been officially banned from the pharmacopoeia in view of its liability to cause renal papillary necrosis and chronic pyelonephritis in addition to occasional blood dyscrasias. *Aspirin* in small dosage acts as a simple analgesic and only exerts its anti-inflammatory effect when given in doses of 3.6g daily or more. It is a traditional domestic remedy but even in low dosage may cause gastro-duodenal hazards especially in patients suffering from gastritis and concurrently taking alcohol, in addition to the much rarer risk of provoking or exacerbating asthma in predisposed patients. The concurrent administration of aspirin with other anti-inflammatory drugs, especially indomethacin, may prove dangerous in the provocation of gastro-intestinal side-effects and is therapeutically inefficient as the drugs act in a competitive rather than a complementary fashion. *Codeine* is commonly used as a mild analgesic, often in combination with aspirin. In the usual dosage of 30–60mg

daily it may cause drowsiness, constipation and occasional vertigo or confusion and it may prove addictive if taken in excessive dosage over long periods of time. However, it is generally regarded as a useful and safe analgesic when properly administered. Its place has been supplanted to some extent by its chemical relative, *dihydrocodeine*, which is a more potent compound with a similar pattern of clinical effect and side-effects. *Dextropropoxyphene* is also frequently used and is approximately equivalent to codeine, with claims that it is non-addictive and has fewer side-effects, but occasional rashes and even hepatotoxicity, have been reported. *Pentazocine* is a more powerful analgesic, reputedly non-addictive but liable to cause drowsiness, vertigo and confusion in patients who are sensitive to its action, or if the inaugural doses are set too high. The most recent addition to the range of plain analgesics is *diflunisal* which is chemically related to aspirin and, like aspirin, has a simple analgesic effect in small dosage but may exercise some anti-inflammatory effect when taken in dosage of 500mg twice daily. It is common practice to add a plain analgesic to a regimen of NSAID, but aspirin and diflunisal should not be used in this role.

Non-steroidal anti-inflammatory drugs with analgesic action (NSAID)

The production of these compounds has been one of the peak activities of pharmaceutical research in the past three decades. There is now a vast number of these compounds many of which are chemically similar and have similar effects but may be presented under a variety of names and in multiple formulations, e.g. tablets, slow-release preparations, capsules and suppositories, or even in combination with analgesics and other drugs. Until 1950, aspirin was the drug of first choice, taken either alone or in combination with phenacetin and/or codeine. Even in those days, the well meant but common mistake of polypharmacy was committed by the concurrent administration of bicarbonate to reduce the gastric side-effects of aspirin, with reduction of the therapeutic effect of the aspirin owing to its ineffectiveness in an alkaline medium. Since 1950, a series of new compounds have been developed and their chemical relationships are shown in Figure 11/1 indicating that many of them are chemically related with acetic, phenyl-acetic or propionic groupings as a common characteristic. Their mode of action remains obscure to a great extent although various effects upon biological systems have been demonstrated to account for their anti-inflammatory properties, e.g. uncoupling of oxidative phosphorylation; inhibition of prostaglandin synthetase activity;

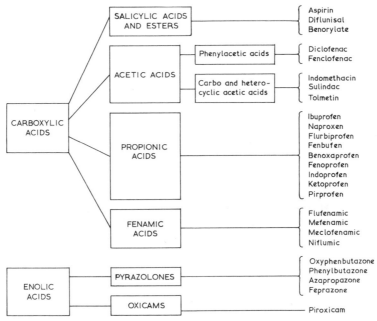

Fig. 11/1 Chemical relationships of non-steroidal anti-inflammatory drugs

displacement of amino-acid, notably tryptophan, from protein binding sites; inhibition of enzyme release and, more recently, inhibition of macrophage activity. All have been advanced as possible mechanisms for their effects, demonstrated chiefly in models of inflammation in experimental animals. In addition to relief of pain and sometimes an anti-pyretic effect, they relieve stiffness and reduce swelling, heat and tenderness in inflamed joints with improvement in function.

There is no automatic first choice of drug for all or even the majority of cases. The initial prescription will depend upon the diagnosis and assessment of the severity of the disease with consideration of previous drug reactions and absolute or relative contra-indications, e.g. dyspepsia or peptic ulceration. In general, it is sound policy to start with the mildest and safest drug in modest dosage, pitched at a reasonable level of therapeutic expectation with the opportunity to change the dosage or the drug according to progress or lack of it. Some cases will cry out aloud for powerful drugs, e.g. severe spondylitis and acute gout, whereas the majority of mild cases of spondylosis and osteoarthritis seen in general practice will manage perfectly well with analgesics alone or with a mild anti-inflammatory drug. It is better for the practitioner to familiarise himself with the use and expected response and side-effects of a *few* drugs than to dabble with many. It is also sound policy to avoid polypharmacy, especially with the anti-

inflammatory drugs, as they are more often competitive than complementary in their actions, and polypharmacy leads to confusion should side-effects develop. One exception used to be the prescription of slow-acting suppositories of indomethacin to provide relief during the night combined with faster acting drugs during the day. There are now several preparations of NSAID in suppository form (ketoprofen, naproxen, oxy-phenbutazone) so that the same drug may be administered day and night within the prescribed dosage limits. The permissible use of NSAID in combination with certain plain analgesics (codeine, dextrapropoxyphene and pentazocine) has already been mentioned.

Aspirin

Traditionally the first choice in the treatment of rheumatic diseases, it is now clear that aspirin has been supplanted by the newer anti-inflammatory drugs although it still occupies a common and important place in the management of milder and non-inflammatory rheumatic conditions, and occasionally proves to be the drug of choice for patients with more severe arthritis who have demonstrated their ability to take it without hazard over many years. Even in small dosage, aspirin may cause superficial gastritis and erosions and the administration of 600mg of aspirin has been shown to cause occult gastro-intestinal blood loss amounting to 4ml or more per day in 70 per cent of patients and volunteers. This effect is quite separate and distinct from the more serious gastro-intestinal hazards that result from the administration of the larger doses of aspirin, 3.6g daily or more, which are required to exercise its full anti-inflammatory effect. With these higher doses there is the risk of massive gastro-intestinal haemorrhage with erosive gastritis in addition to the possible development of gastro-duodenal ulceration and its hazards. Numerous preparations of aspirin have been introduced in an attempt to overcome some of these side-effects, and the commonest of such formulations are enteric-coated tablets (Enseals or Nuseals of aspirin); compound preparations such as aloxiprin (Safapryn) or salsalate (Disalcid); the encapsulation of multiple small coated fragments of aspirin as micro-encapsulated aspirin (Levius) which also has the advantage of slow release so that it need only be taken twice daily.

The concept of chemically combining aspirin and paracetamol to produce a compound which is absorbed unchanged and then metabolises to its active constituents in the bloodstream and liver has been achieved by the introduction of benorylate (Benoral) which is relatively free from gastro-intestinal side-effects and has the advantage of requiring only twice-daily administration to achieve constant therapeutic level. Although some mixtures of analgesic and anti-inflammatory drugs are competitive, in the case of aspirin and paracetamol they exercise a summative effect in such preparations as benorylate and Safapryn, which is a mixture of a central enteric-coated core of 300mg of aspirin enveloped by a further coating of 250mg of paracetamol. The combination of aspirin and paracetamol represents some savings in terms of the administration of tablets. However, benorylate can be taken in the form of a suspension and doses of 2–4g (5–10ml of suspension) b.d. are equivalent to 2.5–5g daily of aspirin. Benorylate may also be taken in the form of tablets or conveniently as sachets each of which contains 2g of benorylate and are easily administered in water, tea and other non-alcoholic beverages.

While these newer formulations have reduced the lesser hazards of mild dyspepsia, superficial gastritis and occult bleeding, they have not overcome the other undesirable side-effects of aspirin including peptic ulceration, tinnitus, deafness, drowsiness, occasional rashes and rarely allergic reactions including provocation or exacerbation of asthma. Furthermore, the newer preparations of aspirin have elevated the cost of the cheapest remedy for arthritis to that of the more expensive and newer preparations. The multiplicity of side-effects, both mild and severe, of aspirin accounts for more than 50 per cent of intolerance in some series,

irrespective of the mode of administration, and this is the outstanding reason why aspirin has had to give pride of place as automatic first choice in treatment to more recently introduced NSAID.

Pyrazole derivatives

The best known of this group is phenylbutazone (Butazolidin) which was introduced into clinical practice in 1951 and is a powerful analgesic and anti-inflammatory drug generally administered in doses ranging from 300–600mg daily. It is especially effective in relief of skeletal and arthritic pain but disappointing in the treatment of neuritic symptoms, so that it can be effective in treatment of a lumbar disc lesion but not especially helpful in the relief of sciatica due to a trapped nerve root. Phenylbutazone provided the first serious challenge to aspirin in the management of rheumatic disorders and was even accepted as a welcome alternative to cortisone as the cumulative hazards of steroid therapy were being recognised in the early 1950s. However, it was known that phenylbutazone was chemically related to amidopyrine which had been largely abandoned because of its risks of inducing bone marrow and hepatic damage. It was soon realised that phenylbutazone had several side-effects, some of which were extremely dangerous. The drug is highly bound to plasma proteins and displaces warfarin if this is being used for concurrent anticoagulant therapy, so that there is a significant potentiation of the anticoagulant effect. It can also interfere with hypoglycaemic drugs and hydantoins in a similar fashion. It may cause oedema with weight retention and aggravation of hypertension to the extent of precipitating cardiac failure, so that its use in elderly patients is very limited. Gastro-intestinal disturbance, including major gastro-duodenal and colitic disasters may occur in addition to rashes and thyroid enlargement due to blockage of the handling of iodine within the thyroid gland. The more serious hazards are fortunately much rarer but include liver damage, sometimes associated with renal changes, and damage to the bone marrow.

The blood dyscrasias induced by phenylbutazone are interesting in that agranulocytosis tends to occur more frequently in the younger age groups and in the early stages of therapy, usually within the first three months and sometimes within the first few days, while in the elderly there is a tendency for the more gradual development of aplastic anaemia after the patients have been taking the drugs for a year or more. Although the early signs and symptoms of blood dyscrasia can be detected at an early stage in many patients by advice concerning the early warning symptoms and by taking periodic blood counts, there are still many cases where severe marrow damage can occur without warning and with a fatal result. This has engendered a great deal of anxiety, and rightly so, in the minds of many clinicians so that phenylbutazone no longer occupies the place it enjoyed in the long-term management of rheumatic disorder in the 1950s and 1960s.

The gross restrictions which limit its use in the elderly have already been stressed and it would be criminal folly to give a potentially dangerous drug like phenylbutazone for minor or self-limiting conditions such as athletic injuries. There must be some degree of acceptable risk in the management of chronic and extensive arthritis and there are some cases who can benefit considerably, if not exclusively, from the use of phenylbutazone. It may be the drug of choice for some patients with severe rheumatoid arthritis, psoriatic arthritis or ankylosing spondylitis but continued vigilance must be maintained in its usage. One derivative of phenylbutazone (oxyphenbutazone (Tanderil)) does not appear to differ significantly from the parent drug in its pattern of clinical effects or side-effects. Such measures as coating the tablet of Butazolidin with alkali (Butacote and Butazolidin Alka) may reduce some of the mild dyspepsia associated with phenylbutazone but do not alter its pattern of side-effects in any other respect.

In general, phenylbutazone is now given a low priority in the prescription for rheumatic disorders and special care must be taken in the elderly or those with hypertension, dyspepsia, diabetes or diseases requiring sedatives, anti-epileptic drugs and anticoagulants. It is customary now to consider or try the vast range of alternative NSAID before resorting to phenylbutazone.

AZAPROPAZONE (Rheumox)
This pyrazolidine drug has recently been introduced and has found a place in the management of chronic arthritis. As it has a plasma half-life of over 12 hours it need only be taken twice daily, and this is an advantage for patients who are working during the day and for the elderly who might otherwise be forgetful. The usual dosage is 300mg capsules three or four times daily; or the 600mg tablet twice daily. Occasional rashes and dyspepsia have been reported and clearly care should be taken, as with all anti-inflammatory drugs, when patients have a known or suspected history of peptic ulceration. No serious side-effects on liver or bone marrow have been recorded but mild fluid retention, rashes and ankle oedema may occur.

METHRAZONE (Feprazone)
Another recently introduced pyrazolidine drug which incorporates a terpene group in its molecule is reputed to have ulcer-healing properties. It is given in a dosage of 200mg twice or thrice daily and may be tolerated by patients who have experienced dyspepsia with other NSAID. While major side-effects on liver and bone marrow have not been reported, it is very liable to cause a rash which is usually florid, extensive, itchy and maculo-papular. The rash usually clears within a few days after withdrawal of the drug but as it is a common occurrence (in at least 10 per cent of cases) it limits the use of the drug. Headaches, nausea and dyspepsia may also occur but are usually mild.

Indole-acetic acid drugs
INDOMETHACIN (Indocid)
This drug was introduced in 1963 and soon gained, and has maintained, a place as one of the most popular of the NSAID. Although it may cause many side-effects, some of them very serious, it does not appear to damage the liver or bone marrow. It seems clear that about 30 per cent of the population just cannot tolerate indomethacin. They are liable to develop cerebral side-effects including headaches, nausea, vertigo, a feeling of 'whooziness' and even confusion, hallucination and occasionally fits. In some patients a more chronic state of insidious depression may develop with loss of insight into the drug-related causation. In some cases the side-effects may develop very early, even after administration of the first dose, so it is wise policy to begin with low dosage of indomethacin and restrict the dosage to that level which produces acceptable clinical response without any side-effects. Other side-effects include dyspepsia and gastro-intestinal lesions; particularly dangerous is the silent development of peptic ulceration with either slow or dramatic blood loss or perforation. Sometimes, single or multiple large pre-pyloric ulcers may develop giving rise to a radiological diagnosis of gastric cancer. Various rashes, furunculosis, breakdown of varicose ulcers and oedema of the ankles have been recorded as well as, in some cases, congestive cardiac failure in the elderly. Renal damage has also been reported and the presence of known renal disease is to be considered a relative contra-indication to its use.

Indomethacin has a short half-life, is usually administered in a dosage of 25mg capsule three or four times daily although some patients may do perfectly well on a small dosage of 25mg b.d.; 50mg tablets are also available and have been used as a night-time dosage to give prolonged pain relief, ensure sleep and reduce morning stiffness. Other methods of inducing a prolonged nocturnal effect are to administer the drug in the form of a suppository (100mg) or as a slow-release capsule of 75mg known as Indocid-R. Some patients prefer to maintain a steady state of pain relief both night and day by the use of suppositories or Indocid-R capsules taken twice daily. Patients with major hand and upper limb arthritis may have difficulties in inserting these suppositories and some patients cannot tolerate suppositories because of haemorrhoids or rectal irritation, or find the administration disagreeable. In these cases, Indocid-R is an acceptable alternative. However, it must be clearly understood that the potential hazards of indomethacin remain, irrespective of the method of administration. Some of the nausea and mild dyspepsia associated with capsules may be due to their retention at the lower end of the oesophagus or irritation of a hiatus hernia, and this will be avoided by the use of suppositories, but the potential for the development of peptic ulceration remains unchanged and several cases of major peptic ulceration have been recorded in patients who were receiving treatment by indomethacin suppository alone.

Indomethacin has certainly maintained a place as one of the front runners in the long-term treatment of arthritic disorders. It is necessary to be alert to the dangers of slow and silent development of peptic ulceration and insidious development of depression but many patients have been able to take indomethacin for many years with benefit and without side-effects. The dosage varies considerably from case to case according to the needs and tolerance of the patient. Severe rheumatoid arthritis, psoriatic arthritis, ankylosing spondylitis and chronic hip disease may benefit from the use of indomethacin. Occasionally, the patients may be able to tolerate a suppository or capsule of Indocid-R but be unable to take any further indocid during the day because of side-effects in the nervous system. In these cases it is reasonable to combine the use of the slow preparation of indomethacin at night with a rapidly acting first-line drug with a short half-life during the day, e.g. ibuprofen or azapropazone.

SULINDAC (Clinoril)
This is an indene-acetic acid derivative, chemically related to indomethacin. It is a pro-drug in that sulindac itself is inactive but when metabolised it is converted in the liver into a sulphide derivative which is the active component and has a long half-life of approximately 18 hours. This means that sulindac is reportedly less liable to cause gastric side-effects and it need only be taken in twice-daily dosage because of the prolonged half-life of the active metabolite. It is supplied in tablets of 100mg and 200mg strength, and dosage is usually 200mg twice daily but some patients may manage with less. It is claimed that sulindac has

little effect on concurrent anticoagulant and antidiabetic therapy and it does not affect platelets or cause significant gastro-intestinal blood loss. Nausea and dyspepsia have been reported and occasional mild central nervous side-effects similar to those seen with indomethacin, especially vivid dreams. Occasional skin rashes have also occurred but in general the drug is safer and milder than indomethacin.

As with many of the first-line drugs, it happens that some patients have a striking preference for a particular drug and certainly it seems that sulindac can be extremely helpful for some patients and well tolerated.

Anthranilic acid drugs
Two chemically related compounds were introduced in the mid-1960s, these being mefenamic acid (Ponstan) and flufenamic acid (Arlef; Meralen). Mefenamic acid is a mild analgesic/anti-inflammatory drug while flufenamic acid has more powerful anti-inflammatory properties but is more liable to cause gastro-intestinal side-effects including peptic ulceration. It seems that these drugs suffered from their untimely arrival on the clinical scene as the much publicised indomethacin had secured a firm foothold and the next two years were to see the introduction of well-regarded propionic acid drugs with ibuprofen as an impressive newcomer. Indeed, mefenamic acid has been referred to as 'the neglected analgesic'. Nevertheless, both of these drugs are effective and mefenamic acid appears to have good analgesic properties in addition to mild anti-inflammatory action. The dosage is one 500mg tablet three or four times daily. The side-effects are chiefly dyspepsia, although this is not too frequent and is usually mild, rashes and diarrhoea. More rarely, mefenamic acid may cause asthma in patients who are predisposed and particularly those who are known to be sensitive, and it may also occasionally cause a Coombs-positive haemolytic anaemia and, very rarely, bone marrow damage.

Flufenamic acid, formerly manufactured in the United Kingdom as Arlef but now known as Meralen is also a short-acting drug and is usually prescribed in doses of 200mg three or four times daily, although lower dosage may be effective. It can be very helpful in terms of pain relief and reduction of inflammation and some patients tolerate it well. The pattern of side-effects is similar to that listed for mefenamic acid but gastro-duodenal hazards and diarrhoea appear to be slightly more frequent with this stronger drug. After some years in the therapeutic wilderness, it seems that both these preparations are now bidding for a place in the range of NSAID used in the management of chronic arthritis. As a distinct class of chemical products, they deserve some consideration in the choice of an analgesic/anti-inflammatory drug.

Propionic acid derivatives

These are an important group of compounds of which the first to be introduced, *ibuprofen*, is the mildest and safest. It suffered from being introduced in a low dosage but is now prescribed at a more effective level of 2g or more per day. Generally speaking it is most useful in treating milder cases of rheumatoid arthritis, osteoarthritis and soft tissue conditions including athletic injuries especially because of its safety. Tablets are supplied in strengths of 200mg and 400mg, but the larger size may not be acceptable to some patients who would have difficulty swallowing it, so a suspension containing 100mg/5ml is available. Its great advantage is its safety with a low incidence of gastric side-effects which is usually mild and settles rapidly on withdrawal of treatment. Occasional rashes have been reported and very rarely an aggravation of asthma and toxic amblyopia, which clears rapidly on stopping treatment. Ibuprofen has proved to be such a safe and useful drug that it has largely supplanted aspirin as the drug of first choice.

More powerful propionic acid drugs have been developed in an attempt to increase the therapeutic effect while maintaining the good safety record. *Ketoprofen* is similar to ibuprofen in its action and side-effects, the dosage being in the region of 50mg capsules four times daily. *Fenoprofen* is similar and is available in tablets of 300mg and 600mg, to a daily dosage of 1.8 to 2.4g daily. *Flurbiprofen* is more powerful but is probably associated with a greater incidence of dyspepsia and gastric erosions. It is supplied in tablets of 50mg and 100mg and the usual daily dosage is between 200mg and 300mg daily.

Naproxen is chemically related to the above drugs as it is a napthyl-propionic acid derivative, and has the advantage that twice-daily dosage is sufficient to maintain a steady rate of therapeutic activity because the drug has a long half-life of 13 hours. It is available in tablets of 250 and 500mg and the usual dosage is between 500 and 1000mg a day.

The propionic acid drugs have played an important part in the treatment of acute and chronic arthritis and rheumatic disorders, and many physicians will use one or other of this group as the drug of first choice. For many patients, there will be a propionic acid derivative which will seem to be especially effective and suitable so it is helpful to go round the houses and try to find the right drug for the right patient before resorting to more powerful and inevitably more dangerous drugs.

Phenyl-acetic acid drugs

This is an important group which is chemically related to the propionic acid group, but generally more powerful and associated in some cases with more side-effects. In fact, two phenyl-acetic acid drugs (ibufenac and alclofenac) had to be withdrawn. *Diclofenac* has a short half-life and is comparable to aspirin, indomethacin and propionic acid drugs in therapeutic efficacy, and it can be taken in conjunction with hypoglycaemic and anticoagulant drugs. Unlike its chemical relative, fenclofenac, it does not appear to interfere with thyroid function tests. It is available in tablets of 25mg and 50mg and the usual daily dosage is between 150 and 300mg. Side-effects are usually mild and include gastro-intestinal disturbances, vertigo, headache and occasionally a rash.

FENCLOFENAC (Flenac)

This is also a rapidly acting phenyl-acetic acid derivative with a plasma half-life in the range of six to eight hours, so that some patients need only to take it twice a day. The usual daily dosage is 300mg tablets, three or four times daily. The most frequent side-effects are gastro-intestinal and rashes which may occur in 7 to 10 per cent of patients. Fenclofenac may also interfere with thyroid function tests and this action appears to be independent of the phenyl-acetic acid radicle and consists of lowering of plasma T_3 and T_4 within 10 days of starting treatment and blunting of the TRH response within 18 days, which may persist for two weeks.

SECOND-LINE DRUGS

The decision to employ a second-line drug should only be taken when the patient has not obtained adequate relief from basic measures of management, of which first-line drugs are but one part. Patients will usually have been given courses of treatments with various drugs of different classes in the hope of finding one that is particularly suitable. Most doctors will have come to know some of these drugs better than others and will know what to expect in terms of therapeutic response. The drugs must be prescribed in safe but adequate dosage and the doctor should be convinced that the patient has complied with the prescription instructions. Polypharmacy is to be avoided in general but NSAID may be combined with a plain analgesic, and a suppository or slow-acting preparation taken at night may be used in conjunction with a short-acting preparation during the day. First-line drugs are relatively safe and essentially symptomatic in their effect and the aim of treatment is to relieve symptoms to the extent of making the patient's life tolerable and comfortable. It is generally unrealistic to seek total abolition of all symptoms as such a goal is likely to lead to over-dosage, polypharmacy and unnecessary side-effects.

In the presence of severe or progressive disease, not controlled by the basic regimen and first-line drugs, consideration has to be given to the use of gold, penicillamine or chloroquine. These are more powerful and more toxic drugs, used especially in the treatment of rheumatoid arthritis and they may exert an effect upon the disease process with arrest or reversal of progressive and destructive inflammation. As these drugs do not have any direct analgesic or immediate anti-inflammatory effect, their use is commonly combined with the continuing administration of a first-line drug and analgesic. Their use involves careful clinical scrutiny and regular blood and urine tests, with ophthalmic tests especially important in patients receiving anti-malarial therapy. Preference for one or other of these drugs will be based upon the clinician's experience but it is common to seek the advice of a specialist rheumatologist in respect of the initial prescription and possibly in relation to monitoring the course of the patient.

Gold

Gold therapy has been used in the treatment of rheumatoid arthritis and also psoriatic arthritis for over 50 years. It has no place in the management of osteoarthritis, is considered to be ineffective in the treatment of ankylosing spondylitis and contra-indicated in the treatment of systemic lupus erythematosus. It is effective as a second-line drug but dangerous, and careful supervision of dosage and monitoring of blood and urine tests with vigilance for the early presentation of side-effects, is essential. Provided these precautions are scrupulously observed, gold therapy may be rendered very much safer and excellent, sustained remission may be obtained in severe and progressive cases.

It is customary practice to give one or two small trial injections of gold of 10mg and 25mg in successive weeks before embarking on a weekly intramuscular dosage of 50mg. The usual preparation is sodium aurothiomalate (Myocrisin) and this is continued until a remission is obtained, usually after about three months of treatment in the region of 600mg total Myocrisin. At this point, or when a conventional total of 1g has been given, the dosage may be reduced to 50mg every three or four weeks according to the patient's progress. It has been shown that gold remissions may be maintained by long-term therapy, but the need for vigilance in respect of side-effects must be

maintained. If no favourable response has been obtained by the time that 1g has been given, it is unlikely that further treatment will produce a remission.

As with other second-line drugs, side-effects are common and may be dangerous, even fatal. The early side-effects of gold include an idiosyncrasy with bone marrow toxicity, especially purpura due to thrombocytopaenia. Proteinuria may also develop early and should be regarded with concern, especially if microscopic examination of the urine shows red cells and casts. Rashes are the most common side-effect and usually develop after 300mg or more have been given, and the rashes may take many forms but one of the commonest presentations is itching round the nailbeds and pruritus with a faint rash. If gold is continued in the presence of cutaneous side-effects there is usually an increase of the rash which may be catastrophic to the point of exfoliative dermatitis. Pleomorphic rashes have been reported but usually the rash is erythematous and with thickened skin and tends to persist for a long time even after withdrawal of gold. Blood dyscrasias may also occur at any time in the course of gold therapy and carry a high mortality as does the occasional appearance of liver damage. Renal damage also occurs, especially when the warning signs of mild proteinuria and microscopic haematuria have been ignored. Rarer side-effects include 'gold lung' and enteritis. Despite these hazards, if gold is given with appropriate care, it can be a most successful remedy and is probably the first choice among the second-line drugs. There is hope that a new oral preparation of gold (Auranofin), which has been shown to be effective clinically, may prove to be safer as oral administration allows a more even method of dosage so that the total dosage of gold is reduced and as little of this oral preparation is excreted by the kidneys, the incidence of renal complications is said to be much less. Auranofin is not yet generally available but is the subject of current clinical trials.

Penicillamine

D-penicillamine is a degradation product of penicillin and has been used since 1953 to increase copper excretion in patients suffering from Wilson's disease. Its use in the treatment of rheumatoid arthritis dates from 1970 and has been validated by a clinical trial which showed that penicillamine could confer significant improvement in patients suffering from rheumatoid arthritis. Side-effects were common and some of them were serious, but it was shown that the high dosage of 1200mg daily or more given in those early days was unnecessary. The majority of patients can manage with doses in the region of 250 to 375mg of the free-base, and rarely is the dose increased beyond 600mg daily. Some patients can manage on even smaller doses. Treatment may be continued for years but the liability to side-effects remains and some side-effects tend to occur after long-term administration.

Gastro-intestinal side-effects are common but rarely serious. Loss of taste can occur quite early in the course of treatment but usually clears up in a few weeks and is rare with the smaller doses of penicillamine currently employed. Other gastro-intestinal symptoms such as anorexia, nausea and dyspepsia are relatively common and occasionally severe vomiting can occur, but there is no firm evidence to suggest that peptic ulceration may be provoked or exacerbated by penicillamine.

Dermatological complications also occur and *previous sensitivity* to penicillin is a complete *contra-indication* to the use of penicillamine. Mild rashes may occur early in the course of treatment and may fade quickly without further trouble but they should always be regarded with care and concern and progression of the rash is a dangerous sign and may lead to exfoliation. Another rash is of a pemphigoid nature and more rarely there may be indolent papular lesions and an unusual condition of *elastosis perforans serpiginosa*. Renal complications vary from the trivial to the most severe. Minor proteinuria may be transient but if progressive or repetitive or associated with microscopic haematuria, then penicillamine should be discontinued as it may lead to more severe nephritis associated with the deposition of immune complexes. Bone marrow damage is particularly serious if caused by penicillamine and, as with gold therapy, careful monitoring of the blood indices must be done at two- or four-week intervals and the drug should be withdrawn if there are three successive falls in the platelet count, irrespective of the level of the platelet count. Similarly, any decrease in red cells or white cells should be checked and the drug withdrawn at least temporarily, and only re-administered with extreme caution.

Various other side-effects, some of them quite bizarre may occur with penicillamine but are fortunately rarer. The development of a lupus erythematosus-like syndrome and occasionally gross myasthenia similar to myasthenia gravis have been reported and the fact that penicillamine may occasionally exacerbate arthritis can be confusing and lead to increasing the dosage when it should be reduced or discontinued.

Although patients on long-term penicillamine therapy for Wilson's disease have been known to have uneventful pregnancies and give birth to healthy children while taking the drug, it is generally considered sound policy to avoid penicillamine therapy and also gold therapy during pregnancy in patients suffering from rheumatoid arthritis.

Anti-malarials

Drugs of this group have been used for over 50 years in the treatment of discoid and sub-acute lupus erythematosus and as they apparently improved the articular component, their use was extended to the treatment of rheumatoid arthritis in the early 1950s. Subsequent control trials confirmed their value in producing a remission and, like gold and penicillamine, their anti-rheumatoid effect is manifested slowly and associated with various side-effects, requiring careful monitoring of their use. Their position in the popularity order of second-line drugs is relegated to third place, largely because of the rare but frightful complication of retinal toxicity with gross risk of progression to complete blindness, adding an almost insufferable additional handicap to an already crippled patient. Despite various tests that have been used to try to detect early retinopathy, none of the proposed tests has been entirely successful in detection and/or prevention. However, it is necessary and sensible to restrict dosage of chloroquine or hydroxychloroquine to 250mg chloroquine phosphate or 400mg hydroxychloroquine sulphate (Plaquenil). Obligatory ophthalmic examination is required at four-month intervals including tests of colour vision, visual fields, tests of retinal sensitivity and electro-oculogram and electro-retinogram. Unfortunately, chloroquine is so cumulative and not amenable to rapid elimination that the presence of early retinopathy is inevitably followed by increasing visual impairment.

Other side-effects of chloroquine include dyspepsia, rashes, blanching of the hair and vertigo. It is considered unwise to treat psoriatic arthritis with chloroquine derivatives as it is alleged that flare-ups of the psoriasis may occur and it is considered unwise to give chloroquine to children because of the occasional risk of cardio-respiratory arrest. Chloroquine is also contra-indicated during pregnancy. Nevertheless, despite the hazards, some authorities consider that chloroquine is a safe and useful second-line drug in the treatment of rheumatoid arthritis when given in low dosage and supervised carefully and therefore is still to be included as second-line therapy. Some consider that hydroxychloroquine (Plaquenil) is better tolerated than chloroquine and it is possible that a safer anti-malarial may be synthesised in the future.

THIRD-LINE DRUGS

Corticosteroids

These are to be considered as a third-line drug although occasionally their prescription may be needed when the second-line drugs are contra-indicated or when some severe complication, e.g. rheumatoid vasculitis or pericarditis, is present. While numerous attempts have been made to discover a 'safe' corticosteroid conferring anti-inflammatory effects without troublesome or dangerous side-effects, none of the newer compounds has fully justified the claims made for it and the basic prednisone or prednisolone remain the most popular in this series. Adrenal stimulation therapy using cortico-trophin (ACTH) or synthetic corticosactrin (Synac-then) has been used to overcome the disadvantage of adrenal cortical suppression when the corticosteroid hormones are given, but ACTH and the like have the disadvantage of causing electrolyte disturbance and water retention with hypertension. The major side-effects of corticosteroid therapy are well known and clearly restrict the use of systemic therapy for rheumatoid and other forms of chronic inflammatory polyarthritis. However, years of experience and clinical trials have given various good guidelines to the proper and safer use of steroid preparations in chronic inflammatory polyarthritis. Generally speaking, the dosage is kept as low as possible commensurate with the required degree of disease control and relief of symptoms.

The use of systemic steroid therapy is mandatory in certain conditions and in certain complications in rheumatic disorders. Thus, for example, control of polymyalgia rheumatica calls for immediate administration of prednisolone in a dosage of 30mg daily, and more if there is associated temporal arteritis, but with time and careful monitoring the dosage may be lowered to 5mg daily or less or even discontinued. Severe vasculitis, occurring as part of rheumatoid arthritis or other disorders, also may require high dosage of prednisolone and other complications of connective tissue diseases including pericarditis, lupus nephritis and severe uveitis will also need high-dosage steroid therapy.

In other cases, the persistence of chronic and unacceptable symptoms despite first-line and second-line treatment may call for the administration of small doses of prednisolone, and in such cases it is advisable to keep the dosage at or as near to 5mg daily as possible, and some favour alternate-day dosage in the hope of reducing side-effects. There is a danger that some patients with a low pain threshold may pressurise the doctor into giving steroids for comparatively mild arthritis,

and this is to be avoided because it is this type of patient who is rarely satisfied with small dosage and will 'dip her hand' into the steroid bottle to the extent of developing severe and dangerous side-effects. Occasionally it is necessary to give a short course of steroid treatment for a few days to tide the patient over a severe exacerbation and then to taper off the dosage over a period of a few weeks. Some doctors would prefer to use adrenal stimulation or an injectable form of corticosteroid so that they have control of the regimen throughout and there is a reduced risk of 'addiction' to steroids. Corticosteroids may be required in juvenile arthritis especially in those patients with involvement of the uveal tract, and alternate-day dosage is advised as there is less pituitary suppression and less interference with growth. Another indication for corticosteroid therapy is the elderly patient whose functional capacity is limited and independence threatened with gross stiffness. A small daily dose of 5mg may be sufficient to maintain mobility and independence with minimal risk of side-effects. The use of locally injected corticosteroid into the most severely inflamed joint is practical and helpful in supporting first-line therapy and may remove the need for considering second-line drugs or systemic steroid therapy. This is a technique which is easily and safely employed in general practice with some training in the techniques and the observance of some elementary aseptic precautions.

Immunosuppressive and cytotoxic drugs

These are by far the most dangerous of the third-line drugs used in the treatment of severe rheumatoid arthritis, often with life-threatening complications, and in the treatment of other major connective tissue disorders. The drugs in this group are commonly used in the treatment of cancer where their potential for causing side-effects is more acceptable. We must not lose sight of the fact that vasculitis is a severe and life-threatening complication in rheumatoid arthritis; in such circumstances these drugs may be required when all else has failed, and their use is therefore justified. However, as with corticosteroid therapy, their use should be limited to such cases and it is not justifiable to consider their use for early cases in the hope of suppressing the disease process. The drugs are both anti-inflammatory and immunosuppressive, and in the case of cyclophosphamide, cytotoxic. The most common drugs in this series are azathioprine, chlorambucil, methotrexate and cyclophosphamide. Azathioprine is usually given in a starting dosage of 100 to 150mg daily, reducing to a maintenance dosage of 75mg daily or less if good control of the disease is obtained. Cyclophosphamide is also given in doses of 150mg daily reducing to 100mg daily if effective.

Among the more severe side-effects of these drugs are the well-recognised risks of chromosomal damage, increased liability to infections and marrow toxicity. An increased liability to develop cancer, especially lymphoma, has also been recorded. Cyclophosphamide may cause loss of hair, haemorrhagic cystitis and subsequent bladder fibrosis, and suppression of cell formation in the gonads. Methotrexate may cause liver damage and azathioprine may aggravate renal damage and produce rashes.

These drugs are essentially desperate measures in desperate situations and their use should only be considered after prolonged thought and consultation. They must be carefully monitored with frequent tests of blood indices, urine and liver function, and as therapy is usually commenced in hospital it is customary to have some measure of hospital control in the follow up.

CONCLUSION

Drug therapy is only one part, albeit an important and sometimes predominant part of the long-term management of patients suffering from chronic rheumatic and arthritic disorders. Advances in our knowledge of the aetiology and pathogenesis of rheumatic disorders should make methods of prevention and treatment more precise, specific and safer. In the meanwhile, it is necessary to plan a programme for each patient and for many this will involve the starting with a mild and safe compound, adjusting the dosage and changing the preparation as necessary to meet the changing needs of the clinical situation. In others it may mean the immediate introduction of a powerful and potentially dangerous drug to control a severe disease state or complication. In all cases, the requisite adjuvant measures of treatment must not be ignored and careful monitoring of the clinical situation to record progress and anticipate or detect side-effects is a necessary part of the therapy.

LONG-TERM MANAGEMENT OF GOUT

This involves control of the serum urate level and co-operation of the patient is essential in regular and prolonged drug administration, in the moderate use of alcohol, some mild dietetic restriction in the avoidance of high-purine foods (liver, kidneys, sweetbreads, fish-roe and tinned fish) and, where appropriate, a gentle weight-reducing regimen. It is also necessary to monitor progress by repeat serum urate estimations.

Following an isolated or a few widely-spaced attacks of gout, and provided that serum urate levels are normal, then it is a matter of judgement in each case as to whether long-term drug control of gout is required. The usual indications for long-term therapy are:

1. Frequent acute attacks
2. Sustained hyperuricaemia after an acute attack
3. Chronic gouty joint changes and/or tophi
4. Renal calculi or renal functional impairment due to gout.

Pharmacotherapy
Two distinct methods are used to control serum urate. Rarely, in severe and refractory cases they may be used concurrently.

1. *Uricosuric drugs*, less popular now, are sulphinpyrazone (Anturan); probenecid (Benemid) and aspirin in high dosage. Aspirin in low dosage causes retention of urate and also antagonises the uricosuric effects of sulphinpyrazone and probenecid. Uricosuric drugs act by partially blocking tubular re-absorption of urate, thereby increasing the urinary outflow. Dosage of sulphinpyrazone should be initially low, say 100mg daily, increasing gradually at weekly intervals to the requisite maintenance level, usually 300 or 400mg daily. Probenecid dosage is 500mg daily initially increasing gradually to 1500mg or 2g daily, or higher if necessary to control the level of serum urate. Side-effects are uncommon but dyspepsia and rashes do occur. The main drawbacks to uricosuric therapy are (a) the liability to provoke acute gouty attacks by mobilising the miscible pool of body urate (urate on the move) which can precipitate in joints, so it is necessary to 'cover' the early weeks of treatment with either colchicine 0.5mg t.d.s. or an anti-inflammatory gout suppressant such as phenylbutazone or indomethacin, and (b) the liability to cause uric acid renal gravel and calculi due to increased urate concentration in the urine. Rarely the uricosuric drugs may cause nephrosis.

2. *Xanthine oxidase inhibitors*, of which allopurinol (Zyloric) is in routine use. This drug acts by preventing the breakdown of xanthine and hypoxanthine to uric acid, so there is an immediate fall in both blood and urinary urate levels. As with uricosurics, treatment must be instituted with low and progressive dosage and 'covered' by colchicine or an anti-inflammatory drug. Usual dosage is 100mg daily increasing to 300 or 400mg, and sometimes doses up to 800mg daily may be needed. Side-effects of dyspepsia, rash and xanthine calculi are extremely rare and the accumulation of xanthine in muscles appears to be harmless.

Allopurinol is becoming the more favoured drug in the long-term treatment of gout, and is especially valuable when renal calculi or impaired renal function preclude the use of uricosurics. Treatment with allopurinol is indefinite, the dose can be adjusted to the urate level, and tophi will recede and damaged joints will heal.

Pitfalls in the long-term management of gout

1. Institute uricosuric and allopurinol therapy gradually, 'go low and go slow'.
2. Cover this therapy with colchicine or anti-inflammatory drugs for the first few weeks.
3. Make all alterations in therapy gradually; only stop suddenly if compelled by side-effects.
4. Be careful with salicylates: small doses as in proprietary medicines cause urate retention and also inhibit the action of uricosurics.
5. Be aware of 'non-gout'. Patients with common musculo-skeletal conditions may have borderline or slightly raised serum urate levels; they may be mis-diagnosed and treated unnecessarily for years.
6. Non-compliance with therapy is common with gouty patients and is responsible for relapses. The single dose 300mg strength allopurinol simplifies therapy and aids compliance.
7. 'Crash diets' to combat obesity may induce acidosis and provoke acute attacks of gout.
8. Dehydration and surgical operations, especially those involving the genito-urinary tract, will also affect urate levels adversely.
9. Diuretics, especially the thiazide groups and frusemide, cause urate retention.
10. Symptomless hyperuricaemia is not uncommon in middle-aged and elderly males. When detected it does not compel treatment unless it is excessively high, say 0.60mmol/litre or more, when the dangers of renal damage and calculi are greater.

Chapter 12   Diabetes

J. D. WARD BSc, MD, FRCP

DIET

The defect in diabetes mellitus is an inability of the body chemistry to control levels of sugar in the blood stream and tissues. Thus the most basic treatment in diabetes is to restrict the intake of carbohydrate food. Unfortunately, it is very difficult for most patients to keep to the limits set for carbohydrate restriction and, as yet, the medical profession with its dietitians and helpers fails in educating and motivating their diabetic patients to this end. Simply speaking, diabetics should avoid as much as possible refined sugars and starches. With the *portion* or *exchange dietary* system 10-gram portions of carbohydrate are described and the total number of such portions prescribed, any one portion being exchangeable for another. It is becoming more common to advise diabetics that they may eat more liberally of the bulky fibre foods such as wholemeal bread, fruit (apples and pears), bran products, beans, jacket potatoes and nuts. Perhaps a more simple approach to broad categories of food with abstention from the refined carbohydrates would be preferable to rigid diet sheets. Lipids should be reduced in diabetics due to their undoubted tendency to an increased incidence of atherosclerotic vascular disease.

Essentially the young diabetic who is not overweight may be allowed approximately 250g of carbohydrate per day, the more overweight patient on insulin 150g of carbohydrate. Patients with marked obesity may well have to be restricted to 100g carbohydrate per day. There are no appetite suppressants of any proven benefit which can help such patients and these drugs should not be used.

ORAL MEDICATION IN DIABETES MELLITUS

Many patients find it difficult to keep to the diet and drugs are available which will assist in reduction of blood sugar levels, but throughout any description of the use of drugs in lowering the blood sugar one must stress that they are an adjunct to, not a substitute for, dietary restriction. However, there are many patients who genuinely keep well to carbohydrate-restricted diets and yet still require the assistance of these drugs to control the blood sugar

The sulphonylureas

These drugs act by directly stimulating the pancreas to produce insulin. They are therefore clearly of no value in the insulin-dependent (deficient) younger diabetic who must be treated with insulin. However, in many older, non-insulin-dependent patients, although there is often an excess of insulin in the blood (indicating a degree of insulin resistance), these drugs can assist in further stimulating the pancreas to produce more insulin which will result in a fall in blood sugar. If possible these drugs should be prescribed after a reasonable period of carbohydrate restriction. There are many proprietary preparations of the sulphonylureas but they are all basically the same. There is little evidence that potency differs from one drug to another and claims that newer sulphonylurea agents also have beneficial vascular results through anti-platelet effects and fibrinolytic mechanisms have yet to be fully substantiated in clinical practice.

Sulphonylureas may therefore be listed as in Table 1.

Table 1 The sulphonylureas (ranking the cheapest drugs first)

chlorpropamide	(Diabinese; Melitase)
tolbutamide	(Rastinon; Pramidex)
acetohexamide	(Dimelor)
glymidine	(Gondafon)
tolazamide	(Tolanase)
glibornuride	(Glutril)
glibenclamide	(Daonil; Euglucon)
glipizide	(Glibenese; Minodiab)
gliclazide	(Diamicron)
gliquidone	(Glurenorm)

It is just as well therefore to use the cheapest drug. In many instances the major attraction of chlorpropamide

(Diabinese) is that its long half-life allows it to be used on a once-daily basis but there are two major objections to chlorpropamide in some patients.

(1) *The elderly patient:* Due to its prolonged half-life this drug is probably more likely to lead to hypoglycaemic episodes, particularly in the elderly patient living alone who is likely to miss a meal or become confused in the taking of tablets; in such patients it is customary to advise the shorter-acting preparations, such as tolbutamide or glibenclamide.

(2) A combination of chlorpropamide and alcohol causes an intense facial flushing in a significant number of patients resulting in considerable social embarrassment and disability. This side-effect of chlorpropamide is very much less common in all the other sulphonylurea agents. Of very great interest is that the ability to flush with chlorpropamide and alcohol is closely linked to genetic factors in diabetes.

The side-effects of sulphonylureas are not common. The most predictable side-effect is indeed *hypoglyceamia*. In the vast majority of ambulant patients who take a regular diet this is a very uncommon complication. However, elderly patients often confused as to the number of tablets they have taken or about meal times, and who even may be unwilling to eat on certain occasions, are at special risk from hypoglyceamia. Once clinical hypoglycaemia with disordered behaviour or unconsciousness has been diagnosed the patient should be immediately admitted to hospital. Intravenous dextrose administered to such patients may well produce good recovery of cerebral function, but due to the continuing and prolonged action of the drug, insulin production is continuously stimulated and the correct treatment is an intravenous infusion of 5 or 10% dextrose which should run for up to 24 hours. There are occasions when minor, less dramatic, symptoms of hypoglycaemia may be due to the sulphonylureas and it is always worthwhile stopping these agents in elderly patients exhibiting manifestations of confusion or poor memory or who do not quite seem to be themselves. Rashes occur and a rare idiosyncratic jaundice has also been reported.

Weight gain is fairly common following the use of sulphonylureas, due to control of glycosuria making a higher percentage of ingested carbohydrate available for metabolism, combined with the known lipogenic action of insulin. In rare instances weight gain may be due to fluid retention related to the antidiuretic hormone-like action of these drugs.

In 1971 the University Group Diabetes Programme (UGDP) produced evidence that tolbutamide (and later phenformin) *increased* the risk of coronary disease in diabetic patients. Subsequently there have been many objections raised to the design and control of this study and its conclusions do not seem to have affected the prescribing habits of diabetic physicians, except perhaps in the younger group of patients.

CLINICAL POINT

It is common to see non-insulin-dependent diabetes in middle-aged or older patients in whom the blood sugar is very high, e.g. 19mmol/litre with some ketonuria. Clearly clinical judgement will be necessary to pick out the occasional such patient who is ill, probably acidotic, and who requires more urgent treatment with fluids and insulin. However, the majority of such patients may be treated either initially with dietary carbohydrate restriction or, sometimes, it would seem reasonable to commence treatment with a sulphonylurea along with the usual dietary advice. On many occasions dietary history will reveal that such patients are not taking an excess amount of carbohydrate, so making it impossible to apply further dietary restriction. Indeed if they exhibit symptoms of neuritis it seems more than reasonable to prescribe the drug along with the diet. In such instances it is quite possible that after many weeks of treatment the dosage of these drugs may be reduced and it is always important to bear in mind the need to stop the drug for a period in order to establish that the patient cannot be controlled with diet alone. All the sulphonylureas should be started at the lower-dose range, the dose building up to the maximum recommended.

The biguanides

Essentially in this group of drugs one is concerned with metformin (Glucophage). Phenformin should no longer be used because of its rare, but undoubted, tendency to produce lactic acidosis. The mechanism of action of these drugs is not fully understood, perhaps relating to improvement in peripheral and muscle uptake of glucose from the blood. They certainly have a tendency to lower the blood sugar and it has also been shown that they are more likely to be associated with weight reduction than the sulphonylureas. It seems logical in the first instance, in the treatment of non-insulin-dependent diabetes, to use the sulphonylureas since they stimulate endogenous insulin production. However, in the obese hyperglycaemic diabetic metformin may be used as a first-line drug in the hope that this will lower the blood sugar as well as assist in weight loss. Cynics suggest that the only reason why there is weight loss in patients treated with metformin is due to the anorectic effect of the drug. Side-effects of this drug consist of gastro-intestinal irritation with anorexia or diarrhoea and occasional cases of lactic acidosis have been reported. Patients with cardiac, renal or hepatic failure should not be treated with this drug.

Combined medication: sulphonylurea–biguanide

A distinct group of middle-aged patients exist who do not respond to diet and tend to fail eventually with diet and sulphonylurea; for these it is customary to add to the sulphonylurea a dosage of metformin. However, at this point it would be reasonable to highlight a distinct *clinical problem* in the middle-aged and older patients. The above sequence has been established with failure on diet and then a sulphonylurea and then the addition of metformin. In his own mind the patient is just about well enough, tends to run blood sugars between 13 and 17mmol/litre and the doctor is reluctant to institute insulin therapy. However, close questioning of such patients commonly reveals a weariness, thirst, nocturia and symptoms which in other circumstances would certainly lead to insulin therapy. Such patients can be greatly helped in their feeling of well-being by institution of insulin injections. Experience has indicated that older patients take very comfortably to the use of insulin and commonly express the comment that they wish the insulin had been given earlier. In such cases, well-being improves dramatically although often the level of blood sugar achieved is only a little less than with the oral agent itself, indicating the many other actions of insulin. The aim of insulin therapy in the older patient however, must be less aggressive in lowering blood sugar for the fear of hypoglycaemia.

The younger non-insulin-dependent diabetic

Another important group of patients are those around the age of 25 to 40 who often present with classical symptoms of diabetes, without significant ketosis and who respond well to carbohydrate restriction. However, this carbohydrate restriction may not lead to totally satisfactory blood sugar levels and the addition of a sulphonylurea in such patients will often produce normoglycaemia. Although as stated above many physicians are sceptical of the results of the UGDP study, one is influenced by the thought of using such agents in patients of this group for anything up to 30 or 40 years. It would therefore seem reasonable policy to use a diet assisted by a sulphonylurea for a period of two or three months and then to observe the effect of dietary carbohydrate restriction alone. There is evidence that after a period of sulphonylurea therapy the pancreas may in fact become more efficient, coupled with the small load of carbohydrate presented to it, and a number of such patients may continue with satisfac-tory blood sugar control with diet alone. However, should they develop intercurrent illness or serious disease they must always be seen as at risk. If such a patient has a rise of blood sugar and the return of symptoms when the drug is stopped it is recommended that they should then be treated with insulin on a life-long basis.

INSULIN TREATMENT

In the insulin-requiring-diabetic insulin is essential and has to be given by injection. This is administered subcutaneously in any part of the body. Many patients seem restricted to small areas of the thighs or upper arm but all parts of the thigh, lower abdomen, arms and even calves may be used if the patient finds it comfortable and convenient. Essentially, a patient will assess his own comforts and although many have an innate fear of abdominal injections, unless the patient is particularly thin, the abdominal wall is an excellent site. More important than the actual site is that many sites should be used so that any individual site is not used more than once every few weeks, avoiding problems of discomfort, fibrosis and impairment of insulin absorption. In some patients speed of absorption will vary from site to site.

The technique should be taught to the patient with some care, indicating an angle of 45° or straight 90° insertion and if possible the patient should administer his very own first injection for confidence and morale. There is no doubt that disposable needles are far more comfortable than the traditional steel needles but unfortunately these can at present only be prescribed by hospital clinics. They may be used more than once and many patients have used disposable needles with comfort for many days. Again, disposable syringes are not available on prescription, either from general practitioners or hospital clinics, but these can also be used on many occasions and multiple use of disposable syringes can still be cheaper than frequent replacement of glass syringes. It is not necessary to boil and sterilise syringes frequently. A simple plastic box containing gauze, dampened with spirit is satisfactory for storage of syringes and needles. The actual glass syringe need only be boiled and sterilised every 10 days or so. As with all other aspects of diabetic management, it is important to achieve a balance of care without obsession or interference too greatly with normal life. Generally speaking, varieties of injection guns to avoid the actual personal introduction of the needle into the skin are not successful and there is no doubt that for the majority of patients, with care and sympathy, the injection can become a routine and not resented.

Types of insulin

Basically, insulin is insulin. The vast proliferation of types of insulin are related to speed of action, developments of purified insulins and the participation of many companies in the manufacture of insulin, so that we have a confusing, indeed bewildering, variety of types of insulin. For both the older and newer types of insulin there are three broad categories:

(1) *Short-acting:* plain insulin which acts fairly quickly.
(2) *Medium-acting:* insulin combined with material to prolong its action to a moderate period of time, around 8 to 12 hours.
(3) *Long-acting:* insulin bound in such a way, *hopefully* to act smoothly over a 24-hour period.

However, the final arbiter in the length and speed of action of all insulins is indeed the patient himself, and whatever the manufacturer may say as to the exact length of action of insulins, the individual variability from patient to patient is so great that it is really only necessary to broadly understand the categories of short-, medium- and long-acting. The older type insulins which have been used for decades and are still widely in use are pancreatic extracts, extracted in such a way that they still contain other proteins and polypeptides as impurities. Over the years companies manufacturing insulin have purified their insulins by changing the method of manufacture to extract as many of these protein polypeptide impurities as possible, producing so called 'mono-component' insulins or highly purified insulins and there is no doubt that many of these insulins now approach a pure simple solution of insulin.

WHY SHOULD WE USE THE NEW INSULINS?

There is no clinical evidence as to the greater benefit of the newer insulins as opposed to the old insulins and they are undoubtedly more costly. To many doctors there is a distinct attraction in giving a pure uncontaminated insulin solution and it is common in this country for most new diabetic patients to be commenced on the more purified insulins. There is a hope that if antibody resistance to pure insulin is less than with older insulins, individual patients will require total doses of insulin which are less than with the older varieties, but this is open to question. In the established diabetic taking the older types of insulin, the indications for changing to new insulins are really only if they are experiencing extreme discomfort at the site of injection (soluble insulin has an acid pH) or where

there is extensive fat atrophy. Fat atrophy at sites of injection, often associated with fat hypertrophy, is extremely uncommon with the new purified insulins, and patients who have suffered such areas of atrophy or hypertrophy, when changed to the newer insulins, experience considerable improvement and remodelling of the subcutaneous tissues. In the case of young girls this is clearly of great importance to them. Often when patients experience difficulties in control or are approaching times of development of complications of diabetes, it is common to change to the new insulins so as to feel that one is applying to the patient the most purified compound. However, there is no firm evidence that the ability to control the blood sugar through the day is any better with the newer insulins. When changing from an old to a new purified insulin the dose should be reduced by 30 per cent. Usually it is necessary to increase the dose back to the previous level but a few patients will have an unpredictable sensitivity to the purer insulin if the original dose is maintained, possibly resulting in hypoglycaemia. (Table 2 gives names of the three groups of insulins as manufactured by a variety of companies.)

WHICH IS THE BEST REGIMEN OF INSULIN DOSAGE?

In the non-diabetic state ingestion of food, particularly carbohydrate food, results in a brisk and short-lived output of insulin thus providing an extremely efficient homeostatic control of blood glucose. In normal individuals the blood glucose is held very tightly between approximately 3.0–6.5mmol/litre. Ideally, therefore, in insulin deficiency an injection of insulin should be applied with each meal, perhaps with a longer-acting insulin to back up the blood glucose control between meals. However, it is difficult, and indeed perhaps unkind, to persuade the majority of diabetics to accept three or four injections each day. Indeed, the average diabetic is very keen to take only one injection a day if this is at all possible.

Daily injections (Lente, Monotard, Lentard, Ultralente)

Quite a few patients will appear to achieve very satisfactory control with one morning injection of a long-acting insulin (Fig. 12/1C). As with all insulins the injection is preferably given approximately 20 minutes before the morning meal, i.e. get up, give insulin, wash, dress, breakfast. Slow release of insulin into the bloodstream should keep the blood sugar reasonably low, but of course regular ingestion of food will have to be taken and indeed this is the major drawback of one injection a day, in that meal-times have to be very accurately spaced and short delays of the regular meal-time can

Table 2 Range of insulin action

Short (2–8 hours)	Medium (3–12 hours)	Long (4–24 hours)
Soluble	Isophane	Lente
Actrapid	Semitard Rapitard	Monotard Lentard Ultralente (24–36 hours)
Velosulin	Insulatard Mixtard Initard	
Neusulin	Neuphane	Neulente
Hypurin	Hypurin Isophane	Hypurin Protamine Zinc Hypurin Lente

produce hypoglycaemia. Many long-acting insulins seem to potentiate the known natural fall in blood sugar during the night, and may be associated with nocturnal hypoglycaemia (see later).

Two injections a day

The conventional compromise of diabetic physicians is to request patients to take two injections a day, one with their breakfast and one with their main evening meal. It seems likely that in many patients two injections of short-acting insulin do not achieve reasonable insulin levels in the latter part of each 12-hour period, so that late afternoon and early morning hyperglycaemia are common. For this reason it is better to recommend that a patient on two injections a day should receive a medium-acting insulin (Isophane, Semitard, Insulatard) (Fig. 12/1B) in the hope that this will provide release of insulin over each 12-hour period. If this is not achieved – particularly if the immediate action is not brisk enough and does not lower the blood sugar for some hours after injection – then one should mix in the syringe a short-acting insulin to cover the first half of each 12-hour period. Twice-daily injections of a mixture of a short- and medium-acting insulin as described in Figure 12/1D is often an efficient method of blood sugar control. This allows the adjustment of four types of insulin during the 24-hour period, such adjustments being based on patients' assessment of their urine or blood sugar. A useful regimen is an injection of short- and long-acting insulin in the morning with a small dose of short-acting insulin in the evening if glycosuria or a high blood sugar is detected. Figure 12/1A demonstrates the use of a very long-acting insulin to provide a constant background of insulin supplemented by short-acting insulin at the two main meals.

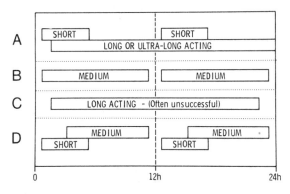

Fig. 12/1 **Suggested Insulin Regimens**
A. Background level of long-acting insulin with short-acting for two main meals
B. Hopefully twelve-hour cover twice per day
C. Cover of insulin throughout the day from one injection
D. Twice daily short and medium mixture to cover each eight-hour period of the day
SHORT: Soluble, Actrapid, Velosulin, Neusulin
MEDIUM: Isophane, Semitard, Insulatard, Neuphane
LONG: Lente, Monotard
ULTRA-LONG: Ultralente

Management of a new patient with insulin-requiring diabetes

Very ill patients with ketosis should be managed in hospital with intravenous fluids and insulin. If the patient is not severely ill in this way strong consideration should be given for the institution of dietary and insulin treatment *without* admission to hospital. Here the specialist diabetic nurse is a valuable, indeed an essential, member of the diabetic team. It is feasible to commence treatment in outpatients with a certain number of home visits to check on injection techniques etc, so resulting in confidence and good morale for the patient who then realises that diabetes should be taken seriously but with minimal interference to his life. The dietary and exercise habits immediately approach a normal life, which cannot be said for hospital admission, and the family are more involved in the establishment of this new condition in their household. It is usual to commence treatment with two injections of a medium- (or short-) acting insulin but not to use doses which are likely to produce a rapid return of blood glucose to normal. In the vast majority of patients moderately small doses, even as small as 8 units twice daily, will produce marked resolution of symptoms and well-being without any dramatic fall in blood sugar. Over the first week or two the patient is instructed in injection techniques, diet, management of urine or blood sugar testing at home, and he gradually gains confidence. Once he is an efficient technical diabetic then the dose of insulin can be increased to produce rather more adequate levels of blood sugar. There is nothing more demoralising in the first week of diabetic insulin treatment than to suffer a profound hypoglycaemic reaction. Careful instruction and description should be given of hypoglycaemia warning symptoms. Many advise that a hypoglycaemic reaction should be induced but this is often difficult to achieve and not really necessary.

It is at this point that we should try and define what we are aiming for in good diabetic control. Urine testing has been heavily used over the last few decades and although of great help there are many inaccuracies due to high or low renal thresholds. Young people have a tendency to a low renal threshold and as patients become older the renal threshold rises. It is easy to demonstrate in many that even with double emptying of the bladder heavy glycosuria may be present in the presence of a relatively low blood sugar. It is possible now by the use of a variety of commercial sticks (Dextrostix) used with an Ames meter, Glucocheck or Hypocount blood glucose meters, or the Boehringer Glycemie 20 to 800 instant visual-reading blood sugar sticks, to have patients perform their own blood sugar estimations at different times of the day. It seems that many patients find this acceptable; indeed, quite a few prefer it to the rather unaesthetic aspects of urine testing. Monolet needles with an Autolet automatic spring loading are far more comfortable than subcutaneous needles or the standard NHS lancets. There is no suggestion here that all diabetic patients should prick their finger many times every day of their life, but at times of poor control, of infections, in pregnancy, and when there are other problems in the diabetic's life it can be extremely useful to study a range of day-time and if possible night-time blood sugars and so allow a more rational adjustment of insulin regimens. Accepting that the normal non-diabetic blood sugar never varies outside 3–6mmol/litre one ideally would be aiming at this range, but any attempt to keep diabetics in this range must run serious risk of hypoglycaemia. One can hardly define any blood sugar above 6.0mmol/litre as adequate but clearly the age of the patient, the presence or absence of complications, and the emotional and co-operative state of the patient will influence how close to that level of blood sugar will the diabetic physician be prepared to achieve. Clearly in the elderly the more serious risks of hypoglycaemia must be balanced and a higher blood sugar tolerated. The attempts to interest diabetic patients in their blood sugar can lead to far better blood sugar control and far greater understanding of diabetes. It can, however, also produce a degree of introspection and neuroticism, and clearly the vigour of attempts to control blood sugar must be always taken as a judgement in individual patients. It is difficult to impress on diabetics the nature and risks of the long-term vascular complications without producing a high degree of fear and unpleasantness in their minds, and indeed no physician can guarantee to any individual patient that he will or will not develop the long-term complications.

In the course of the first few weeks of insulin control of the blood sugar in new young diabetics there seems to be a partial recovery of pancreatic function and it is common to see a definite fall in insulin dosage. In the extreme this may develop into the 'honeymoon period' when blood sugar control can be achieved by simple carbohydrate restriction alone. In the early stages of diabetic management of this sort, therefore, the dose should perhaps be automatically reduced to anticipate the fall in insulin requirement and avoid hypoglycaemia. If a patient should be taken off insulin altogether, strict instructions must be given to the patient and the family that return of thirst, sickness or symptoms suggestive of poorly-controlled diabetes should be reported to the physician immediately.

Almost always such patients eventually require insulin over the next few weeks, months or years.

Strengths of insulin

Perhaps of greater importance than the various types and lengths of action of insulin are the strengths of insulin which are available for use. Hopefully in the not too distant future, as in the United States, Canada and Australia, the British medical profession will achieve the use of a 100 unit strength insulin with a simple syringe so that each mark on a syringe is one unit of insulin. Considerable confusion occurs with doctors, nurses and patients in the use of 40 and 80 strength insulins. With the standard British diabetic insulin syringe *1 mark equals 2 units of 40 strength insulin* and *1 mark equals 4 units of 80 strength insulin*. However, in busy practices and clinics it is surprising how often miscalculations of this simple nature have occurred, and clearly a sudden doubling of the dose of insulin can be very dangerous. Most patients when asked how much insulin they are taking will give a figure of marks on the syringe rather than units of insulin.

Hypoglycaemia

Hypoglycaemia in the insulin-taking diabetic is a common event. Education will lead to patients taking necessary avoiding action and all patients should carry dextrose or other forms of glucose with them. Car-drivers should carry such agents actually in the car isself, and not in their clothing which need not necessarily be with them in the car. As the years of diabetes pass it is possible that a patient can be developing a degree of autonomic nerve damage and as a result he may be less aware of the warning symptoms of hypo-glycaemia. Patients who for 20 years have been able to recognise early warning symptoms often bitterly complain of the sudden onset of virtual complete unconsciousness without warning, and the general level of blood sugar control must be accepted as higher than one would hope to achieve in many younger patients. It is claimed that the beta-blocking agents are likely to produce similar effects although the clinical and published evidence that this is the case is not strong. However, it is certainly well advised to use a more highly selective beta-blocking agent (for example atenolol (Tenormin)) in the treatment of angina and hypertension in diabetic patients.

The reasons for development of hypoglycaemia are an excessive dose of insulin, missed meals, a mixture of both, or additional exercise. Many patients, particularly young people, are extremely exercise-sensitive, and if more strenuous exercise such as football, tennis etc is contemplated, advice should be given to reduce the dose of insulin, even to halve it on the morning of the exercise. It seems bad policy to advise such patients to take extra food but in lean young adults this may be reasonable. Depending on the nature of their work it may be necessary to have different insulin regimens during the week as compared with the week-end. The elderly are particularly prone to hypoglycaemia, particularly because of their age and partly through lack of awareness of the warning symptoms. Also visual impairment, development of arthritis of the hands and an increasing tendency not to bother can lead to excessive doses of insulin being administered and, equally importantly, to food not being taken at the correct times, to balance the insulin injection. As a diabetic patient ages one must therefore accept much higher blood sugar levels.

Once a patient has become severely disturbed or unconscious, the direct method of treatment is the intravenous injection of dextrose. If possible this should be given with some restraint to the patient for partly-treated hypoglycaemia may pass through a rather violent phase. In the management of diabetic children it is common to provide parents with Glucagon, advising intramuscular injection of 1mg. This produces a transient rise in blood glucose which is often enough to allow the patient to rally enough to then take sugar drinks and hence avoid intravenous injections. Glucagon could be used more commonly in the adult diabetic.

Hypoglycaemia may induce epileptic convulsions in susceptible individuals. Great care in avoiding hypo-glycaemia may prevent fits but it is often necessary to use anticonvulsant therapy (phenytoin) in such a patient. Since insulin-taking diabetics who drive are prone, even in the best of circumstances, to loss of consciousness, they should be advised to declare their insulin taking to the licensing authorities. If patients are involved in accidents while hypoglycaemic the authorities will write and question the practitioners and physicians caring for their diabetes, and may suspend them from driving for six months to allow a period of greater stabilisation.

Nocturnal hypoglycaemia

With the ease of frequent blood sugar estimations it has now become apparent that there is a nocturnal fall in blood sugar in many patients whatever insulin regimen they may be taking. This is associated with a natural and uninhibited rise of blood sugar between 8.00 a.m. and 9.30 a.m. Indeed it is very difficult, even with extra addition of short-acting insulin in the morning, to keep the morning blood sugar at a reasonable level and aggressive attempts to lower the 8 a.m. to 9.30 a.m.

blood sugars may lead to unpleasant hypoglycaemia later in the day. The understanding of the natural fall of blood sugars during the night will certainly influence the administration of long-acting insulins and encourage a small intake of food late in the evening.

The pregnant diabetic

All pregnant diabetics should be under the care of a co-operating diabetic physician and obstetrician in a hospital unit. This is the one time in diabetic care when meticulous control of the blood sugar has been proved to result in benefit by producing a perinatal mortality approaching that of the non-diabetic. This needs accurate and regular obstetric assessment. At least two injections of insulin should be administered each day and frequent *blood sugar* measurements should be carried out by the patient at home. In these highly motivated patients it is usually not difficult to achieve near physiological blood sugars and this policy of home monitoring avoids the need for admission to hospital earlier than the last month of pregnancy.

DEVELOPMENT OF DIABETIC KETOACIDOSIS

Although not specifically related to any further drug therapy, the recognition of factors leading to the development of this serious condition which has a high mortality should be well recognised by all those who care for diabetic patients. This condition is most likely to occur in insulin-taking diabetics but patients taking diet alone or diet and tablets may, given sufficient stress or even due to the progression of the natural history of their disease, develop serious ketoacidosis. There is still a serious inability of a percentage of doctors in all areas of medicine to be able to recognise the extremely ill, breathless, dry, sickly ketotic patient. The insulin-taking diabetic is at serious risk of developing ketoacidosis whenever his life is stressed, and this stress may indeed be emotional (with children not taking their insulin or in disturbed family relationships), or infective or traumatic (road traffic accidents, major operations), or indeed any stress from for example a ruptured appendix, myocardial infarction, etc. It is safer to assume potential for major trouble in all diabetics when they are stressed than to hope that they will not develop any serious mal-control of their blood glucose. The vast majority of diabetics with viral infective illnesses (which are by far the commonest reason for the development of ketoacidosis) will become rather thirsty, will often make adjustments in their insulin, and that will deal with the problem well. However, if the condition progresses, education by

their physician should press them to seek medical advice and with the use of home blood sugar measurements the actual measurement of more seriously high blood sugars can be made. Any reasonable diabetic clinic service should have an open-access service for the assessment of such patients, for it is far safer and easier briefly to see a mild ketotic who does not require admission to hospital but who needs a little extra fluid and insulin, than to treat the deeply unconscious acidotic patient.

A great difficulty to the community practitioner is the relatively ill diabetic who is vomiting with a gastro-intestinal illness. The vast majority of these patients will need MORE INSULIN but naturally a practitioner is reluctant to give insulin when the breakfast or latest meal may have been just vomited. Here again blood sugar measurement can be of value but they may need referral to hospital. If the patient is not too sickly, the addition of sugar drinks, milk etc can help maintain the blood sugar in the less seriously ill patients. If referral to hospital can be achieved fairly quickly, there is probably little value in the home practitioner giving an injection of insulin. In most cases of diabetic ketoacidosis, although insulin is central to the treatment, intravenous fluid is perhaps the more important initial step, which will then precede the administration of small doses of insulin.

TREATMENT OF DIABETIC COMPLICATIONS

The vascular complications of diabetes make it the important disease that it is. Regrettably, there is little in the way of drug therapy which can assist the unpleasant complications of diabetes. The question is frequently asked, does the quality of prior blood sugar control influence the speed of onset or the frequency of complications. The answer to this is that the hypothesis has never been tested due to our inability, with conventional insulin regimens, to keep the blood sugar anything near the normal in the majority of patients. Certainly there is circumstantial epidemiological evidence, and animal evidence, to make a good case for aiming at as good a blood sugar as possible, and new delivery systems and pumps for the administration of insulin may allow this question to be answered.

Macrovascular complications

The development of stroke, coronary artery disease and peripheral vascular disease of the ileo-femoral-popliteal axis are more common in diabetics than in the non-diabetic population, but this is probably based on similar aetiological atherosclerotic processes as in the non-diabetic. Therefore, the treatment of these conditions is the treatment of their non-diabetic counterparts. With cerebrovascular disease care should be taken not to overlook the possibility of hypoglycaemia, for neurological features, including hemiplegia, may occur. Cardiac infarction is a potent cause of severe upset of diabetic control in insulin-requiring diabetics. In patients taking sulphonylureas who have suffered a cardiac infarction, the drug should be stopped. There is evidence that the incidence of arrhythmia is increased in diabetics taking sulphonylureas. Such patients, as well as stopping the drug, should be kept on a strict diet with the addition of insulin should it be necessary.

In the treatment of angina or hypertension it is customary to recommend a highly selective beta-blocking agent such as atenolol although it is the experience of most physicians treating a wide variety of diabetics with other beta-blocking agents that little trouble seems to ensue. Finally, in regard to peripheral vascular disease and claudication in the diabetic, it should not be assumed that because they are diabetic they should not be considered for the investigative and surgical reconstruction procedures that would be considered for the non-diabetic. Results of femoro-popliteal by-pass grafts in the diabetic approach those of the non-diabetic. As in the non-diabetic state, there are no peripheral vasodilator drugs of any clinical value.

Microvascular complications

RETINOPATHY

Diabetic patients with developing retinopathy should be encouraged not to smoke and blood pressure should be treated at lower levels than in many non-diabetic patients. Apart from the highly specialised treatment of the diabetic retina with the Argon laser there is no specific drug therapy that can assist this condition. It is the responsibility of all physicians caring for diabetics to examine the fundus regularly so that retinopathy is detected at a relatively early stage and referred for adequate laser treatment. A sympathetic physician and good social service facilities may be all that can be offered in the later stage of the disease.

The cataracts in diabetes are simple senile cataracts at an increased frequency and should be offered for extraction whenever appropriate. True diabetic cataract is rare, usually associated with extremely poorly controlled diabetes, and should be a reason for the most intensive attempts to control the blood sugar to near the physiological range.

Many diabetics when newly presenting to their physician will develop blurring of vision very soon after the institution of treatment. This is probably due to osmotic changes and swelling in the lens which cannot be corrected by the extra-ocular muscles over the first few days of treatment. This is not a serious condition but can cause great concern to the patient who may well be aware of certain visual complications. With time, blurring usually improves although, occasionally, spectacles may have to be prescribed.

NEPHROPATHY

There is no active radical treatment for diabetic nephropathy, other than control of the blood pressure and protein restriction. Once terminal renal failure has developed the patient should be considered for chronic renal dialysis although clearly a very poor vascular state, visual impairment, peripheral neuropathy etc make these patients poor dialysis subjects. Care should therefore be taken in selection although in well-selected instances diabetics can go ahead to adequate home dialysis and renal transplantation.

NEUROPATHY

The most distressing features of symptomatic sensory neuropathy are hardly amenable to drug therapy. The nocturnal pains, tingling and cramps, the hyperaesthesia and the numb cold sensations mainly in the legs and feet of diabetics are extremely difficult to treat. In quite a few instances they are relatively short lived over a period of months or a year or so, but in many other patients they can continue for many years. Simple, fairly acute onset of burning and tingling is not uncommon in newly diagnosed diabetics, or in established diabetics at times of poor blood sugar control, and clearly measures to lower the blood sugar are mandatory. Many drug therapies have been tried in the treatment of painful sensory neuropathy and analgesics of a wide variety may be of some help. Quinine or diazepam for night cramps are certainly helpful; Epanutin as a controller of abnormal sensory discharge has been claimed but in most cases it is of no help; carbamazepine (Tegretol) has likewise been used. Such patients frequently become depressed and there is a distinct place for the use of antidepressants although these drugs are no substitute for a caring physician. The majority of these patients, and indeed many without symptomatic neuropathy, will be impotent and a short time taken to reassure such patients about the nature of their impotence being related to their organic disease can be of some help in settling a patient's mind. Nocturnal symptoms and discomfort from bed clothes are sufficiently common for the use of a simple bed-cradle to be of great therapeutic benefit, so long as it does not press on the foot and produce a pressure sore.

Symptomatic autonomic dysfunction is unusual in diabetes but on a few occasions may present some very distressing clinical features. Gustatory sweating with severe soaking of the head and shoulders after meals, particularly after spicy foods, may respond to big doses of tricyclic antidepressants, but cervical sympathectomy may also be necessary. The classic features of severe postural hypotension in autonomic neuropathy can be assisted by the use of fludrocortisone 0.1–0.3mg daily. The distressing nocturnal diarrhoea of diabetes may be helped by the use of metoclopramide (Maxolon) 10mg t.d.s., and in a few instances the administration of an antibiotic such as tetracycline seems to be of some benefit. For the autonomic paralysis of the bladder there is no specific drug therapy apart from bladder training and regular bladder voiding. Since infections are all too common in the sluggish diabetic bladder, urinary antibiotics and antiseptics have an important part to play. Indeed, in the female diabetic it would seem reasonable to perform regular culture of the urine because asymptomatic urinary tract infections are all too common in the diabetic female.

THE DIABETIC FOOT

This distressing and common condition should be dealt with in a publication of its own. However, no short treatise on the drug management of diabetes with some comment on other aspects of diabetic management can afford to ignore the diabetic foot. We are essentially thinking of the diabetic foot which has a good peripheral blood flow (not an ischaemic foot) but which can so easily break down to ulcerated infection. The reasons for this are the numb painless foot due to neuropathy, the social unawareness of the patient who will allow lesions to develop before taking any action, and the basically poor blood flow and supply to peripheral tissues coupled with the very easy access of infection. With all these factors at play the most serious necrosis, osteomyelitis and gangrene can develop in a foot, and there is no doubt that with education of the patient and family, with regular inspection and attention from doctors and community nurses, the vast majority of these unpleasant neuropathic-type foot ulcers can be prevented. Once they have developed, nursing care, surgical debridement and blood glucose control are of the utmost importance. These together with the judicious use of wide-spectrum antibiotics may achieve very considerable improvement before formal surgical procedures take place. Many simple and even infected foot ulcers can be cared for at home with careful nursing, antibiotics and medical attention, but once more destructive features appear a combined assessment by a diabetic physician and a vascular surgeon should be carried out, for there is an important place for local surgery in its management.

CONCLUSION

Long-term drug therapy in all aspects of diabetes is essentially secondary to the interest of the physician caring for that patient. His team of assistants should include specialist diabetic community nurses, chiropodists and dietitians, and all these aspects of care should take primary place before drug therapy is considered.

Chapter 13 Thyroid disease

C. A. HARDISTY MD, MRCP

INTRODUCTION

In recent years, the management of thyroid disorders has been greatly helped by the widespread introduction of radioimmunoassays which accurately measure the circulating levels of total serum thyroxine (T_4), total serum triiodothyronine (T_3) and thyroid stimulating hormone (TSH). In difficult cases it is useful to test the response of the hypothalamic-pituitary axis by measurements of TSH before and 20 minutes after the intravenous injection of thyrotrophin releasing hormone (TRH). These tests are routinely used both in the diagnosis and in the management of both hypothyroidism and hyperthyroidism.

MANAGEMENT OF HYPERTHYROIDISM

The over-active thyroid gland produces high circulating levels of thyroxine and/or triiodothyronine; the aim of treatment is to lower these hormone levels to within normal limits. This may be achieved by antithyroid drugs, sub-total thyroidectomy or radio-iodine. The actual choice of treatment will depend upon the patient, local expertise and on the underlying pathology producing the thyroid overactivity.

In Graves' disease, stimulation by an abnormal immunoglobulin produces diffuse thyroid overactivity and, occasionally, a spontaneous remission or 'cure' may occur. In contrast, in a toxic nodular gland the excessive production of hormone occurs in over-active nodules and spontaneous remission is infrequent. Rarely, the over-activity is confined to a solitary toxic adenoma, which may preferentially produce triiodothyronine and the natural history is of continuing excessive thyroid hormone production. Clearly, a trial of drug therapy may be appropriate in Graves' disease but not in toxic nodular goitre where sub-total thyroidectomy or radio-iodine would usually be the treatment of choice. In Sheffield, solitary toxic adenoma is treated surgically as the results with radio-iodine have been disappointing.

1. Drug treatment of hyperthyroidism

The two most commonly used antithyroid drugs are carbimazole and propylthiouracil. In both Graves' disease and toxic nodular goitre, they both primarily act by blocking organification of iodide within the thyroid gland and are, therefore, effective in preventing the production of thyroxine and triiodothyronine. The initial dose consists of carbimazole 10–15mg eight-hourly or propylthiouracil 100–150mg eight-hourly. Treatment is reviewed at four-weekly intervals and the dose reduced to maintain euthyroidism. Patients are assessed clinically and by regular measurements of total serum thyroxine and triiodothyronine. Once euthyroid, patients can usually be maintained on carbimazole 5–15mg daily or propylthiouracil 50–150mg daily. Some physicians continue the high initial dose of carbimazole or propylthiouracil and, when hypothyroidism develops, add a thyroxine supplement (100–200 micrograms daily).

Such drug therapy is used on the first presentation of a patient with Graves' disease or in the preparation of a patient with Graves' disease or toxic nodular goitre prior to surgery. Patients undergoing surgery should only require a short period of drug therapy (6 to 12 weeks) to render them euthyroid prior to operation. In Graves' disease, if an elective trial of drug therapy is given then this should be continued for at least one year after the patient has been rendered euthyroid and should rarely exceed two years. When the drugs are discontinued about 50 per cent of the patients will remain euthyroid for at least one year but, ultimately, relapses are seen in most of these apparent cures, sometimes many years after the initial presentation. In these patients and in those who relapse shortly after completing a course of drug therapy, sub-total thyroidectomy or radio-iodine are the treatments of choice. Prolonged repeated courses of antithyroid drugs should not be given in patients with Graves' disease unless there is a specific contra-indication to surgery or radio-iodine. Such treatment would be required, for example, in the occasional young patient who develops recurrent thyrotoxicosis following a sub-total thyroidectomy. The drugs would be required until radio-iodine could safely be administered later in life. Those presenting with a large goitre are less likely to remit after a course of drug therapy and generally should be treated by surgery.

Toxic nodular goitre may be treated with antithyroid drugs but such treatment will usually need to be continued for life and, if possible, such patients should be treated by sub-total thyroidectomy or radio-iodine. Occasionally, in elderly patients, neither operation nor radio-iodine is possible and drug therapy has to be given. Care should be exercised in such patients if there is significant retrosternal extension of the goitre and if there is evidence of tracheal compression as the gland may enlarge.

Complications of drug therapy consist of purpuric or papular rashes which are usually mild and usually respond to a change from carbimazole to propyl-thiouracil or vice versa, cross-reactivity between these two drugs being rare. Leucopenia, thrombocytopenia and agranulocytosis may be seen. These complications are rare and usually occur during the first few months of drug treatment. All patients taking these drugs should be warned to discontinue them immediately and report to a doctor if they develop a sore throat or a fever. A blood film confirms the diagnosis and, if the drug is promptly stopped, then recovery usually occurs; fatalities can occur if the leucopenia persists.

Agranulocytosis can develop at any time and has been seen during a second course of antithyroid drugs. Gastro-intestinal upsets sometimes result in non-compliance but vomiting may be caused by unregulated thyroid over-activity (thyrotoxic vomiting) rather than a side-effect of the drug. Rarely, drug fevers with arthralgia and lymphadenopathy, hepatitis and nephritis may be seen.

Patients on antithyroid drug therapy should be reviewed regularly as severe hypothyroidism may develop as a result of over-treatment. Non-compliance can result in periods of unregulated thyroid over-activity which is not desirable as after some years cardiac complications such as atrial fibrillation and heart failure may develop. As already stated, apart from those few cases to whom no other effective therapy can be offered, prolonged and multiple courses of anti-thyroid drugs should not be given.

THE USE OF β-BLOCKING DRUGS

These are of value in the management of thyrotoxicosis because of their ability to suppress some of the symptoms and signs caused by sympathetic nervous system overactivity. Although propranolol also influences the peripheral metabolism of the thyroid hormones, there is no direct effect upon the thyroid gland and the excessive output of thyroid hormone is not affected by β blockade. Their sole use is, therefore, limited to symptomatic relief in patients with mild thyrotoxicosis. As a prelude to treatment by radio-iodine, β-blockers have the great advantage over carbimazole and propylthiouracil of not interfering with radio-iodine uptake. They are also useful as prompt symptomatic relief in cases of more severe thyroid over-activity while awaiting the full effect of carbimazole or propylthiouracil, which cannot affect the continued release of thyroid hormone formed before drug therapy was commenced. A prolonged course of β-blockade is not recommended as it can mask the effects of continuing thyroid overactivity and delay effective control. Another main use for β-blockers is in the control of atrial arrhythmias in cases with thyrotoxic heart failure and as part of the emergency regimen in the management of thyroid crisis. Although β-blockers have been used as the sole drug prior to sub-total thyroidectomy, the author prefers a period of control with carbimazole and propylthiouracil to eliminate any risk of post-operative crisis. The intrathyroidal store of hormone is unaffected by treatment with β-blockers.

2. Radio-iodine

Radioactive iodine in the form of ^{131}I is a relatively inexpensive and safe means of treating thyroid over-activity. Although a single oral dose is frequently all that is required, it is also important to realise that its full effects may be delayed for many years so that continuing surveillance is needed to detect developing hypothyroidism.

Radio-iodine is reserved for older patients (usually over 45 years of age) with either Graves' disease or a nodular goitre. The latter tend to be more resistant to irradiation and consequently require larger total doses. Opinion and policy regarding dosage varies between different centres, but, in terms of radiation dose to the thyroid, usually lies between 5000 and 10 000 rad/gram requiring the administration of between 4 and 10mCi of ^{131}I. The radiation from ^{131}I therapy can be predicted by a preliminary tracer study so that this is always done in centres which aim to give a precise radiation dose as distinct from others in which a standard number of millicuries (mCi) of radio-iodine is used for all patients.

The therapeutic outcome depends upon the administered dose. Larger doses will tend to control thyroid over-activity more quickly but will result in a greater incidence of early hypothyroidism. Generally, 50 to 60 per cent of patients are cured by the first dose, 20 to 30 per cent by two doses and the remainder require three doses or more. The interval between dose varies depending upon the clinical state of the patient and the policy of an individual department. In some centres, continuing thyrotoxicosis may be retreated after three months but it is usual in Sheffield to wait much longer as progressive gland shrinkage is not completed until two years have elapsed. In patients with continuing thyrotoxicosis antithyroid drugs are commenced but it is necessary to interrupt drug treatment at intervals to see if the patient has become euthyroid. Courses of antithyroid drugs following radio-iodine should not be prolonged beyond two years as, after that interval, it is clear that a second treatment with radio-iodine is needed.

Within ten years following a radiation dose between 5000 and 10 000 rad, at least 50 per cent of the treated patients become hypothyroid. The onset of hypothyroidism may be insidious and can easily be overlooked. Potentially, all patients following radio-iodine can develop hypothyroidism, the increasing prevalence being due to the continued long-term effect of radio-iodine plus, in those cases of Graves' disease, the additional effect of autoimmune destruction of the thyroid. Long-term surveillance is mandatory and is most easily provided by a computer-based register which involves both the hospital physician and the general practitioner in the follow-up.

3. Sub-total thyroidectomy

Following control of thyroid over-activity by antithyroid drugs, sub-total thyroidectomy should be performed in patients with toxic nodular goitres and those with Graves' disease who have a large goitre at initial presentation or choose not to have a prolonged course of drugs. Surgery should be performed in all patients who relapse following an adequate course of drugs and in those few in whom there is a possibility of an associated carcinoma of the thyroid. Solitary toxic adenoma should be treated by operation.

Although operative treatment is usually successful, it may result in hypothyroidism or, in a small proportion of cases, recurrent hyperthyroidism. Recurrent hyperthyroidism is seen in 2 to 15 per cent of patients, the actual rate depending upon the length of follow-up and upon the size of the thyroid remnant left by the surgeon. Recrudescence of thyroid over-activity may be seen even 20 years after operation. If below 45 years of age, these patients are treated with long-term antithyroid drugs or given radio-iodine if older than 45 years.

Hypothyroidism is seen in 5 to 30 per cent of patients; again, the overall prevalence depends on the surgeon. When seen shortly after surgery, it may be temporary and a clinical decision has to be made on the administration of thyroxine replacement therapy. If given in this circumstance, thyroxine should be withdrawn after six months to see if thyroid function has returned to normal. However, even early hypothyroidism may be permanent requiring life-time thyroxine treatment. All patients undergoing surgery should be kept under surveillance for postoperative hypothyroidism which may also be delayed especially in those treated for Graves' disease, who frequently have persisting autoimmune thyroiditis in the remnant.

MANAGEMENT OF HYPOTHYROIDISM

Usually hypothyroidism arises as a result of autoimmune damage to the thyroid gland (Hashimoto's thyroiditis), as a result of treatment for thyroid over-activity (following radio-iodine or sub-total thyroidectomy) or may be idiopathic. Very rarely it is associated with a failure of production of thyroid stimulating hormone (TSH) by the anterior pituitary gland. This is an important differential diagnosis as TSH deficiency is seldom isolated and other life-time hormone replacements may be required.

Replacement therapy with thyroxine is for life and this should be stressed to the patient. In uncomplicated cases, thyroxine is commenced at an initial dose of 50 micrograms daily and the dose is increased at two-weekly intervals to the optimal dose which is usually 150–200 micrograms daily. The effectiveness of treatment is monitored both clinically and biochemically by regular measurements of the circulating thyroid hormones. In elderly patients and in those with cardiac disease, a more cautious approach is used. The initial starting dose should be 25 or even 12.5 micrograms of thyroxine per day and the dose increased in small increments (25 or 12.5 micrograms) every four weeks. Thyroxine has a stimulatory effect on the myocardium and, shortly following the start of treatment, sudden deaths have occurred so that if there is doubt about the cardiac state, referral to a consultant is indicated. Such patients frequently cannot tolerate full thyroxine replacement because of increasing angina and a clinical decision has to be made on the appropriate dose for each individual.

All patients should be kept under surveillance as treatment is for life. Non-compliance is a problem as symptoms of thyroid deficiency may take several weeks to return on discontinuing treatment. Occasionally, in the elderly, the dose of thyroxine has to be reduced in the face of the development of ischaemic heart disease or cardiac failure.

Chapter 14　**Psychotropic prescribing**

JOAN SNEDDON MD, MRCPsych

Many re-admissions to psychiatric hospitals are due to the patient stopping the prescribed medication or taking it as an overdose. If these causes could be prevented, this would avoid family crises, extra work for the family doctor, and the cost of hospital admission, as well as much patient suffering.

It must be emphasised that psychotropic drugs are extremely important in prophylaxis as well as treatment. It is tempting to think that because the patient is well he can stop his medication and need not be seen again. Alternatively, if repeat prescriptions are given without the patient being seen, changes in his condition or drug side-effects may be missed. It is not uncommon to see a patient given a repeat prescription for an antidepressant who takes it as an overdose the same day. It is the difficult task of the general practitioner to recognise *early* signs of recurrence or relapse in these patients. This chapter is an attempt to solve the problems of which drugs to use, their common side-effects and dangerous drug interactions.

SCHIZOPHRENIA

For the acute recurrence of disturbed behaviour chlorpromazine (Largactil) 50–100mg t.d.s., orally or intramuscularly, will control the excitement and eventually the delusions. Admission for observation and assessment is important. Most patients will be discharged on medication. If they stop it they are more likely to relapse.

Major tranquillisers can produce parkinsonian side-effects. These are most marked with trifluoperazine (Stelazine), haloperidol (Serenace); less so with chlorpromazine (Largactil) and thioridazine (Melleril). Though every patient's requirements vary, on average 5mg of trifluoperazine (Stelazine) requires 50mg orphenadrine (Disipal) to minimise these side-effects and 10mg needs 100mg. When using haloperidol (Serenace) these parkinsonian side-effects are common. Three milligrams of haloperidol should be given with orphenadrine 50mg, and if haloperidol is increased, the orphenadrine should be increased up to 100mg t.d.s. Metoclopramide (Maxolon) should not be given with the major tranquillisers as it increases the parkinsonian symptoms.

Dystonic reactions in which the patient becomes suddenly rigid respond to benztropine (Cogentin) 2mg intramuscularly – repeated if necessary. The elderly are especially at risk from parkinsonian side-effects.

A common regimen is chlorpromazine (Largactil) 50mg t.d.s. or for the withdrawn schizophrenic trifluoperazine (Stelazine) 3–10mg t.d.s., given with orphenadrine (Disipal) 50–100mg t.d.s. For the patient who lives alone or is unlikely to take pills, treatment is with fluphenazine decanoate (Modecate) 25mg every two weeks or flupenthixol decanoate (Depixol, Fluanxol) 20–40mg every two weeks. These must be given by deep intramuscular injection into the buttock. If given subcutaneously they cause a hard tender lump at the injection site and the patient then may refuse further treatment. After the acute phase of schizophrenia has been controlled, depression is common. The fortnightly injection gives the doctor a chance to enquire about depressive symptoms and should, except perhaps in the well-controlled case, remain an occasion for face to face contact. An antidepressant, usually the alerting imipramine (Tofranil) 25mg t.d.s. will help but the antipsychotic medication must be continued as antidepressants alone can light up schizophrenic symptoms.

Most chronic schizophrenics living in the community need their medication regularly as a replacement therapy. Of those re-admitted many have stopped it. If they do not attend the surgery, a visit should be made. It is not unusual to find a schizophrenic lying in bed surrounded by pills but too apathetic to swallow them. This, of course, is one good reason for using depot preparations. Some need orphenadrine (Disipal) as both fluphenazine decanoate (Modecate) and flupenthixol decanoate (Depixol) cause parkinsonian symptoms.

A less common side-effect of the major tranquillisers is akathisia. The patient complains of an inner motor restlessness in which he cannot remain still and needs to move about even in bed. He may be mentally well but finds the restlessness very distressing. It is easy to mis-diagnose this as agitation and to increase the medication thus making the symptoms worse. The correct treatment is to reduce the anti-psychotic medication, give an intramuscular injection of 2mg benztropin (Cogentin) and possibly increase the orphenadrine (Disipal).

Pimozide (Orap), although advertised for withdrawn schizophrenics, is more useful in patients with delusions of infestation. It is given as 2–4mg nocte. This must not be stopped prematurely or the insects will certainly return.

In encouraging these patients to continue medication it is important to know why they stop it:

1. They feel well and consider it unnecessary.
2. Their relatives, and sometimes their doctors, tell them to stop it.
3. They have finished their tablets and are too depressed, apathetic or deluded to come to the surgery for more.
4. Doctors give the precise number of tablets, e.g. three weeks' supply, and the patient may run out if he has to miss his appointment
5. They prefer their illness to normal life. The lonely schizophrenic may find company in his voices.
6. The drugs have unpleasant side-effects which have not been properly treated.

MANIC DEPRESSIVE ILLNESS AND RECURRENT DEPRESSIVE ILLNESS

This severe psychotic illness has a 15 per cent mortality from suicide. Patients or their relatives often recognise the early signs and symptoms of recurrence and should be encouraged to consult at this stage.

Acute mania

Chlorpromazine is the best immediate drug treatment in a dose of 100–200mg four-hourly as tablet, syrup or intramuscular injection, depending on the patient's co-operation. Admission is required but may be difficult legally. The chronic hypomanic patient is difficult to control, not ill enough for compulsory admission, but overactive, argumentative and aggressive. Haloperidol (Serenace) 1.5–5mg t.d.s. given with orphenadrine (Disipal) 50–100mg t.d.s. is often more successful and less sedating than chlorpromazine (Largactil) 50mg t.d.s.

Depressive psychosis

This includes true endogenous depression and the depressive swing of manic depressive illness. Patients' early symptoms tend to be initially the same for each attack and may be somatic rather than psychiatric. Pain

is common, headaches, abdominal and low back pain may lead to referral to physician or surgeon. Even a fully developed depressive illness may masquerade as physical disease, dementia or anxiety.

It is vital that relevant questions be asked so that treatment is begun early. Suicide is most likely before the diagnosis has been made or when the patient is beginning to recover, losing his retardation, having enough incentive to kill himself and not sufficiently improved to wish to live. The history should include previously prescribed and present medication as iatrogenic depression occurs with the following preparations:

antihypertensives	physostigmine
steroids	digitalis
oestrogens	sulphonamides
levodopa	phenothiazines
indomethacin	flupenthixol
fenfluramine	β-blockers

The symptoms of depressive illness include:

Low mood with diurnal variation. The patient may feel almost normal by evening, dreads going to bed knowing that in the morning he will feel as bad as ever.
Feelings of guilt, worthlessness and poverty.
Feelings that the family would be better off without him.
Loss of appetite.
Loss of weight.
Loss of concentration.
Loss of energy.
Loss of libido, impotence.

It is very important to ask patients about suicidal thoughts and whether they have made plans to kill themselves. They are often grateful for the question as they have felt guilty about having such thoughts. Patients may admit they would like to go to bed and never wake up even if they have not made suicidal plans. Where there are delusions of poverty, guilt and worthlessness, these patients should be regarded as severe suicide risks. The patient who will not discuss his feelings or plans about suicide should also be considered as a severe risk, especially if he admits to making a will or taking out extra insurance.

If admission is not indicated, treatment should be started with a tricyclic antidepressant, given as one week's supply, preferably to a responsible relative.

Amitriptyline (Tryptizol) is sedative and if given as 75mg nocte also acts as a hypnotic. This can be increased after one week to 100mg nocte and 25mg b.d.

Doxepin (Sinequan) is less sedative than amitriptyline and thought to be less cardiotoxic. 50–75mg at night gives the patient a good night's sleep and is useful for patients who are working as there is little morning hangover. Doxepin is made also in 10mg tablets, and these are valuable when wanting to start with a small dose in the elderly patient.

Imipramine (Tofranil) is alerting and therefore good in retarded and puerperal depression. This should be given as 25mg t.d.s. increasing to 50mg t.d.s after one week, or up to 200mg if the patient can tolerate it. It should not be given in one dose at night and the patient may need a hypnotic for the first few weeks till the depression starts to lift.

It is important to tell the patient that improvement in mood will not occur for 10 to 14 days and that during that time he may feel worse and have such side-effects as dry mouth, blurring of vision, constipation, dizziness due to hypotension, and sweating. He should be reassured that improvement will occur and that the side-effects will become less troublesome. If he is not told these facts, or does not believe them, he may stop the tablets after a few days or take them all as an overdose.

Untreated depressive illness lasts an average three to six months. Antidepressants suppress the illness until natural remission occurs. They should be continued in full dosage till the patient has been well for three months and in half-dosage for the six subsequent months. The dose is then gradually reduced by 25mg every two weeks, and the patient watched carefully over that time. Recurrence of symptoms two to three weeks after reduction of dosage is an indication for increasing it again.

SPECIAL PRECAUTIONS WITH THE TRICYCLIC
ANTIDEPRESSANTS

Tricyclic antidepressants can cause cardiac arrhythmias and should be used with caution in patients with cardiovascular disease and in the elderly. They should not be given within three months of a coronary infarction. For the severely depressed post-coronary patient ECT is safer and may be justified since continued depression and agitation are very bad for the patient with coronary artery disease. Tricyclic antidepressants block the hypotensive action of some drugs, e.g. hydralazine (Apresoline) and debrisoquine (Declinax).

Chlorpromazine (Largactil) is used with tricyclics in treating the very agitated depressed patient. The addition raises the plasma tricyclic level but increases the risk of anticholinergic side-effects, especially hypotension and constipation, of special importance in the elderly patient. The combination of benzodiazepines and tricyclics has no effect on the tricyclic level. Both tricyclics and chlorpromazine (Largactil) can cause convulsions, especially in overdose and should be used with caution in epileptics.

Tricyclics and pimozide (Orap) are useful in patients whose delusions of infestation are treated with pimozide but are then found to be depressed.

Other antidepressants

Mianserin (Bolvidon) is sedative and useful when the anticholinergic effects of the older tricyclic drugs would be harmful. It is said also to be less cardiotoxic. Initially, it is given as 30mg nocte or in divided doses increasing to a maximum of 90mg daily. Nomifensine (Merital) is alerting also and has fewer side-effects than the older established tricyclics. It is relatively safe in overdose, even in patients with cardiac disease. It does not increase the chances of a seizure in epileptic patients. The starting dose is 25mg b.d. (usual range 50–200mg daily). It must not be prescribed with the MAOIs. Flupenthixol (Fluanxol) is also effective in low doses (0.5–1.0mg t.d.s.) so that side-effects are fewer. This can be especially helpful for rather withdrawn depressives, but severe parkinsonian side-effects, even on this low dosage, can be dangerous for the elderly. This drug should not be given after 4.00 p.m. or to confused or over-active patients.

Monoamine-oxidase inhibitors have not been found useful in endogenous depression but will be discussed later in relation to neurotic depression and phobic states (p. 152).

Lithium

Lithium is valuable as a mood normaliser in patients with manic depressive psychosis and in many patients with recurrent depressive illness. While taking lithium, patients who previously had one or two attacks of psychosis a year remain well. The main indication for using lithium is the patient who has had two attacks in the last year or three attacks in the last two years, as without lithium the frequency of attacks will increase at the rate of 10 to 20 per cent per year.

The usual practice is for the attack of mania or depression to be treated with the appropriate drugs and sometimes ECT. Lithium is started when the patient is improving but before discharge, as blood levels need to be done every few days until the patient is stabilised on the drug. A healthy adult needs about 1000mg of lithium carbonate daily to obtain a serum lithium of 0.8–1.4mmol/litre which is the usual therapeutic range. This is given as 250mg or 400mg of Camcolit in divided doses. Priadel is also lithium carbonate 400mg in a controlled-release tablet.

Patients should carry a card describing the side-effects and the signs of overdose and know to stop the drug if signs of overdose occur and report to their doctor or to the lithium clinic. A serum lithium (with the blood specimen in a plain tube) should be requested urgently.

Common side-effects include: fine tremor of the hands, nausea and polyuria.

Signs of toxicity include: marked coarse tremor of the hands, nausea, vomiting and diarrhoea. Late signs of ataxia, tinnitus, confusion and coma appear in cases with severe toxicity.

The biological half-life of lithium is 18 to 30 hours so the psychiatrist may be able to restart the lithium at a lower dose after a few days.

CONTRA-INDICATIONS AND PRECAUTIONS

Lithium should be stopped in the following circumstances:

1. Twenty-four hours before surgery involving an anaesthetic.
2. In medical illness: it may cause profound electrolyte disturbance, especially in heart failure, Addison's disease or when using diuretics. In patients who are slimming, a normal salt intake must be maintained.
3. Lithium and diuretics should not be prescribed together. The thiazide diuretics, such as bendrofluazide, cause the lithium to rise to toxic levels (Kerry, Ludlow and Owen, 1980).
4. If possible lithium should be avoided during the first three months of pregnancy. A review by Schou (1968) makes the following points:

Pregnancy occurring during the use of prophylactic lithium is not in itself an indication for the termination of pregnancy.

If pregnant, more frequent serum lithium estimations should be made and the lower end of the therapeutic range should be used.

At the time of childbirth, stop lithium because of the associated electrolyte and hormonal changes.

Breast-feeding should be avoided. The information concerning this is limited and that which is available shows that important amounts of lithium (30 to 100 per cent of the mother's serum level) are present in breast milk. One or two reports have suggested that 'floppiness' in babies was the result of the toxic effects of lithium via breast milk.

INTERACTION OF LITHIUM WITH OTHER DRUGS

When haloperidol (Serenace), fluphenazine decanoate (Modecate) and flupenthixol were combined with lithium adverse reactions, neurological in character,

have been suspected. As previously mentioned, diuretics should not be prescribed.

Given sensible precautions, lithium can be used safely, preventing many hospital admissions and is far less dangerous than the 15 per cent mortality from attempted suicide. Minor mood changes may still occur and are more safely handled with lithium alone. The tricyclics may cause hypomania; the major tranquillisers tend to produce a downward mood swing.

Puerperal illness (Including all types of puerperal psychosis)

Acute psychotic puerperal illness occurs in 1:500 births and 80 per cent of patients are admitted in the first 28 days postpartum. Recurrence in successive pregnancies is at least one in five. The woman is normally well until the fourth to fifth day postpartum and then after one or two sleepless nights becomes acutely psychotic. Most need admission, preferably to a mother and baby psychiatric unit. In those less severely ill or prior to admission, chlorpromazine (Largactil) and tricyclic antidepressants are safe in moderate doses in women who are breast-feeding. However, lithium is contra-indicated as it is excreted in the breast milk and can cause a floppy baby. Puerperal psychotic illness waxes and wanes over the six months or longer following delivery, and it is very important that medication be continued and the patient carefully monitored after discharge from the ward.

In milder neurotic depressions seen in women after childbirth, it is better to avoid diazepam. In lactating women, it makes the baby drowsy and slow to feed and benzodiazepines are known to release aggression possibly leading to child abuse. Tricyclic antidepressants work well. Imipramine (Tofranil) 25mg t.d.s. is the first choice for the puerperal girl who often complains of the lethargy, apathy, fatigue and loss of libido, that are difficult to differentiate from the fatigue common to all women looking after a new baby.

There are some women who present in the first few months with what appears to be a neurotic depression with complaints of family disharmony but who do not respond fully to antidepressants. They respond well to ECT and should certainly be referred for a psychiatric opinion as suicide and infanticide are avoidable with treatment (Sneddon et al, 1981).

PSYCHOTROPIC DRUGS IN THE ELDERLY

These should start with very small doses, if possible once daily, preferably, and more safely, at bedtime.

Depression: doxepin (Sinequan) 30mg nocte.

Paraphrenic schizophrenia: trifluoperazine (Stelazine) as Spansule 2mg nocte.

Dementia needing tranquillisers:
  promazine (Sparine) 25mg b.d. or 50mg nocte.
  haloperidol (Serenace) 0.5–1.5mg b.d. with orphenadrine.
  thioridazine (Melleril) 25–50mg b.d. or nocte.

Night sedation:
  promazine (Sparine) 25mg.
  temazepan (Normison) a short-acting benzo-diazepine will avoid morning hangover and falls.
  chlormethiazole 250–500mg. This should not be given if the patient is already taking phenothiazines and haloperidol.
  Welldorm is no longer popular. It is contra-indicated where there is hepatic or renal dysfunction and causes skin rashes.
  chlorpromazine (Largactil) is best avoided especially in those living alone because of its hypotensive and hypothermic effects.

The sudden onset of a confusional state may be due to:

1. Too high a dose of the drug, e.g. diazepam and nitrazepam in a patient with poor renal and hepatic function. Stopping the drug may be all that is needed for recovery.
2. Drug interactions.
3. Physical illness (symptoms of which may not be complained of), e.g.
   chest infection
   urinary tract infection
   undiagnosed coronary or CVA
   fractured neck of femur.

Depressive illness in the elderly is often recurrent and if they become withdrawn and have depressive paranoid delusions they may refuse to allow the doctor into the house. Fortunately, these patients often present to the surgery earlier while they are still amenable to treatment. A common presenting symptom is insomnia. In an elderly person presenting with insomnia with early morning wakening not due to pain, questions about depressive illness should be asked. Doxepin (Sinequan) 30mg nocte is better treatment than a hypnotic. Seventy per cent of prescriptions for hypnotics in general practise are written by the receptionist compared with 22 per cent for other drugs (Oswald, 1979). Depressed elderly patients may appear demented, but after treatment they function normally. If the diagnosis is in doubt, it is vital to treat them as depressed.

THE NEUROTIC PATIENT

It is difficult to differentiate between unhappiness where understanding and reassurance are helpful, and neurotic anxiety and depression due to life circumstances which may be helped by medication.

The patient who presents regularly at the surgery requesting tranquillisers with a variety of psychosomatic complaints is well known. Many find illness a more attractive way of life than health, but because of their constant complaints, they are given tranquillisers followed by repeat prescriptions. Thus, they often increase the dose without anyone noticing and if they are clever, they persuade both the general practitioner and the hospital doctor to prescribe at the same time.

The most commonly noted tranquillisers are the benzodiazepines and they all have the same actions so there is little point in changing from one to another:

diazepam (Valium) as 2–10mg t.d.s and chlordiazepoxide (Librium) 5–20 mg t.d.s. have stood the test of time.

nitrazepam (Mogadon) 5–10mg nocte is a good safe hypnotic.

In those who complain of hangover, temazepam (Normison) with a shorter half-life can be tried.

The benzodiazepines are relatively safe in overdose but all can be addictive and sudden withdrawal can cause increased anxiety, insomnia and attacks of shaking. The importance of this is shown when a patient who has been taking diazepam 5–10mg t.d.s. for some months, takes it all as an overdose, is sent home from hospital, goes to the doctor for some more and is refused them. They should be reduced and hopefully withdrawn over two to three weeks.

Anxiety, phobic attacks and neurotic depression may be impossible to distinguish clinically. Whereas minor tranquillisers may make depression worse, amitriptyline (Tryptizol) or doxepin (Sinequan) as 50mg nocte are helpful and avoid the use of a hypnotic and day-time drug taking.

For the chronically anxious patient the phenothiazine, trifluoperazine (Stelazine), often helps when the benzodiazepines have failed. At doses of 1mg t.d.s. or 2mg Spansule nocte, parkinsonian side-effects are rare. Neither tricyclics nor phenothiazines are addictive but unfortunately they are more dangerous in overdose than benzodiazepines.

The monoamine-oxidase inhibitors have been found helpful in patients with severe phobic anxiety states, especially agoraphobia. Though some respond to behaviour therapy alone, the more severely ill patient requires both methods together. Phenelzine (Nardil) as 15mg t.d.s. is the drug of choice but the dose can be increased to 60mg daily in rapid acetylators of the drug. The treatment should be continued for at least six months while the patient has regular exposure to the phobic situation or symptoms will return.

The patient is given a printed sheet stating that he is taking MAOIs and it is shown to any medical and dental staff who may need to treat the patient. The following foods should not be taken:

Cheese
Pickled herring
The pods of broad beans
Bovril, Oxo
Alcohol except for the occasional glass of wine.

MAOIs are contra-indicated in liver disease, cardiac failure, cerebrovascular disease and epilepsy. They should not be given with:

1. The tricyclic antidepressants or within 14 days of ceasing treatment with the tricyclics.
2. Amphetamine, fenfluramine, ephedrine.
3. Barbiturates, pethidine and morphia.
4. Antihypertensives.
5. Antihistamines.
6. Hypoglycaemic agents.

Failure to observe the above precautions can lead to a dangerous rise of blood pressure. Deaths have occurred.

Barbiturates, stimulants like dexamphetamine (Dexedrine), appetite suppressants like diethylpropion (Apisate) and hypnotics like methaqualone and diphenhydramine (Mandrax) should never be prescribed. All are addictive and the middle-aged addict for whom they are prescribed is difficult to treat. When these drugs are available, youngsters take them knowingly for 'kicks'.

ALCOHOL DEPENDENCE

Alcohol dependence is a serious illness with an overall mortality two and a half times that of the average population and a suicide rate 80 times above normal in men (Kessell and Grossman, 1961).

It is an important differential diagnosis in a patient of any age and either sex presenting with a history of:

Repeated accidents, especially road traffic accidents
Epigastric pain and loss of appetite
Requests for sick notes for Monday and Tuesday after a weekend drinking
Depression in the patient or the spouse

Disturbance in the children, or the possibility of child abuse
Family violence
Impotence, especially if associated with pathological jealousy of the spouse
Peripheral neuritis
Poor sleep with nightmares and sweating
Chest infection – they have five times the national average.

Heavy drinking may be associated with a true psychiatric illness. The depressed drowns his sorrows, the obsessional finds solace from his doubts and ruminations and the schizophrenic blocks out the voices. There may be a family history of heavy drinking. Most patients deny their heavy drinking or give a modest estimate of their consumption. Early help is more likely to be successful because family life and job will still be intact. Every doctor, whether general practitioner or specialist, should watch out for early signs of this new epidemic.

Having made the diagnosis, the next problem is for the patient to accept it and co-operate in treatment. For complete withdrawal from alcohol, admission is usually necessary as it is very difficult to assess how severe the reaction will be and epileptic fits may occur. In hospital the commonly used tranquilliser during this stage is chlormethiazole (Heminevrin) as 500–1500mg t.d.s. This is both tranquilliser and anti-epileptic. Nitrazepam (Mogadon) 5–20mg nocte will help with the insomnia and Parentrovite high-potency-paired ampules is given daily for five days. The dose of Heminevrin is reduced to nil hopefully by the end of the first week as it is an addictive drug. Its effects are also potentiated by alcohol and no patient should be discharged while still taking it.

After discharge the patient often becomes depressed and may need treatment with tricyclics. It is at this stage, when for the first time for months the patient soberly sees his real problems, that suicide may occur.

The patient who continues to drink despite admissions for drying out and follow-up support may, if well motivated, remain abstinent while taking disulfiram (Antabuse) 200mg daily or as a subcutaneous implant. If he drinks alcohol with this drug he feels ill, sweaty and vomits and may have cardiac arrhythmias. Antabuse is contra-indicated in cardiac, renal or hepatic disease and in patients with diabetes, epilepsy or psychosis. This limits its use to the young fit patient.

SEVERE PERSONALITY DISORDERS
(Psychopaths)
Where possible they should not be given drugs of any

kind. They abuse them, sell them, mix them with alcohol and take them as overdoses. Requests for barbiturates, dihydrocodeine (DF 118), dipipanone (Diconal) and chlormethiazole (Heminevrin) by temporary residents should be refused. All are addictive.

Drug addicts requesting heroin should be referred to the licensed psychiatrist. If showing signs of withdrawal, methadone (Physeptone) as linctus should be prescribed, 5–20mg, and the patient should be watched while he takes it.

Barbiturate withdrawal can be fatal. Admission may be required as barbiturates must be withdrawn gradually under supervision. Rapid withdrawal may cause epileptic fits.

Patients with severe personality disorders often complain that they feel anxious, tense and aggressive. Many also abuse alcohol. Diazepam may increase their aggressive urges. Small doses of intramuscular flupenthixol 10mg every two to three weeks act as a good tranquilliser, reduce aggressive feelings and avoid the risk of overdose or other antisocial misuse.

REFERENCES

Kerry, R. J., Ludlow, J. M., and Owen, G. (1980). Diuretics are dangerous with lithium. *British Medical Journal*, 2, 371.

Kessell, N. and Grossman, G. (1961). Suicide in alcoholics. *British Medical Journal*, 2, 1671–2.

Oswald, I. (1979). The why and how of hypnotic drugs. *British Medical Journal*, 1, 1167–8.

Schou, M. (1968). Lithium in psychiatric therapy and prophylaxis. *Journal of Psychiatric Research*, 6, 67–95.

Sneddon, J., Kerry, R. J. and Bant, W. P. (1981). The psychiatric mother and baby unit. *The Practitioner*, 225, 1295–1300.

Chapter 15 Cancer chemotherapy

JOHN RICHMOND MD, FRCP, FRCP(Ed)

Since World War II there has been an explosion of interest in the application of drugs that are variously known as nucleotoxic, cytotoxic, radiomimetic and anti-mitotic to the management of malignant disease. Some have their origins in folklore, some are chance discoveries and some have been deliberately synthesised because of a calculated chemical effect on cell division. Much of the improvement in the treatment of cancer in the past 25 years stems from more sophisticated surgical and radiotherapy techniques and better general medical support to control infection and during marrow depression. It is, however, the advent of cytotoxic chemotherapy that has made the greatest change by the aggressive use of drugs, usually in combinations, so that they have a complementary effect to achieve a maximum kill of malignant cells by interfering with mitosis. Unfortunately, dividing healthy cells are also killed and the balance between destroying the tumour and serious adverse effects on the patient can be very fine.

Although chemical treatment of leukaemia was tried empirically more than 100 years ago it was the study of mustards that led to the initial breakthrough. Sulphur mustard was synthesised in the 1850s and its vesicant action was known before the turn of the century. Interest in its biological and chemical properties was intensified between World War I and II and its marked cytotoxic action was observed. The cytotoxicity was apparently due to an alkylating effect, the formation of covalent linkages with critical structural moieties in nucleic acid synthesis, e.g. guanine residues of DNA. This led to trials of the effect of nitrogen mustards in animal tumours and human malignancy. The first of the latter were mainly in the lymphoreticular malignancies, the leukaemias and lymphomas; they were conducted in conditions of military secrecy and the first reports of striking, if temporary, effects were published in 1946. There then followed a period of intense activity. A whole series of alkylating agents was developed. More or less concurrently, interest started in the cytotoxic properties of antimetabolites, analogues of naturally occurring compounds. Then it transpired that certain antibiotics had significant anti-

tumour activity and simultaneously miscellaneous compounds were discovered that could not be classified easily.

Although hundreds of drugs have been shown to have cytotoxic activity only a score or so are widely used. Before looking at the common cytotoxic regimens it will be helpful to summarise the individual drugs and to discuss how they have been selected for therapeutic application; an important part of the selection process is of course the acceptability of a drug's adverse effects.

Table 1 Classification of common cytotoxic drugs

1. Alkylating agents	
mustine	busulphan
cyclophosphamide	thiotepa
chlorambucil	dacarbazine
melphalan	nitrosoureas
2. Antimetabolites	
methotrexate	6-mercaptopurine
thioguanine	cytarabine
3. Antibiotics	
actinomycin	bleomycin
doxorubicin	
4. Miscellaneous	
corticosteroids	L-asparaginase
vinca alkaloids	cisplatin
procarbazine	

CLASSIFICATION OF COMMON CYTOTOXIC DRUGS (Table 1)

Alkylating agents

Mustine (nitrogen mustard, mechlorethamine) was the first to be established. It is given intravenously and into serous cavities and usually causes unpleasant nausea and vomiting in the six to eight hours after administration. It is still a first-line drug in the management of Hodgkin's disease and can also give worthwhile palliation of recurrent effusion from metastatic carcinoma in the pleural and peritoneal spaces.

Cyclophosphamide (Endoxana) can be administered orally and intravenously. It is a very effective drug in regimens used in the non-Hodgkin's lymphomas and it features in combinations being tried as adjuvant therapy for solid tumours. It is also a satisfactory drug for chronic lymphocytic leukaemia; however, for this particular leukaemia, the favoured drug is another mustard *chlorambucil* (Leukeran) which can be given orally and has lower toxicity. *Melphalan* (phenylalanine mustard) has found favour in the palliation of multiple myeloma but perhaps its best success has been as an adjuvant to surgery in the management of malignant melanoma. *Busulphan* (Myleran) differs from the mustards in being a sulphonic acid ester. It is given orally and is the drug of first choice for chronic myelocytic leukaemia. Although not able to cure the disease it produces a striking first remission in more than 80 per cent of patients. The *nitrosoureas* BCNU (carmustine) and CCNU (lomustine) have their best effect in the malignant lymphomas and in some solid tumours. In that they are among the few cytotoxic drugs which cross the blood-brain barrier they are potentially useful in the management of meningeal leukaemia and brain tumours.

Less frequently used drugs are *thiotepa* which is sometimes given in adjuvant therapy for carcinoma of breast and ovary and by intracavitary injection to control malignant effusion and *dacarbazine* (DTIC); the latter is relatively new and has found a place in a second-line regimen for Hodgkin's disease.

Antimetabolites

The development of antimetabolites is historically just as significant as the discovery of the effect of alkylating agents. When folic acid was synthesised in 1945 it was quickly discovered to have an aggravating effect in childhood leukaemia. This led to the deliberate preparation of folic acid antagonists, the first being aminopterin, and to the report in 1948 of the first worthwhile remission in acute leukaemia. *Methotrexate* (amethopterin) followed quickly and remains one of our most important drugs in the maintenance therapy of acute leukaemia. It can be given by mouth and parenterally and since it does not cross the blood-brain barrier very readily it is fortunate that the drug can also be given intrathecally. Since the 1950s it has been known that given alone methotrexate has striking effects in choriocarcinoma. It also features in many solid tumour regimens.

The other antimetabolites, mainly purine and pyrimidine antagonists also act by interfering with nucleic acid synthesis. *6-mercaptopurine* features in the maintenance therapy of acute leukaemias. *Azathioprine* (Imuran), although closely related to 6-mercaptopurine, is more used for its immunosuppressive effects in transplant work and in enhancing the effects of corticosteroids. *Thioguanine* (an antipurine) is being used successfully in acute myeloblastic leukaemia in conjunction with *cytosine arabinoside* (cytarabine) an anti-pyrimidine. *Fluorouracil* features as a main agent in adjuvant therapy combinations for some solid tumours and in palliation of advanced carcinoma, particularly of breast, bronchus, gastrointestinal tract, female genital tract and head and neck.

Antibiotics

A series of actinomycins were the first to be shown to have cytotoxic activity. Interest has centred mainly on *actinomycin D* (dactinomycin) which came into therapeutic use in the 1950s. The actinomycins, usually given intravenously, are effective in a number of neoplasms but they have been mainly applied in childhood tumours of mesodermal origin, e.g. nephroblastoma, resistant ovarian and testicular tumours, in choriocarcinoma and as immunosuppressive agents in transplant work. Subsequent antibiotics of interest have had strange origins, e.g. organisms obtained from Sardinian sewage and from soil obtained from a Japanese coal mine. *Daunorubicin* (rubidomycin) was one of the first drugs, along with cytarabine, to be effective in acute myeloblastic leukaemia. *Doxorubicin* (Adriamycin) has largely replaced daunorubicin of which it is the hydroxylated analogue. It is given intravenously and has a wide spectrum of activity, mainly in acute myeloblastic leukaemia, in non-Hodgkin's lymphoma and as a second-line drug in Hodgkin's disease. *Bleomycin* has a valuable role along with doxorubicin in advanced Hodgkin's disease; it is also used in palliation of miscellaneous solid tumours particularly testicular teratoma and head and neck cancer.

Miscellaneous agents

(a) *Corticosteroids* suppress mitosis in lymphocytes and have found their main place in acute lymphoblastic leukaemia and the malignant lymphomas; they are also combined in some solid tumour regimens. They may have effects other than anti-mitotic effects which are important; they help to reduce cerebral oedema and hypercalcaemia from metastatic disease, probably reduce the bleeding tendency in thrombocytopenic patients and, for reasons not understood, may reduce bone marrow suppression caused by the more myelotoxic drugs.

(b) The *vinca alkaloids* derived from the periwinkle *Vinca rosea* help to illustrate the fascinating beginnings of some of our most important agents. From Indian folk medicine it was believed that the periwinkle might have hypoglycaemic activity. This proved to be groundless but the original experiments showed a cytotoxic effect which led to the extraction of five active alkaloids. Two proved to be interesting, *vincristine* (Oncovin) and *vinblastine* (Velbe) and they have become most useful agents. They have a comparable spectrum of activity in malignant lymphoma and solid tumours where, although similar chemically, they seem to show little cross-resistance. Vincristine is the better drug in acute lymphoblastic leukaemia, a condition which now has a dramatically improved prognosis. Vinca alkaloids are among the few compounds to act on cell microtubules and to interfere with the mitotic process itself as spindle poisons.

(c) *Procarbazine* (Natulan) was developed during the search for new monoamine-oxidase inhibitors. It is a methylhydrazine, given by mouth and is one of our main agents in the combination chemotherapy of Hodgkin's disease.

(d) *L-asparaginase*, although not fulfilling early promise, illustrates an important principle in the relentless search for effective anti-cancer remedies. Certain neoplastic cells including the lymphoblast of acute childhood lymphoblastic leukaemia have L-asparagine as an essential growth requirement; unlike normal cells they cannot synthesise it for themselves. L-asparaginase acts as a cytotoxic drug because it effectively cuts off the neoplastic cell from environmental L-asparagine. Some day another discovery like this may suddenly transform the whole face of cancer management. L-asparaginase is only used at present in the complicated protocol for acute lymphoblastic leukaemia.

(e) *Cisplatin* compounds particularly DDP are still being evaluated. They originally attracted interest in experiments with bacterial proliferation in an electrical field. They are toxic, especially to the kidney, but have an established place in the treatment of testicular teratomas.

SELECTION OF DRUG COMBINATIONS

The early use of cytotoxic drugs was empirical but now most treatment regimens have been carefully assembled and the following principles apply to selection and combination:

1. Effect of an individual drug in vitro, on animal tumours and then in human malignancy.
2. Acceptability of adverse effects and degree of separation between worthwhile therapeutic effect and toxic effect.
3. Evidence of synergism of combinations based both on trial and error and knowledge of pharmacokinetics.

Procarbazine is, for example, a very effective drug when given alone in Hodgkin's disease but disappointing in the non-Hodgkin's lymphomas. Prednisolone alone and vincristine alone will each induce complete remission in about 50 per cent of children with acute lymphoblastic leukaemia; given together they have the remarkable effect of inducing complete clinical and haematological remission in more than 90 per cent of children.

However, it is our detailed knowledge of the mechanism of action of individual drugs on the cell cycle that has led to a rational basis for many of the present combinations. Each cell reproduces itself in mitosis (Fig. 15/1) and then proceeds to the so-called

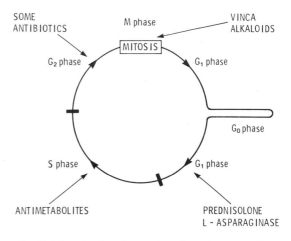

Fig. 15/1 Site of action of some phase-dependent cytotoxic drugs in cell cycle

G_1 phase, a period of RNA and protein synthesis; this phase can last from a few hours to many years and it is this phase which separates the rapidly dividing from the slowly dividing cells and tissues. During the G_1 phase there is a resting G_0 phase during which the cell is out of the active cycle and not responsive to any cytotoxic attack. The next phase, the S phase is the period of DNA replication and it lasts for some six to eight hours. Then finally there is the premitotic or G_2

phase which lasts for about two hours; in this period there is further synthesis of RNA and cytoplasmic proteins. Some drugs like the alkylating agents and nitrosoureas act at several points in the cycle and are said to be phase-independent; others act at a specific point and are phase-dependent, e.g. antibiotics and antimetabolites. Hence in choosing a combination drug regimen it would be sensible to mix a selection from these classes of alkylating agent, antimetabolite, antibiotic, vinca alkaloid and corticosteroid and indeed that is exactly what many effective recipes embrace.

Apart from the combination of drugs for synergistic effect it has been found that doses of individual drugs can be reduced with some mitigation of adverse effect. The other practice that has evolved is the giving of drug therapy in pulses with rest periods between. The intervals between these pulses are calculated from a knowledge of the division time of tumour cells and the division time of particularly vulnerable normal cells, e.g. haemopoietic stem cells. It is possible with serial pulses to expect progressive destruction of the mass of tumour cells with complete recovery of healthy tissues in the intervals.

Although the host's immune mechanism must be important it cannot be relied upon and the objective has to be total tumour kill. The problem is forbidding. When an individual has clinical disease, e.g. in acute leukaemia, he could be carrying a burden of 10^{12} tumour cells or 1kg of neoplastic tissue. Tumour cell kill seems to occur by what is termed first-order kinetics; each pulse of treatment destroys a constant percentage of cells, not a constant number. This means that if we kill 99.99 per cent of cells, 10^8 tumour cells, about 100mg of neoplastic tissue still remain. The patient may well appear to be cured but every single remaining cell is capable of inducing relapse and killing the patient. This is why modern cancer chemotherapy has to be so protracted and so demanding on the patient.

ADVERSE EFFECT OF CYTOTOXIC DRUGS (Table 2)

For the doctor who is not directly concerned in cancer chemotherapy it is usually the more unpleasant aspects of patient management that have to be coped with, the failures and the adverse effects. The adverse effects can be very severe and in an individual patient their potential development has to be weighed very carefully against the chance of cure or the chance of useful palliation with a good quality of life before deciding on the wisdom of aggressive treatment. There are non-specific effects common to all the cytotoxic drugs and

resulting from anti-mitotic action on healthy tissues and specific effects peculiar to a particular drug.

Table 2 Main adverse effects of cytotoxic drugs

A. Non-specific
  Bone marrow depression
  Gastro-intestinal disturbance
  Alopecia
  Suppression of pituitary-adrenal function
  Depression of immunity
  Hyperuricaemia

B. Specific
  Neuropathy – vinca alkaloids
  Cardiotoxicity – doxorubicin
  Lung fibrosis – bleomycin, busulphan
  Haemorrhagic cystitis – cyclophosphamide
  Renal and liver toxicity – methotrexate

Non-specific effects
These are seen preferentially in those tissues with the most active cell turnover and the main ones are as follows:

1. *Bone marrow depression.* This is most troublesome with mustine, cyclophosphamide, the antimetabolites and doxorubicin. It is least troublesome with vincristine and bleomycin; indeed vincristine sometimes improves the platelet count. Many patients have to be tided over the worst effects of bone marrow depression with blood transfusion or special concentrates of white cells and platelets.

2. *Gastro-intestinal* distress due to interference with mucosal cell division. There may be diarrhoea but the most usual problem is nausea and vomiting. Mustine is the worst offender but there is considerable individual patient variation. In that infusions of mustine are invariably given in hospital the patient's discomfort can generally be controlled with sedation and/or an antiemetic. The folic acid antagonists are prone to cause oral mucosal ulceration.

3. *Alopecia.* The cells of the hair follicles are also rapidly dividing. Cyclophosphamide, doxorubicin and vincristine are the drugs which cause most hair loss and it can be distressing to women and to children. Fortunately hair returns usually after three to four months and most patients can cope with the provision of a wig. Children with acute lymphoblastic leukaemia now routinely have prophylactic cranial irradiation at an early stage and this is another cause of total but, fortunately, temporary hair loss.

4. *Endocrine function.* The on-off use of large doses of corticosteroids is surprisingly well tolerated. There is, however, evidence that successive pulses of cytotoxic therapy do have a depressive effect on pituitary/adrenal function. This should be remembered when a patient, after protracted chemotherapy, is stressed by an acute infection or trauma including surgery; for the occasional patient will need temporary corticosteroid support. Amenorrhoea is usual and so is infertility. Impotence is probably more related to the severity of illness than to drug therapy. It is not at present clear what long-term mutagenic effects there might be from cytotoxic drugs. Many women have recovered fertility and given birth to apparently normal children. In addition there are now several reports of women 'cured' of childhood leukaemia after the usual extensive treatment and who have given birth to normal children. The most difficult issue arises when chemotherapy may be necessary during pregnancy. In early pregnancy, abortion can be considered by the criteria that are used for any serious illness; otherwise, in order to save the mother's life, the risk that the fetus will be injured has to be accepted.

5. *Immunity and infection.* Some diseases, notably the malignant lymphomas, may have significant depression of immunity as a feature of the condition. Cytotoxic therapy regularly causes neutropenia and poor white cell response to infections. More important than either of these factors is, however, a general reduction of humoral and cell-mediated immunity. This is expressed in a variety of ways. There is first, a proneness to common fungal, bacterial and viral infections. Many patients on a long course of chemotherapy will have candidiasis which, in the early stages, responds to local nystatin or amphotericin; occasionally systemic candidiasis complicates the patient's terminal illness. Zoster and zoster-varicella are commonly seen particularly in the lymphomas. Zoster tends to be extensive and to leave deep scars. Viral warts may be more evident than in the healthy population and pudendal warts can be particularly troublesome. Bacterial skin and pulmonary infections are more frequent than in the healthy population and recrudescence of tuberculosis particularly during corticosteroid therapy is well recognised. Infections constitute a serious management problem and need to be treated promptly and energetically. In the severely immunosuppressed patients it is necessary to give patients broad-spectrum antibiotics, e.g. gentamicin/cloxacillin/cephalosporin immediately. A particularly vulnerable group that all doctors need to be aware of is the patients who have had a splenectomy as part of the staging process for Hodgkin's disease. They are prone to sudden fulminating bacteremia and meningitis particularly from the meningococcus and pneumococcus and can die within hours. Immuno-depressed patients are also prone to bizarre infections with organisms that normally have low pathogenicity – 'opportunist infections'. Examples are pulmonary infections with *Pneumocystis carinii* which fortunately gives a characteristic radiographic picture and is very responsive to co-trimoxazole and CNS infections such as torulosis and cryptococcosis. In relation to the latter the possibility of one of these strange infections should be considered in the event of grumbling headache or meningism or unexplained behaviour disturbance.

6. *Hyperuricaemia.* Because of the rapid turnover of cells particularly in the lymphoreticular diseases many patients have a raised blood uric acid level; this may rise alarmingly when there is rapid destruction of tumour tissue with real danger of uric acid nephropathy and renal failure. Gout is seldom a problem but does occur. Hyperuricaemia can be controlled by allopurinol and this is used routinely in patients at risk.

Specific effects

Patients at risk need to be regularly monitored, total cumulative doses need to be set, and change to an alternative drug has to be prompt if there is any suspicion of damage. The main effects to be aware of are as follows:

1. The *vinca alkaloids* regularly cause peripheral neuropathy, vincristine more so than vinblastine. When neuropathy develops during vincristine therapy change to vinblastine is the usual course. Most patients on long courses of vincristine lose deep reflexes and some have troublesome paraesthesiae in hands or feet which are slow to clear. Also well recognised is an autonomic neuropathy, which may be as bad as is seen in diabetic patients, with marked postural hypotension – this may also explain the constipation which some patients suffer in the early stages of therapy. The neuropathic effect of the vinca alkaloids is thought to relate to their action on microtubules.

2. *Doxorubicin* produces cardiomyopathy and the total dose must be limited. The effects, probably due to avid myocardial DNA binding, include arrhythmias, ECG changes and rapidly progressive congestive cardiac failure.

3. *Cyclophosphamide* occasionally causes haemorrhagic cystitis.

4. *Bleomycin* regularly causes lung fibrosis with high total doses. Fortunately adverse effects can be detected at an early stage with simple respiratory function tests before the lungs show radiographic abnormality. *Busulphan* can also cause lung fibrosis but this occurs

rarely; this drug may also cause increase in skin pigmentation and has been described as causing a clinical syndrome resembling Addison's disease.

5. *Methotrexate*. Apart from gastro-intestinal toxicity, methotrexate is prone to cause renal damage, particularly in patients already suffering renal impairment, and a chronic hepatitis leading to cirrhosis. Because its main action is to antagonise an enzyme (dihydrofolate reductase) in the metabolism of folic acid, megaloblastic change in the bone marrow has to be prevented by giving folinic acid some hours after high dosage methotrexate therapy.

COMMON CYTOTOXIC REGIMENS (Table 3)

The most successful combination chemotherapy regimens have been applied to the lymphoreticular malignancies. These are rare diseases and the average general practitioner may only see one new case every 10 to 15 years. However, with improved life expectancy and with the size of group practices, most doctors in the UK must be associated with patients who are having or have had protracted chemotherapy for leukaemia or malignant lymphoma. Unfortunately, cytotoxic chemotherapy has as yet little part to play in the management of the common solid tumours affecting breast, bronchus, gastro-intestinal tract and female

Table 3 Common cytotoxic regimens

A. The leukaemias

Acute lymphoblastic leukaemia
Prednisolone, vincristine → cranial irradiation + intrathecal methotrexate → prednisolone, vincristine, 6-mercaptopurine, methotrexate, cytosine arabinoside.

Acute myeloblastic leukaemia
Doxorubicin, thioguanine, cytosine arabinoside

Chronic lymphocytic leukaemia
Chlorambucil, prednisolone

Chronic myelocytic leukaemia
Busulphan

B. The lymphomas

Hodgkin's disease
MOPP – mustine, Onvocin/vincristine, procarbazine, prednisolone
or
MVPP – mustine, Velbe/vinblastine, procarbazine, prednisolone
ABVD – Adriamycin/doxorubicin, bleomycin, vincristine, dacarbazine

Non-Hodgkin's lymphomas
COP or CVP – cyclophosphamide, Oncovin/vincristine, prednisolone
CHOP – COP with the addition of doxorubicin
or COPAd

C. Solid tumours

Choriocarcinoma – methotrexate
Wilms' tumour – actinomycin D, vincristine
Neuroblastoma – cyclophosphamide, doxorubicin, vincristine
Lung – BCNU, cyclophosphamide, vincristine, procarbazine
Breast – cyclophosphamide, vincristine, fluorouracil → cyclophosphamide, vincristine and methotrexate
Head and neck – vincristine, doxorubicin, bleomycin, 5-fluorouracil, 6-mercaptopurine
Testicular teratoma – cisplatin, vinblastine, bleomycin

reproductive tract. This contrast between the major therapeutic advance seen in the lymphoreticular disorders on the one hand and the disappointing progress with the solid tumours on the other is probably a reflection of the rate of cell division in the different diseases; in the leukaemias, for example, the cells are multiplying rapidly and dividing within hours whereas in the solid tumours the malignant cells are known to spend long periods of weeks and months in the G_0 resting phase when they are inaccessible to cytotoxic drugs.

The leukaemias

The most exciting developments have been in the management of *acute lymphoblastic leukaemia* in children. Beginning with the first remissions in the late 1940s after the introduction of folic acid antagonists the picture has steadily improved. Now the average survival time is beyond five years and a high proportion of children, some 50 per cent, are getting protracted remissions and are disease-free at 10 years suggesting the possibility of 'cure'. The picture with adults is less impressive but still very gratifying. The treatment protocols have become progressively more sophisticated and in Britain have evolved through collaborative studies supervised by the Medical Research Council. It is possible only to give a general outline. Remission is induced mainly with prednisolone and vincristine and currently L-asparaginase and 6-mercaptopurine are also given in this period. Then, as a prophylactic measure, remission induction is followed by a series of intrathecal injections of methotrexate with cranial or cranio-spinal irradiation. Maintenance of remission then depends upon a series (usually eight) of 12-week cycles of treatment comprising prednisolone, vincristine, 6-mercaptopurine, methotrexate and cytosine arabinoside. The patients require close hospital supervision including regular bone marrow review. Now that meningeal relapse has become unusual with prophylactic therapy, a new problem has emerged, testicular relapse.

Acute myeloblastic leukaemia by comparison remains a more difficult condition to treat. Various regimens are under trial and one effective combination embraces doxorubicin, cytosine arabinoside and thioguanine. Some 60 per cent of patients go into complete remission but the average survival time is still in the region of one year; however about 20 per cent of the complete responders are achieving lasting remission beyond five years. Because of the poor prognosis for the majority of patients acute myeloblastic leukaemia is being studied as a condition possibly justifying bone marrow transplantation.

The treatment of the chronic leukaemias has changed little in the last 10 to 15 years. The lasting disease-free remission now being seen in some patients with acute leukaemia is not yet possible in the chronic group. In *chronic lymphocytic leukaemia* it is normal practice to withhold treatment until systemic disturbance or large nodes or marrow depression demand some action. Remission is usually induced with chlorambucil, often initially together with prednisolone. Partial remission can then be maintained with small doses of chlorambucil continuously; alternatively some experts choose to give intermittent courses of chlorambucil. Because of the immunodepression which characterises chronic lymphocytic leukaemia, long-term use of prednisolone is usually not advocated.

Chronic myelocytic leukaemia is best treated with busulphan which in most patients produces striking reduction of splenomegaly and improvement in the blood picture; again, maintenance can be either by regular busulphan therapy or intermittent courses. In the end the patients transform into an acute myeloblastic leukaemia and need to be treated as above but the prognosis is generally poor. In chronic myelocytic leukaemia the average survival time is around three to four years; in chronic lymphocytic leukaemia it is somewhat longer, particularly in the older age groups.

The lymphomas

The malignant lymphomas are another group of conditions where striking progress has been made using cytotoxic chemotherapy; the most consistent results are being achieved with Hodgkin's disease. In the management of the malignant lymphomas and particularly with Hodgkin's disease careful staging of the disease is required at the outset. This involves detailed haematological and radiographic assessment including abdominal lymphography. In a proportion of patients full staging may include laparotomy and splenectomy. The early stages of disease are best treated by radical radiotherapy. The more disseminated disease is treated mainly by combination therapy.

For *Hodgkin's disease* the MOPP (mustine, Oncovin/vincristine, procarbazine, prednisolone) or the MVPP (mustine, Velbe/vinblastine, procarbazine, prednisolone) regimen is used. The combination of drugs is usually given in two-week courses initially at four to six week intervals and then three monthly later. The necessary duration of treatment is uncertain but 6 to 10 courses are usually advised. About 75 per cent of patients with advanced disease get complete remission and about two-thirds of these are disease free at five years. When there is failure of therapy or relapse after satisfactory remission various alternative regimens may be applied. One example is the ABVD combination, Adriamycin/doxorubicin, bleomycin, vincristine and dacarbazine. This mixture needs careful supervision because of the cardiotoxicity of doxorubicin and the lung toxicity of bleomycin.

The *non-Hodgkin's lymphomas* are a miscellany of conditions. The well-differentiated small cell lymphocytic group may be slowly progressive and can be managed in the same manner as chronic lymphocytic leukaemia; sometimes no treatment is advised at first and then chlorambucil (initially with prednisolone) is introduced. The very aggressive poorly-differentiated lymphomas may respond initially to a regimen similar to that used in acute lymphoblastic leukaemia. For the majority in the intermediate group the favoured combinations are COP or CVP (cyclophosphamide, Oncovin/vincristine and prednisolone) sometimes with the addition of doxorubicin (COPAd or CHOP). The treatment is given in pulses over 6 to 10 courses as in Hodgkin's disease.

Solid tumours

In choriocarcinoma the treatment of choice is methotrexate (with folinic acid rescue to mitigate the antifolate effects on the bone marrow); the results are excellent with a 90 per cent complete remission rate and a high proportion of apparently permanent remissions in the complete responders. In general the chemotherapy of all other solid tumours is unsatisfactory although short-lived palliation can often be achieved and occasional unexpected long remissions are seen. The best results are being obtained in the embryonal tumours of childhood. For *Wilms' tumour* surgery and radiotherapy are followed by cyclical courses of actinomycin D and vincristine. In advanced cases of *neuroblastoma* initial radiotherapy is required for bulky primary disease and worthwhile remissions have been achieved using cyclophosphamide, doxorubicin and vincristine.

For *lung cancer* at present only the oat (small) cell carcinoma is showing much responsiveness but remission and prolongation of life is averaging only a few months. There are several regimens under trial, e.g. BCVP, a combination of BCNU, cyclophosphamide, vincristine and procarbazine. Likewise for advanced *breast cancer* a regimen combining cyclophosphamide, vincristine and fluorouracil followed after four to six days by cyclophosphamide, vincristine and methotrexate has been shown to give an average remission time of around six months. For advanced inoperable *head and neck cancer* similar results are obtained using several agents, e.g. vincristine, doxorubicin, bleomycin, fluorouracil, and 6-mercaptopurine. In extensive *testicular teratoma* the PVB combination (cisplatin, vinblastine and bleomycin) appears to be the most effective and manageable at present. Provisional reports suggest 80 to 90 per cent complete remissions with 50 per cent of these being sustained. If this is confirmed this could prove to be a major development.

Perhaps the most difficult topic is the use of adjuvant chemotherapy in the management of early cancer, e.g. early breast cancer. It has to be emphasised that this still has to be thoroughly evaluated. Prolongation of remission can be achieved but it is still not clear if the natural history of the disease is significantly affected. CMF (cyclophosphamide, methotrexate and fluorouracil) and similar combinations are being studied. The loss of hair and marrow depression which attends such treatment regimens has to be weighed against any possible advantageous effect.

Malignant effusions

The rapid re-accumulation of fluid in the pleural or peritoneal space can be a distressing problem in patients with terminal malignant disease who may yet have many months to live. Various procedures have been tried including the instillation of radioactive isotopes and of talc; of the cytotoxic agents, nitrogen mustard and thiotepa produce relief in some cases. Recently, the instillation of both bleomycin and doxorubicin have been reported as being effective but tetracycline (not generally regarded as having antitumour activity) is described as producing benefit in a similar proportion of patients. Most patients are likely to get some temporary benefit from one of the foregoing procedures but it remains to be determined which is the best and the safest.

CONCLUSION

Great advances have been made in the last 25 years and particularly in the last 10 years. The lymphoreticular malignancies are now very rewarding conditions to treat. For the common forms of cancer cytotoxic chemotherapy still has only a limited contribution to make and because unpleasant toxic effects are not too far removed from worthwhile therapeutic benefit careful judgement must be exercised in deciding when to treat and when not to treat.

Chapter 16 Symptom-control in terminal cancer

R. G. TWYCROSS MA, DM, FRCP

INTRODUCTION

In cancer, symptoms are not necessarily caused by the malignant process. Even when they are, different mechanisms may be operative and treatment for the same symptoms may vary considerably from patient to patient. Moreover, many symptoms are multifactorial in aetiology; it is necessary, therefore, to identify the various factors involved and then to seek to correct those that are reversible. In this way, though the underlying pathological process remains unaltered, it is generally possible to relieve a symptom either completely or to a considerable extent.

Treatment begins with an explanation by the doctor of the reason(s) for each symptoms. To learn that the doctor understands what is going on is reassuring and does much to reduce the impact of the symptom on the sufferer. If explanation is omitted, the patient continues to think that his condition is totally shrouded in mystery, and this is frightening. Sometimes it is appropriate to discuss treatment options with the patient and to decide together on the immediate course of action. Parallel explanation and discussion with the relatives is also important.

GENERAL CONSIDERATIONS

Treatment should not be limited to drugs. For example, hand cream or lanolin applied to dry, itchy skin two or three times a day and the use of emulsifying ointment instead of soap will relieve pruritus in most patients (Table 1, p. 176). When a drug is indicated, it should be:

1. Individually determined in terms of choice of medication and dose.
2. Administered prophylactically on a time-contingent basis related to the modal duration of action, and not 'as required'.
3. Carefully supervised to maximise benefit, to minimise unwanted effects, and to achieve optimum compliance.

Choice of drug

The choice of drug to relieve a given symptom is governed by a number of considerations. For example, the choice of an anti-emetic depends on:

1. the underlying pathological mechanism
2. whether used purely prophylactically
   (e.g. when a narcotic is prescribed for the first time)
3. the severity of vomiting
4. the degree of co-existent anxiety
5. whether the patient is drowsy
6. the desirability of anti-cholinergic side-effects
   (e.g. the drying up of saliva in patients with troublesome drooling).

Timing

Narcotic analgesics should usually be administered every four hours. Most other drugs, however, do not need to be given so frequently. Yet, to avoid an excessively complex regimen – one drug four-hourly, another drug six-hourly – and so on – it may be sensible to give a six-hourly drug every four hours, though possibly in smaller dosage, because the patient is receiving a narcotic. Although the duration of the effect of the drug is positively correlated with its plasma half-life, the relation is not linear. When taken regularly, methadone has a half-life of between 20 and 60 hours, compared with 2 to 2.5 hours for morphine. However, the duration of the analgesic effect of methadone is generally only some 6 to 8 hours, that is, 1.5 to 2 times that of morphine. Even so, generally drugs with a long plasma half-life need to be given less frequently. The severity of the symptom also tends to affect frequency of administration. Thus, although for most patients prescribed diazepam, a single daily (bedtime) dose is adequate, in those with overwhelming anxiety more frequent administration is often necessary. Similarly, with oral doses of morphine above 120mg or injections of diamorphine above 60mg, it is sometimes necessary to reduce the interval between administration from four to three hours.

Supervision

With narcotic analgesics, psychotropic drugs and laxatives in particular, it is not usually possible to predict the optimum dose exactly. Dose adjustments will therefore be necessary, especially over the first week or two. This should be anticipated and arrangements made for continuing close supervision and follow-up. Whenever the prescription of an additional drug is considered, it is important to ask:

1. Is it possible for the patient to stop one or more of the preparations he is already taking?
2. Is it possible to substitute one drug for any two of those presently or about to be prescribed?

It is useful discipline to try to keep the number of drugs to be taken regularly to four or less; this tally not including once a day drugs such as laxatives and night hypnotics.

It follows from what has been said that precise guidelines are necessary to achieve maximum patient co-operation, particularly when narcotic analgesics are prescribed. 'Take as much as you like, as often as you like' is a recipe for anxiety, poor symptom-control and maximum side-effects. When morphine is prescribed, the need for a regular administration every four hours must be emphasised. The first and last dose of the day should be 'anchored' to the patient's waking- and bed-times. The best additional times during the day are generally 10 a.m., 2 p.m., 6 p.m., unless the patient wakes or goes to bed exceptionally late. The drug regimen should be written out in full for the patient and his family to work from, stating times to be taken, names of drug, reason for use, ('for pain', 'for bowels', etc) and dose (*x*ml, *y* tablets; (Fig. 16/1)). The patient and the family should be warned about possible initial side-effects and follow-up arrangements confirmed.

Expectations

Although most symptoms respond completely or to a large extent to a combination of drug and non-drug measures, it is sometimes necessary to compromise in order to avoid unacceptable unwanted effects. For example, anti-cholinergic effects such as dry mouth or visual disturbance may occasionally be limiting factors; and, in relation to bowel obstruction, it is often better to aim to reduce the incidence of vomiting to once or twice a day rather than to seek absolute control.

Increasing weakness, although it may be associated with hypercalcaemia or paraplegia (Table 2, p. 177), generally means that the battle against the malignant process has been lost. It is at this stage that the patient is forced to face the fact that death is inevitable. Equally, it is a time when support and com-

NAME ...... Mr John D. .... DATE ...... 28 March 1980 ..

On Waking	PAIN MEDICINE (20mg in 10ml)	10ml
	NYSTATIN	2ml
	FLURBIPROFEN (50mg)	1 tablet
10.00 a.m.	PAIN MEDICINE	10ml
	DIOCTYL FORTE (for bowels)	1 tablet
	DORBANEX (for bowels)	2 capsules
	PREDNISOLONE (5mg, for appetite)	1 tablet
	NYSTATIN	
2.00 p.m.	PAIN MEDICINE	10ml
	PREDNISOLONE	1 tablet
	NYSTATIN	2ml
	FLURBIPROFEN	1 tablet
6.00 p.m.	PAIN MEDICINE	10ml
	PREDNISOLONE	1 tablet
	NYSTATIN	2ml
Bedtime	PAIN MEDICINE	10ml
	NYSTATIN	2ml
	FLURBIPROFEN	1 tablet
	CHLORPROMAZINE (25mg)	3 tablets

If awake in the night with pain –
PAIN MEDICINE 10ml

If you get pain between times –
PAIN MEDICINE 10ml

Fig. 16/1 Example of written instructions given to outpatients

panionionship are of paramount importance. Although the doctor may feel powerless in the face of death, his continued attendance, indicating that he will stand by the patient no matter what happens, is of inestimable value to the patient, the family and other staff.

PAIN CONTROL

Assessment

Pain may be limited to one site or be multifactorial. Each site where pain is felt should be recorded. A body image is of value as a baseline for future reference and in considering the underlying pain mechanisms (Fig. 16/2) because treatment varies with the cause of the pain. Moreover, a diagnosis of cancer does not necessarily mean that the malignant process is the cause of pain. Constipation, peptic ulcer, pressure sores, cystitis, and musculo-skeletal disorders may be responsible, and each benefits from specific treatment (Table 3, p. 177).

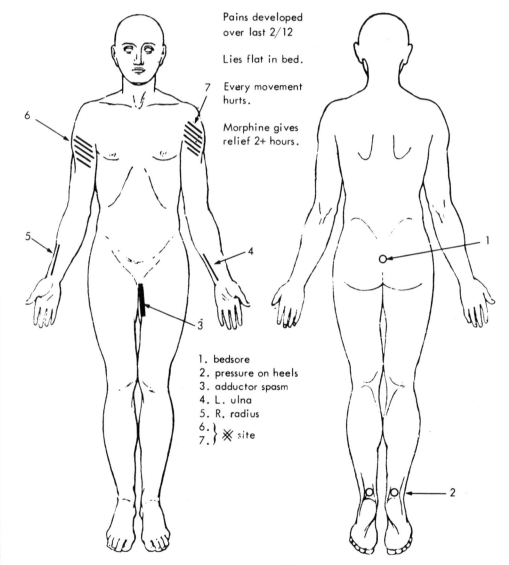

BODY CHART	Hospital No. Surname First Names
Ca. Prostate	R.M. age. 65 13.7.77

Path✻ L. femur 26/5, R. humerus 30/5, L. humerus 20/6 ⟶ all pinned etc.

Pains developed
over last 2/12

Lies flat in bed.

7 Every movement
hurts.

Morphine gives
relief 2+ hours.

6

5

4

3

1

2

1. bedsore
2. pressure on heels
3. adductor spasm
4. L. ulna
5. R. radius
6. }
7. } ✻ site

<u>Note</u> jumps when touched.   Use analgesics + diazepam.

Fig. 16/2 Pain chart of 65-year-old male with carcinoma of prostate. Note, adductor spasm is usually protective, i.e. secondary to involvement of the pubis; treatment is as for bone pain, though sometimes diazepam may also be necessary

Patients often put on a brave face for the doctor; moreover, although in severe pain, they may not look distressed. Accordingly, intensity of pain should be assessed not only by the patient's description but also by discovering what drugs have failed to relieve, whether sleep is disturbed, and in what way activity is limited ('How long is it since you went out?' 'What are you doing around the house?'). In addition, the patient's spouse should be interviewed. Often only his or her comments give the true picture though, when the pain is relieved, the patient frequently concurs spontaneously with the spouse's earlier opinion.

A patient who is obviously in pain and who says or implies that 'it's all pain, doctor' is best thought of as having overwhelming pain; that is, very severe pain compounded by anxiety, depression, and loss of morale. In this situation, detailed assessment is difficult. The patient should be given an appropriate dose of diazepam and diamorphine by injection and reviewed later. The probability that the initial prescription will be inadequate increases with pain intensity. Hence, patients should be reassessed within an hour or so if the pain is overwhelming, or after one or two days if it is severe or moderate. Should troublesome or unacceptable side-effects result, it may be necessary to change the treatment. In addition, relief of a major pain may allow a second, less severe pain to become apparent.

Treatment
Relief of pain may be achieved by one or more of the following methods:

1. Modification of the pathological process.
2. Elevation of the pain threshold.
3. Interruption of pain pathways.
4. Immobilisation.

MODIFICATION OF PATHOLOGICAL PROCESS
Osseous metastases is the main cause of pain in the majority of patients with carcinoma of the breast, bronchus, or prostate. Bone pain is also common in carcinoma of the kidney and thyroid and multiple myeloma. Modification of the pathological process by radiation, chemotherapy, or hormone treatment should be considered, even in far-advanced cancer, though it is important to ensure that the treatment is not worse than the disease. Moreover, because androgens or oestrogens have been prescribed, this does not mean that analgesics should be withheld; a combined approach should be employed. If relief is obtained and there are no complaints of 'breakthrough' pain, the drug regimen can then be modified –

a less potent preparation prescribed or the analgesic withdrawn completely.

Radiation therapy gives partial or even complete relief in 90 per cent of patients experiencing bone pain, and generally it may be administered in a single, non-fractionated dose. A recent study showed that, although patients treated by a single dose commonly had more nausea and vomiting, many of those receiving fractionated treatment were exhausted by the end of the course (Penn, 1976). Fractionation is probably necessary only when there is a high risk of nausea and vomiting despite prophylactic anti-emetics, e.g. when irradiating in the region of the stomach and when treating half or more of the pelvis.

ELEVATION OF PAIN THRESHOLD
Pain is a dual phenomenon, one part is the perception of the sensation and the other is the patient's emotional reaction to it. This means that attention must be paid to non-drug factors that modulate pain threshold, such as anxiety and depression, as well as to the correct use of analgesics and other drugs (Table 4, p. 178). The use of analgesics is best seen as but one way – generally a powerful way – of elevating the pain threshold, though a failure to allow the patient to express his fears and anxieties can cause otherwise relievable pain to remain intractable.

Most patients fear the process of dying – 'Will it hurt?', 'Will I suffocate?' – and many fear death itself. These fears tend to remain unspoken unless the patient is given the opportunity to express them. The doctor must provide time and opportunity for the patient to talk about his progress or lack of it. One group of general practitioners discovered that 'as the doctor-patient relationship improved, many doctors found they could reduce the drugs. As the true diagnosis of the patient's pain became clear and the patient was helped to deal with the pain of dying, there was less need for sedatives, tranquillisers and analgesics. This almost certainly reflected the doctor's own feelings. Once he was able to deal with his own pain of the patient dying ... the need for drugs became less. In many instances there was, at the same time, an increased demand on the doctor's time. A number of well-documented cases bear this out' (Harte, personal communication).

Tranquillisers have only a limited place in terminal cancer care, though patients who are markedly anxious usually require a combination of a tranquilliser and an analgesic in the same way as the patient with overwhelming pain.

INTERRUPTION OF PAIN PATHWAYS

A discussion of this aspect of cancer pain control is beyond the scope of this article. It should be noted, however, that analgesics alone are often effective in relieving pain due to nerve compression. If the response is poor, however, the use of prednisolone is recommended, initially 10mg three times a day. This reduces the degree of nerve compression by decreasing inflammatory swelling around the growth. In patients with a prognosis of only a few weeks, this may be sufficient to circumvent the need for chemical neurolysis. In those with a longer life expectancy, the pain may return as the tumour continues to grow; in these a nerve block will be required. In patients whose morale is low or precarious, it is advisable to warn that a block may become necessary in order to avoid loss of confidence should the pain return.

IMMOBILISATION

Some patients continue to experience pain on movement despite analgesics, other drugs, radiotherapy, and nerve blocks. In these, the situation may be improved by suggesting commonsense modifications to daily activity. For example, a man may continue to struggle to stand when shaving unless the doctor suggests that sitting would be a good idea. Such a suggestion is accepted more readily if accompanied by a simple explanation of why weight-bearing precipitates or exacerbates the pain. Individually designed corsets or plastic supports for patients with multiple collapsed vertebrae or Thomas' splints for femoral pain are occasionally necessary to overcome intolerable pain on movement in bedridden patients.

Internal fixation or the insertion of a prosthesis should be considered if a pathological fracture of a long bone occurs, as these measures obviate the need for prolonged bed rest and pain usually is relieved. The decision whether or not to treat surgically depends on the patient's general condition; whereas in bronchial carcinoma or malignant melanoma pathological fracture often presages death, in breast cancer this is not generally so, particularly if the tumour is hormone-sensitive. The median survival after the first or only pathological fracture associated with breast cancer is about six months, with a range of two months to four years (Twycross, 1977).

Analgesics

'Four-hourly as required' has no place in the treatment of persistent pain; continuous pain requires regular preventive therapy (Fig. 16/3). The initial dose should be increased progressively until the patient becomes pain-free, and the next dose given before the effect of the previous one has worn off. In this way, it is possible to erase the memory and fear of pain. As patients do not like taking tablets or receiving injections constantly, a four-hour interval between doses should be regarded as the norm, though occasionally more frequent

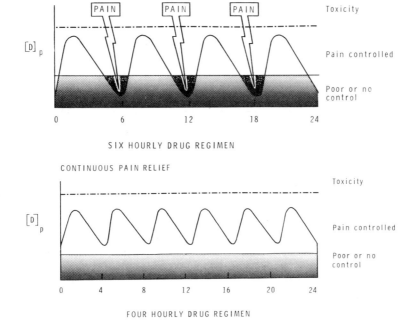

Fig. 16/3 Diagram to illustrate the result of 'as required' and overspaced time-contingent medication compared with regular four-hourly morphine sulphate

administration may be necessary. Many patients do not require a dose in the middle of the night, particularly if a larger dose is given at bedtime. If necessary, however, a patient should be wakened to take it (or set his alarm) rather than let him wake later complaining of pain.

The effective analgesic dose varies considerably from patient to patient (Table 5, p. 178); the right dose of any analgesic is that which gives adequate relief for at least three or preferably four or more hours. 'Maximum' or 'recommended' doses, derived mainly from postoperative parenteral single-dose studies, are not applicable in advanced cancer. Patients usually will accept two, sometimes three, analgesic tablets per administration together with additional medication; four or more tablets of the same preparation are not generally acceptable. Thus, if two tablets are not adequate, a more potent alternative should be prescribed. Pain unrelieved by other measures, not short-life expectancy, is the primary criterion in far-advanced cancer for the prescription of morphine or other potent narcotic analgesic.

CHOICE OF ANALGESIC

When the non-narcotic analgesics, aspirin and paracetamol, fail to relieve, a weak narcotic such as codeine, dihydrocodeine or dextropropoxyphene should be prescribed alone or with aspirin or paracetamol (Table 6, p. 178). However, if the patient is clearly incapacitated by pain, for example, housebound or bedbound, a more potent narcotic almost certainly will be necessary. In these circumstances, the weak narcotics should be bypassed.

When one of the weak narcotics fails to relieve adequately, a more potent analgesic should be given. To move laterally from one preparation to another of approximately equal efficacy is bad practice and, as new tablet after new tablet fails to achieve the hoped for relief, is likely to lead to despair in both patient and doctor.

Pethidine and pentazocine should not be used. The former has a relatively short duration of action – some two or three hours – and by mouth in the doses usually given (25–50mg) is not a potent analgesic. Pentazocine shares these disadvantages but, in addition, is an agonist-antagonist. If used in association with another (more agonistic) narcotic, it will have an antagonistic rather than an additive effect. Moreover, the incidence of psychotomimetic effects is unacceptably high.

Pharmacologically, oral morphine is the next logical step and, indeed, is the strong analgesic of choice at most hospices (Table 7, p. 179 and Fig. 16/4).

Yet, many doctors feel reluctant to prescribe it at this stage because of fears of tolerance, addiction, impair-

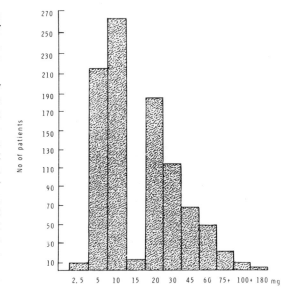

Maximum dose of oral morphine sulphate

Fig. 16/4 Histogram of maximum four-hourly doses of orally administered morphine sulphate in 955 patients at St Christopher's Hospice (1978–79). Median dose = 10mg. *Note*: 75+ means 75, 80 or 90mg, and 100+ means 100, 110 or 120mg

ment of mental faculties, and respiratory depression. However, when used within the context of total patient care, tolerance is not a practical problem even if morphine is prescribed for several months (Fig. 16/5). Physical dependence may develop, but it does not prevent the downward adjustment of dose should this become feasible as a result of non-drug treatment. The majority of patients may experience drowsiness when morphine is prescribed initially, but unless the patient is extremely ill, this usually passes within a few days of being stabilised on a steady dose. Significant or troublesome respiratory depression is a rare problem. Moreover, at equi-analgesic doses, the degree of respiratory depression does not vary significantly from strong narcotic to strong narcotic.

The only valid reason for using intermediates, such as papaveretum and dipipanone, is convenience; if the patient is still at work, he may find a bottle of medicine more cumbersome than tablets. On the other hand, the use of tablets introduces a 'rigidity' factor, as the dose can be only a certain number of tablets. By varying the strength or volume of a solution to be taken, it is much easier to balance the dose more precisely against the patient's needs. Similarly, levorphanol, and

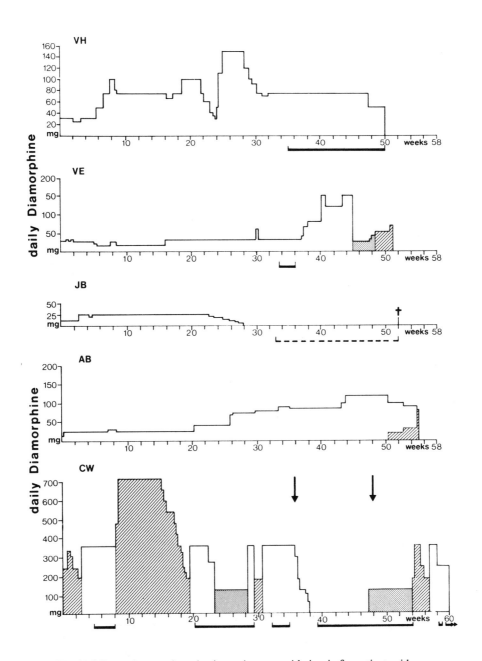

Fig. 16/5 Change in narcotic analgesic requirements with time in five patients with advanced cancer. *Open areas:* diamorphine by mouth; *hatched areas:* diamorphine by injection; *dotted areas:* other narcotic analgesic (V.E., C.W.); *arrow:* phenol-in-glycerine nerve block; *horizontal bar:* time spent at home. V.H., V.E., and A.B. received diamorphine up to the time of death; C.W. is still alive. Similar patterns are seen with morphine

phenazocine should be regarded simply as convenient alternatives to morphine. By mouth, on a weight-to-weight basis, they are several times more potent than morphine (Table 8, p. 180), and tend to have a longer duration of action. Methadone, because of its prolonged plasma half-life, should be used with care, if at all, in the elderly or extremely debilitated.

The practice of combining narcotic analgesics cannot be recommended, as a higher dose of one of the preparations will be equally efficacious. The custom in some hospitals of administering a potent narcotic such as morphine alternately with a weak narcotic such as codeine or dihydrocodeine (so that the patient receives something every two hours) is to be condemned. It stems from a gross lack of understanding of narcotic analgesic clinical pharmacology and ties a patient unnecessarily to a two-hourly regimen when, in practice, a four-hourly one almost certainly will be as effective.

DIAMORPHINE

Diamorphine (diacetylmorphine, heroin) enjoys a vogue in some centres but is no more efficacious than morphine when given by mouth. *In vivo*, deacetylation to monoacetylmorphine and morphine occurs rapidly. Despite this, oral diamorphine is about 1.5 times more potent than oral morphine because of more complete absorption. Diamorphine is unstable in solution and has a shelf-life ($t_{10\%}$) of about six weeks in simple solution at room temperature. On the other hand, if dispensed in combination with a phenothiazine syrup (particularly chlorpromazine), the $t_{10\%}$ is shortened to 10 to 14 days. However, since the degradation products are pharmacologically active and not more than a two-week supply usually is dispensed, the limited shelf-life of diamorphine is mainly of theoretical importance, even in this situation.

Co-analgesics (Table 9, p. 181)

CORTICOSTEROIDS

Corticosteroids are widely used in far-advanced cancer (Table 10, p. 181). Inclusion in this list does not imply that their use is the sole or most important treatment in these situations. It simply means that the use of corticosteroids may be of benefit and should be considered as a treatment option to be tried alone or in association with other recognised measures. In the majority of patients with, for example, incipient paraplegia, superior vena caval obstruction or haemoptysis, a corticosteroid should be given in association with radiation therapy. Similarly, a corticosteroid is not generally the treatment of choice for malignant effusions but, where other measures have failed or seem inappropriate, it may be tried with or without a chemotherapeutic agent.

The use of a corticosteroid as a co-analgesic should be considered wherever there is a large tumour mass within a relatively confined space. There is often an oedematous area around a tumour, and pressure on neighbouring veins and lymphatics may lead to further local or regional swelling. In other words, the total tumour mass = neoplasm + surrounding hyperaemic oedema. Corticosteroids reduce this oedema, thereby reducing the total tumour mass.

The classic situation is that of headache caused by raised intracranial pressure in association with cerebral neoplasm. A combination of an analgesic and a corticosteroid, with or without a diuretic and elevation of the head of the bed, relieves the headache. Other central nervous symptoms or signs often improve as well; the improvement lasting for weeks or months after starting treatment. As already indicated, corticosteroids also help to relieve the pain of nerve compression.

Metastatic arthralgia (Table 10, p. 181) refers to the pain caused by metastatic involvement of the acetabulum (relatively common) or glenoid fossa (relatively uncommon). In addition to radiation therapy, maximum relief is sometimes obtained only by the combined use of a narcotic, a non-steroidal anti-inflammatory drug, and a corticosteroid. Alternatively, injections into the joint space of a long-acting preparation of either methylprednisolone or triamcinolone hexacetonide may be considered.

Patients with cerebral oedema usually are given 4mg dexamethasone three or four times a day initially. This drug is seven times more potent than prednisolone and has less mineralo-corticoid activity. No controlled comparisons, however, have been made. In other situations, prednisolone usually is given in a dose of 5–10mg three times a day. The dose needed to achieve maximum benefit varies from patient to patient. It is often advisable to begin with a higher dose to avoid missing a treatment effect; the dose can be adjusted downward after one or two weeks, or sooner if unacceptable, unwanted effects occur.

NEUROLEPTICS

This term refers to the phenothiazines and butyrophenones. In terminal cancer, the main indication for a phenothiazine is as an anti-emetic. However, in patients with an appreciable psychological component to their pain – for example, the patient with lung cancer experiencing both pain and dyspnoea who fears death by suffocation, or the woman who feels that her fungating breast cancer is jeopardising her relationship with her husband – chlorpromazine used in conjunction with oral morphine often yields better results than a higher dose of morphine alone. If chlorpromazine causes troublesome anti-cholinergic side-effects (Table 11, p. 182), it may be necessary to use prochlorperazine or haloperidol with diazepam, though in the absence of nausea and vomiting, diazepam can, of course, be used alone. In addition, phenothiazines have a definite place in the relief of a number of less common pain states and other symptoms associated with malignant disease.

ANXIOLYTIC SEDATIVES

From Table 12, p. 182, it will be seen that at Sir Michael Sobell House diazepam commonly is preferred to chlorpromazine in many situations. Diazepam generally is used as the drug of choice where there is muscle spasm or tension and chlorpromazine in the less well-defined discomforts of rectal and bladder 'tenesmoid' pain caused by unresected primary tumour, or by local recurrence after abdomino-perineal resection or total cystectomy. Other centres use chlorpromazine more widely, stressing the depressing tendency of diazepam. In our experience, neither drug is notably depressing, possibly because of the counteracting effect of the symptomatic relief. However, it is important to be aware that patients receiving these drugs may become depressed and that an anti-depressant may be required.

ANTIDEPRESSANTS

The need for an antidepressant increases the longer a patient is maintained on a narcotic analgesic. Whether the onset of depression is precipitated by the protracted terminal illness itself or is a side-effect of long-continued treatment with a narcotic and a phenothiazine is not clear. It is important to be aware that depression not only can, but frequently does, supervene in patients receiving so-called 'euphoriant' drugs, and a trial of therapy should be initiated when it does. Amitriptyline is the most commonly used anti-depressant. Treatment should be started with half the usual adult dose, as debilitated patients commonly become confused and disorientated if a high dose is given initially, particularly if they are receiving a narcotic or another psychotropic drug.

As might be expected, not all patients respond to an antidepressant. If no effect is noted after a reasonable trial of therapy, treatment should be stopped. Alternative measures to be considered include:

1. Use of corticosteroids, e.g. prednisolone
2. Prescription of dexamphetamine
3. Change of environment, e.g. temporary admission to a hospice or similar unit.

Support and companionship are always necessary particularly in cases where the depression is more properly described as sadness at the thought of leaving behind family, friends, and all that is familiar.

Tricyclic antidepressants are of benefit in terminal care in other ways (Table 13, p. 182), particularly as the main analgesic agent in managing superficial dysaesthesia and post-herpetic neuralgia. Either amitriptyline or clomipramine may be used beginning with a dose of 25mg at night and increasing every few days until unacceptable side-effects occur (dry mouth, drowsiness, confusion), or the pain is alleviated.

PSYCHOSTIMULANTS

Two controlled trials have recently shown that there is no benefit in the routine use of cocaine with morphine. The addition of cocaine made no difference to pain, mood or drowsiness (Twycross, 1979; Melzack et al 1979). Many physicians, however, have seen patients – usually elderly – who have become restless, agitated and confused when prescribed a morphine-cocaine mixture and whose symptoms have persisted until the cocaine was withdrawn. In view of this cocaine should not be prescribed concomitantly as was former practice. Instead, the patient is told that he may feel drowsy for two or three days following the start of treatment, but the drowsiness will lessen. If drowsiness persists and is troublesome to the patient it is occasionally worth prescribing 2.5–5mg dexamphetamine once or twice daily. First, the patient's existing medication should be reviewed. If a second drug (e.g. chlorpromazine, diazepam, nitrazepam, flurazepam) is being used which can cause drowsiness, the dose should be reduced or a less sedative alternative prescribed.

Results

With time, attention to detail, and close supervision, it is always possible to relieve the pain of terminal cancer, either completely or considerably. However, whereas relief is obtained within two or three days in some patients, in others it may take three or four weeks of inpatient treatment to achieve satisfactory control, particularly in those whose pain is made worse by movement and in the very anxious and depressed. Even so, it is possible to achieve at least some improvement within one to two days in all patients.

Since some pains respond more readily than others, improvement should be assessed in relation to each pain. The ultimate aim is complete freedom from pain, but there will be less disappointment and, paradoxically, more success, if one sets a series of targets in practice. The initial target should be pain-free, sleepful nights. Many patients have not had a good night's rest for weeks or months and are exhausted and demoralised. To sleep through the night pain-free and wake refreshed is a boost to both the doctor's and patient's morale. Next, one aims for relief at rest in bed or chair during the day. The final goal is freedom from pain on movement. The former is always possible eventually; the latter is not.

Cancer is a progressive pathological process, so new pains may develop or old ones re-emerge. It should not be assumed that a fresh complaint of pain merely calls for an increase in a previously satisfactory analgesic regimen; it demands reassessment, an explanation to the patient and, only then, modification of drug therapy or other intervention.

CONFUSION

The ability of a family to cope with a death in the home depends in large measure on the doctor's ability to help patient and family understand and cope with the confusional symptoms that ultimately occur in most cases. Confusional states are characterised by 'clouding of consciousness', are usually associated with drowsiness, and manifest as one or more of the following:

1. poor concentration
2. impairment of recent memory
3. disorientation
4. misperceptions (often) ± paranoid delusions
5. hallucinations (sometimes)
6. rambling and incoherent speech
7. restlessness ± noisy/aggressive behaviour.

Confusional states tend to be variable in degree and intensity. In some patients, symptoms are never more than mild and remain intermittent. Those associated with metabolic disturbances (renal failure, hepatic failure, intestinal obstruction) tend to be more prolonged and more marked than those associated with terminal pneumonia which by definition is self-limiting.

Disorientation for time and, to a lesser extent, for place, is eventually the norm for the dying. Explanation and reassurance is all that is usually necessary:

'When someone is not well, the mind often works more slowly, and doesn't always manage to stay in gear.'

'Most patients are like you – they lose track of time. After all, when you are not up and about and working, time is not so important, is it?'

Misperceptions are common too. A similar type of explanation is generally all that is necessary:

'It is something we all do at times but, when you are ill, it tends to happen more often'.

'You are not losing your mind/going mad; this sort of thing can happen to any of us when we are poorly'.

Most complaints of hallucinations, whether from the patient himself, the family or nurses, turn out in practice to be misperceptions, nightmares or vivid daydreams (Stedeford, 1978, 1980). It is necessary therefore to ask the patient and/or the family about the 'hallucinations'. Commonly, if they are misperceptions, explanation by the doctor is all that is necessary by way of treatment. However, when these phenomena are clearly expressions of anxiety about dying and death, anxiolytic medication is often helpful, together with continuing discussion about the experiences and possible psychological precipitating factors. Blunderbuss therapy with chlorpromazine – a common medical response to this situation – may help to suppress hallucinations but may also increase the tendency to misperceive by causing further clouding of consciousness. It is important to remember that most confusional states in the dying are multifactorial in origin (Table 14, p. 183). In each case, consider which factors are operative as some may be readily correctable (Table 15, p. 184).

DYSPNOEA

Careful assessment will usually indicate the main reason(s) for a patient's breathlessness. Specific causes such as heart failure benefit by traditional measures. In most patients, though, dyspnoea is the result of a number of factors, some of which are quite clearly irreversible, for example, chronic obstructive airways disease, anaemia of chronic disease and weakness. Explanation always helps, and discussion with both patient and family about ways in which the patient's lifestyle may or should be modified is an important part of treatment.

For patients with carcinomatous lymphangitis, or who are wheezing because of neoplastic pressure on one or more major bronchus, a trial of corticosteroids should be instituted. In many cases dyspnoea is secondary to pleural effusion and paracentesis may be necessary. If, because of irreversible compression atelectasis, paracentesis results in a little benefit, or the patient is too ill for such treatment, symptomatic measures should be used. Phenothiazine and benzodiazepine tranquillisers help reduce the anxiety and fear that accompany dyspnoea. Morphine, with its direct depressant effect on the respiratory centre, is of particular value when the patient is markedly tachypnoeic, e.g. 2.5–15mg every four hours by mouth.

ALIMENTARY SYMPTOMS

Dry mouth

Many patients, if asked, complain of a dry mouth. While it may be an indication of hypercalcaemia, it is more usually multifactorial in aetiology (Table 16, p. 184). Control of nausea and vomiting, encouraging the patient to drink more (what is his favourite beverage?), and treating moniliasis if present, will go a long way to easing the discomfort. In some patients who are sensitive to the anticholinergic effects of psychotropic and other drugs, it may be possible to modify their medication.

When modification is either not possible or fails to relieve, measures to stimulate the flow of saliva and/or to lubricate the mouth should be considered, including smoking, chewing gum, sucking acid (lemon) drops or ice chips, sucking glycerine and blackcurrant lozenges, and the avoidance of dry food.

Other treatments include the use of vitamin C effervescent tablets in a glass of water with meals, and also a mixture of one part simple syrup with four parts olive oil and a few drops of lemon essence, to use as a lubricant for the mouth two or three times daily. Regular oral toilet is especially necessary in the very ill. Artificial saliva (Glandosane), available as a convenient aerosol spray in two tastes (plain and lemon), is a great help in patients who have lost most or all salivary function as a result of surgery or radiotherapy.

Hiccup

Although, strictly speaking, this is a respiratory symptom, it is dealt with here because the commonest cause is gastric distension (Table 17, p. 185). Most traditional remedies rely on a 'gating' mechanism which is triggered by pharyngeal stimulation. In Oxford, Asilone – an antacid preparation containing dimethicone (a defoaming agent) – is regarded as the treatment of choice but, at other hospices, drinking from the 'wrong' side of the cup or the use of granulated sugar have pride of place (Table 17, p. 185). It is rare to need to prescribe chlorpromazine but, in 'squashed stomach syndrome' (*vide infra*) or if gastric stasis is thought to be relevant, metoclopramide is prescribed either t.i.d. and nocte, or with morphine four-hourly.

Anorexia

Anorexia may be caused by the fear of precipitating vomiting by eating; it may also be the prodrome of nausea and vomiting. Careful history-taking will indicate if it is the former; the latter may have to be assessed by a therapeutic trial of an anti-emetic. Being offered too much or pressed to eat more by an over-anxious spouse may also provoke anorexia. Often it is possible to achieve improvement in appetite by attending to the various contributory factors (Table 18, p. 186). It is often worth considering a 7- to 10-day trial of prednisolone 5–10mg t.i.d. However, when close to death, giving the patient 'permission' not to eat and the family 'permission' not to force-feed is often the most appropriate form of management:

'Just eat what you fancy – and not too much. Whatever you do, don't eat for Science's sake, my sake, or even your wife's sake. Trying too hard is only counter productive'.

'Provided you are taking plenty of fluid, I shall be happy; solid food is not important for you at the moment'.

One cause of anorexia is early satiation. This occurs commonly in patients with hepatomegaly and, if only to help in doctor-patient communication, can be described as 'squashed stomach syndrome' (Table 19, p. 187). The aim of treatment is to avoid relative overdistension of the stomach, this being the cause of the patient's symptoms.

Nausea and vomiting

Vomiting occurs in about 25 per cent of patients with terminal cancer. The treatment varies according to the underlying cause(s) (Table 20, p. 188). If the cause is intracranial, cyclizine (50–100mg four-hourly) is the drug of choice as this acts directly on the emetic centre. If related to stimulation of the bowel, metoclopramide (10mg four-hourly) is often the best anti-emetic as it enhances peristalsis in the upper gastro-intestinal tract, speeds gastric emptying and increases lower oesophageal sphincter tone. It has no anti-cholinergic properties and is ineffective against vomiting of intracranial aetiology. For nausea or vomiting of chemical origin, (neoplastic, toxic, biochemical, pharmacological, chemotherapeutic, radiological), metoclopramide is often efficacious. However, the anxious patient will respond better to a drug with sedative properties such as a phenothiazine.

In Oxford, haloperidol 0.5mg two or three times daily is regarded as the drug of choice for chemically induced vomiting. In this dose, it is non-sedative and generally does not cause dryness of the mouth. If the patient is experiencing radiation induced emesis, a higher dose (e.g. 1.5mg b.i.d./t.i.d.) is indicated, with or without pyridoxine. If associated with chemotherapy, 1.5mg four-hourly (or 3mg eight-hourly) may be necessary. In doses of 3mg or more a day, there is a danger of parkinsonian side-effects. If these occur, try to reduce the dose and/or prescribe orphenadrine 50–100mg b.i.d. Cyclizine is of little value in radiation induced vomiting (Stoll, 1962).

When the bowel is obstructed, anti-emetics are generally of little value (unless the vomiting is partly due to chemical factors), though chlorpromazine seems to help on occasion. The right approach is partly to paralyse the bowel in order to prevent the painful peristaltic contractions which commonly precede obstructive vomiting (Table 21, p. 188). Unfortunately, no two obstructed patients are alike, and it is therefore necessary to consider each patient individually, weigh up the many factors relating to that patient's particular obstructive syndrome and then proceed on the basis of trial and error. If the obstruction is in the pylorus, duodenum or jejunum, it may be necessary to pass a nasogastric tube. This can be aspirated before drinks and meals and possibly left on free drainage overnight. The patient will be much relieved despite the negative fluid balance and often remains remarkably well for several days before deteriorating rapidly as a result of accumulated fluid and biochemical losses.

Constipation

Constipation is the commonest alimentary symptom in patients with advanced cancer (Table 22, p. 189). Prevention is always better (and less traumatic) than the subsequent correction of impaction of faeces with or without obstructive features. The use of a laxative is usually necessary for patients receiving narcotic analgesics and for those taking drugs with anticholinergic side-effects. Adequate fluids, bran with breakfast cereal, fruit juice, improving appetite and mobilisation all play their part in both prevention and correction. However, for many patients, some or all of these measures cannot be employed. It should, therefore, be the general rule to prescribe a laxative in patients who have been commenced on a narcotic analgesic regimen. The use of Dorbanex syrup – a combination of a colonic stimulant and a softener – is recommended, beginning with 10ml either at night or in the morning. If the patient can tolerate this preparation it is easy to adjust the dose over a wide range because of the availability of a stronger (forte) syrup. This is *three times* as strong as the ordinary syrup. If the liquid preparation is unacceptable, capsules can be used; these are not so versatile but the use of Normax as a 'strong Dorbanex' capsule (*twice* as potent) give a useful extra dimension to the capsule range.

For patients who do not respond to Dorbanex forte 20ml daily or to 6 capsules of Normax a day in divided dosage (=danthron 300mg+softener), it is worth adding a small bowel flusher such as Epsom salts (magnesium sulphate) or Milpar (25% liquid paraffin and 6% magnesium hydroxide) before concluding that oral laxatives are not going to work. Even so, at least a third of all terminal cancer patients will require, in addition, rectal measures, i.e. suppositories, enemata or manual removal.

TEAMWORK

Terminal care cannot be done by individuals, only by individuals working together as a team. The composition of the team may vary, but includes the patient himself, the immediate family, friends, doctor(s), nurses, social worker, other ancillary staff, chaplain and, on occasion, lawyer. The team is collectively concerned for the total well-being of the patient and the family – physical, psychological, spiritual and social. In this situation, roles may become blurred, at least at the edges. Moreover, unless the community nurses and the family actively participate in symptom control, the lead given by the doctor will be seriously undermined. Indeed for every step forward there may be a step backwards unless, for example, nurses are encouraged to:

1. Support the patient through the period of initial side-effects commonly seen with morphine-like drugs
2. Advise the patient when to increase the dose of an analgesic.
3. Contact the doctor rather than wait for his next visit if the patient becomes less well when a new treatment is started.
4. Contact the doctor if the patient fails to get a good night's sleep.
5. Advise about diet and fluid intake.
6. Encourage the patient by quietly emphasising that his symptom(s) will soon be better controlled.
7. Give the patient the opportunity to express anxieties and fears.

Without this degree of involvement, the doctor's task is made considerably more difficult and, occasionally, impossible. On the other hand, the doctor should expect no more than about 25 per cent of his prescriptions to be immediately both acceptable and efficacious. Doses will need to be adjusted and, not uncommonly, changes will have to be made.

The need to review, adjust and revise regimens may make considerable demands on the general practitioner in time and energy. It is not enough to instruct the family to contact the surgery, or even your home, if they are worried. Nor is it enough to emphasise that you are happy to make home visits (despite being so busy). It is necessary to recognise that unless one initiates and maintains contact with the patient and the family, unacceptable delays will occur, and the situation may in fact completely break down. Ultimately, it is often appropriate and necessary to simplify drug regimens, and possibly to convert to injections or suppositories when the patient is no longer able easily to swallow. Anticipation and preparation of the family for this eventuality is important. After all, for most people, home still remains the best place to die.

REFERENCES

Harte, J. D. Personal communication.

Melzack, R., Mount, B. M. and Gordan, J. M. (1979). The Brompton mixture versus morphine solution given orally: effects on pain. *Journal of the Canadian Medical Association*, **120**, 435–9.

Penn, C. R. (1976). Single dose and fractionated palliative irradiation for osseous metastases. *Clinical Radiology*, **27**, 405–8.

Stedeford, A. (1978). Understanding confusion. *British Journal of Hospital Medicine*, **20**, 694–704.

Stedeford, A. (1980). *Confusional States*. In The Continuing Care of Terminal Cancer Patients, (eds Twycross, R. G. and Ventafridda, V.). Pergamon Press, Oxford.

Stoll, B. A. (1962). Radiation sickness. *British Medical Journal*, **2**, 507–10.

Twycross, R. G. (1977). *Care of the Terminal Patient*. In *Breast Cancer Management – Early and Late*, (ed Stoll, B. A.). William Heinemann Medical Books Limited, London.

Twycross, R. G. (1979). *Effect of Cocaine in the Brompton Cocktail*. In *Advances in Pain Research and Therapy*, Vol 3, pp. 927–32, (eds Bonica, J. J., Liebeskind, J. C. and Albe-Fessard, D. G.). Raven Press, New York.

ACKNOWLEDGEMENTS

Tables 3, 4, 5, 7, 8, 9, 21 and Figure 16/2 are reproduced by permission of Pitman Medical, Tunbridge Wells; Table 6 is reproduced by permission of Edward Arnold, London; Tables 10, 11, 12 and 13 are reproduced by permission of the American Society of Regional Anesthesia; Figure 16/5 is reproduced by permission of Raven Press, New York.

The author also acknowledges his indebtedness to many colleagues past and present, but particularly to Dr Sylvia Lack.

APPENDIX OF TABLES

APPENDIX OF TABLES

Table 1 Pruritus in terminal cancer

AETIOLOGY
1. Dry, flaky skin
2. Drugs
3. Disease process
4. Obstructive jaundice
5. Renal failure
6. Co-existent skin disorder (including scabies)

TREATMENT

General
1. Discourage scratching (cut nails if necessary)
2. Allow gentle rubbing
3. Discontinue use of soap (use Oilatum or emulsifying ointment)
4. Avoid very hot, long baths
5. Dry skin gently by 'patting' with towel
6. Avoid overheating and sweating

Topical measures
1. 'Oil' dry itchy areas after bath and each evening (lanolin cream, emollient creams (Boots E45), hand cream)
2. Use vioform-hydrocortisone cream b-t.i.d. (if inflamed)
3. Crotamiton (Eurax) cream b-t.i.d.
4. Antihistamine creams b-t.i.d.* (e.g. Anthisan, Caladryl)

Oral drugs
1. Antihistamines
   e.g. chlorpheniramine (Piriton) 4mg b-t.i.d. and promethazine (Phenergan) 25–50mg nocte
2. Prednisolone 5–10mg t.i.d.
   if skin red and 'angry' as a result of scratching and not apparently infected.
3. Norethandrolone (Nilevar) 10mg t.i.d., *or*
   methyltestosterone sublinguet 25mg b.i.d.
   only of value in obstructive jaundice.
4. Cholestyramine (Questran) 4g q.i.d.
   Not recommended; only of value in obstructive jaundice but not liked by patients and unnecessary if other measures implemented.

---

* Not recommended for long-term use as a significant number of patients develop sensitivity reactions.

Table 2 Generalised weakness

Causes	Treatment options

Secondary to surgery
        chemotherapy
        radiation	

Anaemia	Haematinics Blood transfusion
Fever	Antibiotics Corticosteroids
Dehydration	Hydration
Malnutrition	Nutrition IV alimentation
Hypokalaemia	Potassium supplements
Hypercalcaemia	Hydration Corticosteroid Phosphate, etc.
Neuro-myopathy	Corticosteroid
Insomnia	Night sedative
Exhaustion	Rest

Prolonged bed rest
    Pain
    Dyspnoea
    Malaise
	Alleviation of causal symptoms
	Mobilisation (if possible)
	Physiotherapy

Depression	Antidepressants
Progression of disease	Modification of lifestyle

Table 3 Pain in terminal cancer

1. Caused by cancer:	2. Related to cancer:	3. Related to therapy:	4. Unrelated to cancer or therapy:
Soft tissue infiltration	Constipation	Postoperative neuralgia	Migraine
Visceral involvement	Pressure sore	Post-radiation fibrosis	Tension headache
Bone±muscle spasm	Lymphoedema	Post-chemotherapy neuropathy	Osteoarthritis
Nerve compression	Candidiasis	Phantom limb pain	Rheumatoid arthritis
Raised intracranial pressure	Herpetic neuralgia	Post-radiation myelopathy	Musculo-skeletal
Ulceration±infection	Deep vein thrombosis		
	Pulmonary embolus		

Table 4 Factors affecting pain threshold

Threshold lowered	Threshold raised
Discomfort	Relief of symptoms
Insomnia	Sleep
Fatigue	Rest
Anxiety	Sympathy
Fear	Understanding
Anger	Companionship
Sadness	Diversional activity
Depression	Reduction in anxiety
Boredom	Elevation of mood
Introversion	....
Mental isolation	Analgesics
Social abandonment	Anxiolytics
	Antidepressants

Table 5 Reasons for variations in effective analgesic dose of oral morphine sulphate

1. Differences in pain intensity
2. Differences in alimentary absorption
3. Differences in plasma half-life
4. Age
5. Hepatic dysfunction
6. Fundamental differences in patient's pain tolerance threshold (relates to CNS endorphin stores)
7. Acquired differences in patient's pain tolerance threshold (relates mainly to mood and morale)
8. Previously *induced* tolerance
   (a) by needless increases in dose
   (b) initial use of morphine by injection in excessive amounts
9. Previous inadequate use of strong narcotics, especially 'PRN' injections
10. Previous use of strong narcotics
11. Duration of treatment (overall *tendency* for dose to increase)
12. Use or non-use of 'co-analgesics'

Table 6 Weak narcotic analgesic preparations

	Content (mg)		
	Narcotic	Adjuvant	Proprietary preparation
Dextropropoxyphene 1	65	–	Doloxene
2	150	–	Depronal SA
+ aspirin 1	(50)*	500	Napsalgesic
2	(100)*	325	Dolasan
+ paracetamol	32.5	325	Distalgesic
Codeine phosphate	15,30,60	–	–
+ aspirin	8	500	Codis
+ paracetamol	8	500	Neurodyne Panadeine
Dihydrocodeine tartrate	30	–	DF 118
+ aspirin	10	300	Onadox – 118
+ paracetamol	10	500	Paramol – 118

* Weight refers to dextropropoxyphene napsylate; equivalent to 32.5 and 65mg of hydrochloride, respectively.

Table 7 Use of morphine sulphate solution

1. Strong narcotic of choice at most hospices.
2. Administered in simple aqueous solution (10mg in 10ml).
3. No advantage in giving as Brompton Cocktail.
4. Usual *starting* dose 10mg every 4 hours.
5. 5mg may be adequate if previously only had a weak narcotic analgesic (Table 6).
6. With frail elderly patients, may be wise to start on sub-optimal dose in order to reduce likelihood of initial drowsiness and unsteadiness.
7. If changing from alternative strong narcotic (e.g. levorphanol, dextromoramide, methadone) may need considerably higher dose (Table 8).
8. Adjust upwards after first dose if not more effective than previous medication.
9. Adjust after 24 hours 'if pain not 90 per cent controlled'.
10. Most patients satisfactorily controlled on dose of between 5 and 30mg four-hourly; some patients need higher doses, occasionally up to 200mg (Fig. 16/4, p. 168).
11. Giving a larger dose at bedtime (1.5 or 2×daytime dose) may enable a patient to go through the night without waking in pain.
12. Use co-analgesic medication as appropriate (Table 9).
13. Either prescribe an anti-emetic concurrently or supply (in anticipation) for regular use should nausea or vomiting develop.
14. Prescribe laxative, e.g. Dorbanex (danthron + softener).
    Adjust dose according to response.
    Suppositories may be necessary.
    Unless carefully monitored, constipation may be more difficult to control than the pain.
15. Write out regimen in detail with times to be taken, names of drugs and amount to be taken.
16. Warn all patients about possibility of initial drowsiness.
17. Arrange for close liaison and follow up.
18. It is almost never necessary to resort to parenteral administration for pain control *per se*.

Table 8 Approximate oral narcotic analgesic equivalents

Analgesic	Proprietary Name	Unit Size	Potency Ratio with morphine sulphate	Oral dose (mg) morphine sulphate	Oral dose (mg) diamorphine hydrochloride[2]	Duration of action (hrs)[3]
pethidine/meperidine	Demerol	50mg	1/8[4]	6	4	2–3
		100mg		12	8	
pentazocine	Fortral, Talwin	25mg	1/6[4]	4	3	2–3
		50mg (caps)		8	5	
		50mg (supp)		8	5	
*dipipanone	Diconal	10mg (+ 30mg cyclizine)	1/2	5	3	3–5
papaveretum	Omnopon	10mg	1/2	5	3	3–5
*oxycodone pectinate	Proladone	30mg (supp)	2/3	20	13	6–8
*Nepenthe[5]		1ml (solution)	1	12	8	3–5
*dextromoramide	Palfium	5mg	(2)[6]	10	7	2–4
		10mg		20	13	
		10mg (supp)		20	13	
methadone	Physeptone, Dolophine	5mg	(3–4)[7]	15–20	10–13	4–8
levorphanol	Dromoran,	1.5mg	5	8	5	4–6
*phenazocine	Narphen	5mg	5	25	16	4–6

* Not availabe in USA

1. Tablets unless stated otherwise.
2. By mouth diamorphine hydrochloride is 1.5 times more potent than morphine sulphate, i.e. 5mg is equivalent to 7.5mg of morphine sulphate.
3. Dependent to a certain extent on dose, often longer lasting in very elderly and those with considerable liver dysfunction.
4. Experience suggests that, compared with *regularly* administered morphine sulphate, these preparations are not as potent as these ratios would indicate.
5. Nepenthe is a standard solution of morphine (as base) and opium. 1ml contains the equivalent of about 12mg of morphine *sulphate*, and is usually prescribed as a 10% (1ml diluted in 10ml) solution.
6. Dextromoramide single 5mg dose is equivalent to diamorphine 10mg/morphine 15mg in terms of PEAK effect but is generally shorter acting; overall potency rate adjusted accordingly.
7. Methadone – single 5mg dose is equivalent to diamorphine 5mg/morphine 7.5mg. Has a prolonged plasma half-life which leads to cumulation when given repeatedly. This means it is several times more potent when given *regularly*.

Table 9 Additional analgesic measures

	Type of pain	Co-analgesic	Non-drug measures
1.	Bone pain	aspirin 600mg 4-hourly *or* flurbiprofen 50–100mg t.i.d.	Irradiation
2.	Raised intracranial pressure	dexamethasone 2–4mg t.i.d. diuretic (?)	Elevate head of bed Avoid lying flat
3.	Nerve pressure pain	prednisolone 5–10mg t.i.d.	Nerve block Irradiation
4.	Post-herpetic neuralgia	amitriptyline 25–100mg nocte	
5.	Superficial dysaesthetic pain		
6.	Intermittent stabbing pain	valproate 200mg b-t.i.d. *or* carbamazepine 200mg t-q.i.d.	
7.	Gastric distension pain	asilone 10ml p.c. and nocte *and* metoclopramide 10mg 4-hourly	
8.	Rectal tenesmoid pain	chlorpromazine 10–25mg 8–4-hourly	
9.	Bladder tenesmoid pain		
10.	Muscle spasm pain	diazepam 5mg b.i.d. *or* baclofen 10mg t.i.d.	Massage
11.	Lymphoedema	diuretic *and* corticosteroid (?)	Elevate foot of bed Elastic stocking Compression cuff
12.	Infected malignant ulcer	metronidazole 400mg t.i.d. *or* alternative antibiotic	
13.	Activity precipitated pain		Modify way of life (if possible)

Table 10 Corticosteroids in terminal cancer

Non-specific uses
1. To improve appetite
2. To reduce fever
3. To enhance sense of well-being
4. To improve strength

Co-analgesic
1. Raised intracranial pressure*
2. Nerve compression
3. Hepatomegaly
4. Head and neck tumour*
5. Intrapelvic tumour
6. Abdominal tumour
7. Retroperitoneal tumour
8. Lymphoedema*
9. Metastatic arthralgia

Other specific uses
1. Hypercalcaemia
2. Carcinomatous neuromyopathy
3. Incipient paraplegia
4. Superior vena caval obstruction
5. Airway obstruction
6. Carcinomatous lymphangitis
7. Haemoptysis
8. Leuco-erythroblastic anaemia
9. Malignant effusion*
10. Discharge from rectal tumour**
11. To minimise radiation-induced reactive oedema
12. To minimise the toxic effects of radiation or chemotherapy
13. As an adjunct to chemotherapy

* May benefit by concurrent use of a diuretic
** Given rectally

Table 11 Common anticholinergic side-effects

1. Blurred vision
2. Dry mouth
3. Oesophageal reflux
4. Tachycardia
5. Urinary retention
6. Constipation

Table 12 Tranquillisers in terminal cancer

	Chlorpromazine	Diazepam
Nausea and vomiting	+	−
Insomnia	+	+ +
Overwhelming pain	+	+ +
Anxiety	+	+ +
Tension headaches	+	+ +
Muscle spasm pain	+	+ +
Rectal 'tenesmoid' pain	+ +	+
Bladder 'tenesmoid' pain	+ +	+
Urethral spasm pain	+ +	+
Agitated, confused state	+	+ +
Coma + restlessness*	+	+ +
Coma + rigidity	+	+ +
Coma + twitching	+	+ +
Convulsions	−	+

This table summarises the use of tranquillisers at Sir
Michael Sobell House, Oxford.
* May indicate unrelieved pain, full bladder, or over-
loaded rectum. A tranquilliser is appropriate only
when these aspects have been dealt with and the rest-
lessness persists
− Not used for this indication
+ + Generally regarded as drug of first choice
+ Also used but less often than drug of choice, or if
latter fails to relieve

Table 13 Need for antidepressants in terminal
cancer

1. Depression
2. Insomnia
3. Nocturnal frequency
4. Nocturnal enuresis
5. Superficial dysaesthetic pain
6. Post-herpetic neuralgia
7. Rectal 'tenesmoid' pain

Table 14 Aetiological factors in confusion

1. unnecessary
   unfamiliar } stimuli {
   excessive
	too hot, too cold
	wet, crumbs in bed
	creases in sheets
	full bladder
	constipation
	pain, itch

8. vitamin deficiency
9. drugs
   - narcotics
   - psychotropic
   - antiparkinsonian
   - barbiturates
   - digoxin

2. change of environment

10. age/dementia
11. tumour
    - systemic effect
    - cerebral involvement
12. cerebro-vascular accident

3. cerebral anoxia
   - anaemia
   - cardiac failure
   - hypoxia
4. hypercapnia
5. sepsis
6. metabolic failure
   - liver
   - kidney
7. biochemical
   - hypercalcaemia
   - hyponatraemia

13. severe anxiety
14. severe depression
15. alcohol
    - intoxication
    - withdrawal

Table 15 Treatment of confusional states

NON-DRUG MEASURES

1. Explanation to patient, family, nurses
2. Stress that patient is not going mad
3. Stress that almost always there are lucid intervals
4. Continue to treat patient as a sane, sensible adult
5. Appreciate that hallucinations, nightmares and misperceptions may reflect unresolved fears and anxiety

DRUGS

Generally use drugs only if symptoms are marked, persistent and cause distress to patient and/or family. Review sooner rather than later if a sedative drug is prescribed, as may exacerbate symptoms.

Specific

1. *reduction* in present medication
2. *oxygen* if hypoxic/cyanosed
3. *dexamphetamine* (2–4mg t-q.i.d.) if cerebral tumour
4. *cerebral stimulant* (RARELY appropriate) if not agitated and if associated with drug induced drowsiness*
   (a) cocaine 10–20mg 4-hourly
   (b) dexamethasone 2.5–5mg daily or b.i.d.

* usually better to reduce and/or modify existing medication.

General

1. *diazepam* (Valium) 5–10mg by mouth or parenterally, especially if agitated and generally restless
2. *haloperidol* (Serenace) 1.5–5mg by mouth or intramuscularly, especially if hallucinations and paranoia, and if diazepam fails to relieve
   (a) Initial dose depends on previous medication, weight, age and severity of symptoms
   (b) Subsequent doses depend on initial response
   (c) Daily or b.i.d. maintenance doses usually adequate
   (d) Sometimes more frequent administration is necessary
3. chlorpromazine (Largactil) ⎤
4. promazine (Sparine)   ⎥ useful alternative preparations
5. thioridazine (Melleril)   ⎥
6. chlormethiazole (Heminevrin) ⎦

Table 16 Causes of dry mouth in advanced cancer

Local	Mouth-breathing
	Non-functioning salivary glands
	Moniliasis
General	Poor fluid intake
	Excessive fluid loss ⎧ Vomiting ⎫ ⎧ diuretic
	⎨ Diarrhoea ⎬ ⎨ hypercalcaemia
	⎪ Polyuria ⎪ ⎨ diabetes insipidus
	⎩ Pyrexia ⎭
Drugs	(Narcotic analgesics)
	(Cocaine)
	Phenothiazines
	Tricyclic antidepressants
	Cyclizine
Psychological	Anxiety
	Depression

Table 17 Hiccup in terminal cancer

DEFINITION

Involuntary inspiratory muscular efforts associated
with a closed glottis

AETIOLOGY

1. Gastric distension
2. Diaphragmatic irritation
3. Toxic
   (a) uraemia
   (b) infection
4. CNS tumour
   (a) intracranial
   (b) medullary
5. Phrenic nerve irritation

TREATMENT

1. Rebreathing into paper bag (or inhalations of 5%
   CO_2)
2. Pharyngeal stimulation
   (a) drinking from 'wrong' side of a cup
   (b) granulated sugar (2 heaped teaspoons)
   (c) liquor (2 glasses)
   (d) cold key down back of neck
       (acts via hyperextension of neck)
   (e) nasopharyngeal tube
3. Correction of gastric distension
   (a) peppermint water (relaxes oesophageal
       sphincter)
   (b) defoaming agent (e.g. Asilone 10ml *after* meals
       and nocte)
   (c) metoclopramide (10mg 6–4 hourly; hastens
       gastric emptying)
   (d) nasogastric intubation
4. Drugs
   (a) chlorpromazine 25mg IV + 25mg IM initially if
       patient distressed and other measures have
       failed.
   (b) chlorpromazine 10–25mg up to 4-hourly
   (c) methylamphetamine 5–10mg IV if (a) fails
   (d) phenytoin 100mg b-t.i.d. or carbamazepine
       200mg b-q.i.d. if related to cerebral lesion
5. Phrenic nerve block/crush (never necessary in
   terminal cancer in author's experience)

Table 18　Failure to eat (anorexia)

Causes	Treatment options
1. fear of vomiting	1. anti-emetics
2. unappetising food	2. choice of food *by patient*
3. offered too much food	3. small meals
4. early satiation	4. snacks between meals
5. dehydration	5. rehydrate
6. constipation	6. laxatives
7. mouth discomfort	7. mouth care
8. pain	8. analgesics
9. fatigue	9. rest
10. malodourous ulcer	10. prevention of malodour
	(a) irrigation of ulcer b.i.d.
	(e.g. hydrogen peroxide)
	(b) local antiseptic
	(e.g. povidone iodine)
	(c) air fresheners:
	Nilodor
	Saltair (for colostomy bag)
	(d) adsorbent dressing:
	Bandor
	Actisorb
11. biochemical:	11. correction of hypercalcaemia:
hyponatraemia	increase fluid intake
hypercalcaemia	corticosteroids
uraemia	phosphate
	mithramycin
12. secondary to treatment:	12. modify drug regimen
drugs	
irradiation	
chemotherapy	
13. disease process	13. trial of corticosteroids
	(e.g. prednisolone 5–10mg t.i.d.)
14. anxiety	14. anxiolytic
15. depression	15. antidepressant
	16. getting up
	17. getting dressed
	18. change of environment

Table 19 'Squashed stomach syndrome'

DEFINITION

Dyspeptic symptoms associated with inability of stomach to distend normally because of hepatomegaly. Similar symptoms may be seen with carcinoma of stomach, linitis plastica, or post-gastrectomy ('small stomach syndrome')

SYMPTOMS

1. Early satiation
2. Epigastric fullness
3. Epigastric discomfort/pain
4. Flatulence
5. Hiccup
6. Nausea
7. Vomiting
   (especially post-prandial)
8. Heartburn

TREATMENT

1. Explanation
2. Dietary advice
3. Defoaming agent
   (e.g. Asilone 10ml after meals and bedtime)
4. Metoclopramide
   (4-hourly if also receiving morphine)
   (or after meals and bedtime)
5. Cyclizine 50–100mg 4-hourly is occasionally also necessary

Table 20 Vomiting in terminal cancer

Is the patient vomiting? – exclude expectoration
                                    regurgitation

CAUSES

1. Reactive – pain
              anxiety
2. Intracranial – raised intracranial pressure
                  direct stimulation of vomiting centre
                  (vestibular disturbance)
3. Chemical (mediated via chemoreceptor trigger
   zone (CTZ))
   (a) Toxic   – infection
                     carcinoma
                     radiation
   (b) Drugs   – digitalis
                     narcotics
                     oestrogens
                     chemotherapy
   (c) Biochemical – uraemia
                     hypercalcaemia
4. Cough-induced
5. Pharyngeal stimulation
6. Gastric irritation
   (a) Chemical   – expectorants
                    iron
                    blood
                    antibiotics
   (b) Physical   – aspirin
                    non-steroidal anti-inflammatory
                    agents
                    corticosteroids
                    alcohol
   (e) Distension – overeating
                    gastric stasis
7. Obstruction
   (a) constipation
   (b) mechanical
   (c) paralytic ileus

TREATMENT

1. Dietary advice
2. Specific measures
   (a) analgesic
   (b) anxiolytic
   (c) cough sedative
   (d) antibiotic
   (e) modification of drug therapy
   (f) correction of hypercalcaemia

   (g) corticosteroid – if raised intracranial pressure
       (e.g. dexamethasone)
   (h) corticosteroid in breast cancer if no response to
       other measures
       (e.g. prednisolone)
3. Antiemetic
   (a) depress vomiting centre
       i. belladonna alkaloids:
          hyoscine, atropine*
       ii. antihistamines:
          cyclizine (Valoid)
          dimenhydrinate (Dramamine)
          diphenhydramine (Benadryl)
          promethazine (Phenergan)
   (b) depress chemoreceptor trigger zone
          phenothiazines
          (e.g. prochlorperazine)
          butyrophenones (e.g. haloperidol)
          metoclopramide (Maxolon)
          hydroxyzine (Atarax)
   (c) 'normalise' upper bowel function
          metoclopramide (Maxolon)
   (d) other
          pyridoxine
          marihuana analogues

* Useful when patient moribund.

Table 21 Medical management of bowel
obstruction

1. Explanation and dietary advice:
   small meals, less roughage
   eat earlier rather than later in day
   eat only if want to, etc.
2. Do not use peristaltic stimulants by mouth
3. Reduce peristalsis:
       diphenoxylate   ⎫ Choice depends on the
       codeine phosphate   ⎬ presence or absence of
       morphine sulphate   ⎭ background pain.
4. Soften bowel contents:
       Dioctyl forte tablets 100mg b-t.i.d.
5. Enemata/suppositories:
       e.g. bisacodyl 10mg 1–2 times a week.
6. Trial of corticosteroids:
       prednisolone 10mg t.i.d.
       dexamethasone 2–4mg t.i.d.

Table 22 Constipation in terminal cancer

DEFINITION

Infrequent motions associated with difficulty of defaecation

CAUSES

1. Inactivity
2. Poor nutrition   – decreased intake
                            low-residue diet
3. Poor fluid intake
4. Dehydration   { vomiting
                     – polyuria
                     fever
5. Drugs – anticholinergics { phenothiazines
                              tricyclic antidepressants
                              cyclizine
       aspirin-like
       narcotic
6. Biochemical   – hypercalcaemia
                         hypokalaemia
7. Weakness
8. Inability to reach toilet when urge to defaecate

TREATMENT

1. Mobilize, if possible
2. Correct anorexia inducing factors (Table 18)
3. Add bran to diet
4. Increase fluid intake
5. Encourage fruit juices
6. Laxatives (*vide infra*)
7. Rectal measures   { suppositories
                         – enemata
                         manual removals

Laxatives

1. *Regulators* (hydrophilic bulk-forming agents)
   (a) bran
   (b) methylcellulose (Celevac, Cologel)
   (c) mucilloids – psyllium (Metamucil)
                    ispaghula (Isogel)
                    sterculia (Normacol)

2. *Softeners*
   (a) lubricants – (e.g. liquid paraffin)
   (b) wetting agents – dioctyl (in Normax)
                        poloxamer (in Dorbanex)

3. *Small bowel flushers*
   (a) salts:
       magnesium compounds
       sodium picosulphate (Laxoberal)*
   (b) non-absorbable sugars:
       lactulose (Duphalac)*
       sorbitol
       mannitol

4. *Colonic stimulants*
   (a) bulk
   (b) sodium picosulphate (Laxoberal)*
   (c) non-absorbable sugars (via organic acids
       produced when metabolised by gut bacteria)
   (d) polyphenolics – phenolphthalein
                       bisacodyl (Dulcolax)
   (e) anthracenes – senna
                     danthron (in Dorbanex,
                     Normax)

* Stimulate both small and large bowel but not as efficacious as Dorbanex in comparable amounts.

Chapter 17 Principles of prescribing for the elderly

J. N. AGATE CBE, MA, MD, FRCP

INTRODUCTION

The elderly are above all people – individuals, deserving of proper care and concern. Ninety-five per cent or so are at home, the rest in homes or hospitals. Those in the latter are to be found in almost every ward, not simply isolated in geriatric departments. They have no less right to accuracy of diagnosis and appropriate treatment than any other group, and they are undeniably rewarding to treat, provided the therapeutics are well conducted. In the case of the elderly treatment must of course comprise far more than drug therapy; reassurance, prevention of complications, maintenance or restoration of mobility and self-confidence, are all primary objectives. Even though therapeutic success may be limited, if a doctor cannot bring himself to believe the truth of these assertions then his care of old people is likely to be a sterile and passive exercise tinged sometimes with a touch of cynicism. The elderly are seldom well served by pessimistic doctors and nurses. A few of our colleagues frankly believe that old people are 'not worth treating'; a small minority consider that it is just a waste of their expertise. They will not have reached even this point in this chapter.

In the past 50 to 60 years particularly, drugs have played a major part in the eradication of old people's diseases and the relief of their distress. One need only consider highly successful modern treatment of heart failure or megaloblastic anaemia, or our more modest successes with parkinsonism and depression in older people. Drugs may even have added a few years to some individual elderly lives, though this is not the primary objective of geriatric medicine, where the quality of the life which may be prolonged should be of more concern than its actual prolongation. There are no drugs yet for the extended treatment of natural senescence; and indeed if there were, most serious ethical problems would have to be faced. Naturally, many acute medical conditions arise in old people, and the quicker they are treated the more successful will be the outcome. However, in this volume, concerned with long-term use of drugs, the 'acute' happening must be largely disregarded. So also must that perplexing, often

present, dilemma: how far is it justifiable actually to treat a new, life-threatening acute disorder in a very frail, aged and deteriorated individual who seems already to have run his natural race? Any physician worth his salt must be ready to face these urgent ethical conundrums – but not here. At some stage in most longer-term treatment it may eventually seem best just to let events take their course; but that is a decision to be arrived at without hurry.

Because of an increasing general expectation of life – as yet still rising – and because more younger people are surviving early health hazards and growing old, the numbers of the elderly have been multiplying for more than 150 years. In round figures retired people now comprise 17 per cent of the population of these islands. Forward projections suggest that the numbers of the retired may have declined a little by the year 2000, but within their ranks the proportion who will live beyond 75 years is expected still to be rising. It is this group, the 'old old', exhibiting frailty together with a multiplicity of disorders, which will present us for several decades with Medicine's most pressing practical and logistical problems. Already the elderly occupy well over twice their 'share' of hospital beds, and for longer periods than the average stay. Because of this high bed-occupancy there could eventually arise a crisis when younger people with acute illness could be denied the use of a hospital bed. In addition it is believed that older people's medical problems give rise to 30 per cent of the total expenditure on drugs in this country. It is therefore essential for all doctors in hospitals to consider the efficient use of beds – which means resolving to discharge at once older people who are cured or relieved. This, and not just custodial care, is the first intention of any geriatric department. Likewise, simple economics place on all who ever prescribe for the elderly a duty to consider most critically their own use of drugs from the dual standpoints of effectiveness and cost. Further, every prescriber owes it to his patients and the community as a whole to ensure that his treatments do not increase the chance of morbidity, the risk of patently iatrogenic disorders, or even the possibility of side-effects brisk enough to endanger patients' lives.

Patients often have to be admitted to hospital just because of drug reactions. The proportion of such admissions was found in one series to be 2.9 per cent for all age-groups, but 4.8 per cent in the group aged 71–80 (Caranasos et al, 1974). However, more recent work from the Professorial Department in Edinburgh indicates a figure as high as 7.7 per cent of all geriatric admissions being attributable to this cause (Williamson and Chopin, 1979). Iatrogenic disorders did not happen on this scale 25 or so years back. It is hard to see it as other than a sharp reminder of the toxicity (and potency) of modern drugs, or an indictment of the methods of many modern prescribers. It will be a principal aim of this chapter to show how easily these disasters could arise – old people not being quite the same as young people – and how undoubted risks might be lessened.

NORMAL AGEING AND DRUGS

Ageing, that is normal senescence, is an inevitable process, though it does not proceed at the same rate in all people, nor yet at a steady rate even in one individual. General considerations of age-related physiological change should take full account of individual variation, while the patient's stated age may be quite unimportant in deciding how to tackle his treatment, and with what dosage of which drugs. Much more important than age are the patient's configuration, speed of response, outlook and general viability. These are necessary value judgements. However, age changes might be expected to modify drug absorption, availability in the serum, metabolism and excretion, just as they measurably affect old people's overall physical and mental performance.

Intelligent deduction from a rapidly increasing corpus of knowledge about senescent changes would lead anyone to expect peculiarities of response to drugs. It is (or should be) well known that abnormal drug responses and interactions are exceedingly common in elderly patients. Indeed, adverse drug reactions were noted in from less than one per cent to 35 per cent in various reported series, depending on whether these were retrospective or prospective investigations. Adverse reactions to drugs among hospital inpatients in general have been observed in some 12 per cent of those treated, but in the age-group 70 to 79 the figure can be above 20 per cent (Hurwitz, 1969). The incidence of drug reactions in elderly patients treated at home might well be higher, because there cannot be such close control of the drug administration. At present the behaviour of only a limited number of

specific drugs has so far been experimentally investigated, and much more research is called for. There is generally prolongation of the transit time through the gut of food taken by old people, gastric acidity tends to decline with age, and some pathological conditions and certain drugs reduce intestinal motility. These changes and delays might reasonably be expected to alter drug absorption. However, experimental evidence does not suggest there is either poor absorption or enhanced absorption because of relative stasis. One must therefore look elsewhere for explanations of increased plasma concentrations of drugs in elderly people. This might be because of changes in the apparent volume of distribution of the drugs, itself consequent upon the known decrease in lean body mass and total water content of the aged body. Again, the amount of a drug freely available in plasma might presumably vary inversely with the amount of it which was bound to albumin, and upon whether there are other drugs in use which could compete for the plasma-binding sites or the final receptor sites. At all events, it has long been known that older people have a reduced plasma albumin level (Woodford–Williams et al, 1968). Experimental evidence on these points of distribution and availability nevertheless tends to be conflicting, and it is likely that any such abnormality in old people accounts for only a minor part of the total picture.

With the metabolism and final excretion of drugs there is more certainty. Some, e.g. phenobarbitone and paracetamol, are metabolised in the liver by its microsomal enzymes. These drugs have increased plasma half-lives in old people, consistent perhaps with the reduced liver weight and blood flow, and a decrement in microsomal enzyme activity. However, certain other drugs like chlorpromazine have the effect of increasing hepatic enzyme activity, thus promoting the breakdown of drugs like the tricyclic antidepressants, causing a reduction in their therapeutic activity. O'Malley et al (1980) have reviewed and compared for several common drugs the responses of old and young subjects in these respects.

The excretion of some drugs is via the bowel after degradation in the liver, but more are excreted by the kidneys. Classical early studies of kidney function have shown that there is a steady reduction in glomerular filtration rate (as indicated by creatinine clearance), and also of tubular secretion – and this in the absence of renal disease. The decline has been estimated at roughly one per cent per year after 40, so that at 90 'normal' renal function is reduced by at least half, when compared with a young middle-aged person. There is already experimental evidence of a reduced rate of excretion in old people of such commonly used drugs as phenobarbitone, digoxin, sulphamethiazole, benzyl-penicillin and kanamycin. No doubt many others will eventually be added to the list.

Age-related factors apart, temporary or prolonged functional renal impairment from pathological extra-renal causes is common in old people; for example, they are liable to hypotensive episodes, congestive heart failure, and dehydration from many causes. Additionally, kidney pathology such as ascending pyelonephritis is regrettably a commonplace. Many substances which are excreted by the kidneys are therefore found to have higher-than-expected plasma levels and much prolonged half-lives. With some drugs such as penicillin this can be of therapeutic advantage. However, with other antibiotics like streptomycin and gentamicin the effect is greatly to increase the risks of ototoxicity and of nephrotoxicity itself. Similarly, there are increased risks from relative renal impairment when such common drugs as chlorpropamide and digoxin are in use. Tubular function is the excretory pathway for a number of drugs like thiazide diuretics, sulphonylureas, salicylates and the various penicillins, and any of these given together may compete for the pathway, thus mutually elevating their various plasma levels beyond the toxic limit. Such considerations should give us pause whenever prescribing several drugs together, and dosage levels in general need particular attention when renal function is already compromised or even suspect – which is not an easy matter to be sure about, especially since the normal range of the blood urea is much wider in old people than it is in the young. A sound principle in geriatric work is to be wary of any drug which is excreted by the kidneys, and keep the dose as small as practicable.

Whatever events may or may not derive from changes in drug absorption, distribution, metabolism and excretion in the elderly, there are in practice common effects which pre-suppose some age-related alterations in actual tissue sensitivity. Furthermore, homeostatic responses are well known to be impaired as part of ageing. This is never better illustrated than by the proclivity of old people to hypothermia and hypotension (both sometimes drug-induced), as well as by the high probability of mental confusion being the earliest indicator of some physical disorder. The aged brain, perhaps with a recently compromised blood supply or already under threat from progressive and irreversible histological changes, cannot compensate for an altered internal milieu which is further disturbed by a higher plasma level of drugs than expected. The consequence would be a greater risk of unwanted drug effects, causing increased confusion, agitation, hallucinosis and restlessness, together with dizziness and a tendency to fall about. Adding 'sedative' drugs to such a patient's drug schedule will simply cause even greater problems and perhaps compound some earlier unwise choice of preparation or dose. In practice, one of the commonest causes of falling about of aged people is a 'toxic' manifestation of an occult chest infection; a second is postural hypotension from impaired baro-receptor reflexes (often aggravated by drugs); and a third is the toxic effect of too high and too regular a dosage with nitrazepam and similar drugs. These favourite hypnotics are often poorly excreted, become cumulative with a high plasma level, and produce a muddled hangover effect – since the brain cells may already be showing reduced functional efficiency. A simple mental score test, taking only a few minutes, would alert one to this possibility. It has been pointed out that hypnotic and sedative drugs impair higher cerebral function, not enhance it. Thus to exhibit them for patients with known progressive impairment of cognitive function is illogical. Even the patient with an acute confusional episode may thus be rendered more confused till the drugs take charge; and having taken charge they make the patient stuporose and render him immediately vulnerable to pressure effects and all the other sequelae of even short-term immobility. Unfortunately, the doctor is often caught between, on one side, the demand of relatives to have calm and peace after a trying episode, and on the other side the interests of his aged patient, which require as little sedation as possible. Besides, there is a greatly increased likelihood of respiratory tract infection in old people under sedation.

It happens commonly that an old person has been provided with a certain type of drug regularly over a number of years. He is habituated, psychologically dependent upon it, and often exerts a kind of moral blackmail to ensure that he gets it. Hypnotics are a case in point. As he has grown old, so that particular drug may have become unsuitable for him on other grounds, and a change is called for. This requires persuasion and courage. As an example, phenobarbitone and most other barbiturate drugs are highly likely to produce adverse side-effects, and must be considered unsuitable for old people, except perhaps in the treatment of epilepsy. The old medical adage that 'One should not change the established habits of anyone over 40' always was specious nonsense, and in the matter of drug regimens it is a counter-productive and dangerous principle. It is a poor outlook if the habits of even the young middle-aged cannot be influenced. Most very old people can eventually be persuaded to accept change if it is in their interests to do so.

COMPLIANCE IN DRUG TAKING

Physicians like to believe patients take the drugs they prescribe for them, at the correct dosage and intervals. That this is not so has been demonstrated many times. It can never, of course, be easy to get at the facts, for people are unlikely to be frank about their errors of commission and omission even to a disinterested research worker. How many doctors or nurses who have been ill could say they always took their drugs precisely as ordered? Patients are often positively devious in this matter, and the elderly no less so than others. In hospital it is assumed that drug administration is tightly controlled. Yet elderly patients frequently hide away their tablets and go to some lengths to dispose of them elsewhere, into the upholstery or plumbing, out of windows, into their handbags or laundry. Modern hospital drug-recording methods make for a little more certainty, though what is handed out does not necessarily reach the patient's stomach. Commonly, hospital patients just refuse doses of their drugs, but this is at least recordable. It is far more difficult to get even reasonable compliance from patients in their own homes, and the elderly exhibit various disabilities which make self-administration of drugs difficult even when they are keen to comply (see below). Experience of domiciliary visiting in consulting practice shows how remarkably uncommon it is for elderly patients to be receiving the drugs which their doctors confidently claim they are 'on'. Indeed, one cannot be certain of this even when a relative is supervising the regimen, though it is a little more likely when one sees the daily schedule has been written out in bold letters and put on the mantelpiece. Dosage is often mistaken by at least 100 per cent, and timing highly erratic. It is just as common to learn that the patient has spontaneously stopped taking a drug, saying it 'upsets' her in some way or other; at times the drug is one which ought not to be stopped suddenly. Often a patient confidently and sometimes angrily attributes to a drug an accession of symptoms which should be attributed to a new turn in the illness, and so will have stopped taking it when a larger dose might be required. Be it noted that this is usually done without consulting the prescriber again, for confidence may have been unjustly undermined. Unless the prescribing doctor from time to time actually rehearses with an elderly patient the intended schedules, and has the bottles actually in his hands, he cannot be sure his instructions are being complied with. Repeat prescribing without seeing the patient and his drug containers leads to bizarre and potentially dangerous circumstances, especially with older patients whose compliance is uncertain. The writer has more than once discovered a patient at home taking three times her supposed dose because she possessed three half-full bottles of the identical drug, on each of which the label indicated 'One tablet to be taken twice daily'. In one case the drug was digoxin. This apparently was an unexpected level of compliance following upon a period of non-compliance! To quote another example, an elderly countrywoman was admitted to hospital because of unexplained confusion; she had not seen her doctor for several months but had had repeat prescriptions by post. On admission she was found to have in her handbag seven containers and envelopes, each full of drugs, but all mixed. In aggregate they numbered 773 tablets and capsules; five types were identifiable, but three types were unidentifiable white tablets. When these were confiscated and no drug treatment was ordered the patient became mentally clear within a week. Naturally, the more preparations ordered, the greater the chances of mistakes and non-compliance.

According to a review of this problem (Blackwell, 1972) various studies have suggested that some 25 to 50 per cent of patients do not take their drugs at all, and in another American survey of drugs given long term, about one half of the patients were found to take their drugs as advised (Sackett, 1976). In prescribing for older patients, therefore, one must say with regret that it is more realistic to assume non-compliance than compliance, until the latter can be demonstrated. The practical implications of this are however profound. This is a fruitful field of work for health visitors. Non-compliance will usually result in an accumulation of tablets and medicines in the house, for old people seldom throw drugs away even when they have neglected or rejected them. Adherence to the doctor's own instructions is one thing, but there are also many elderly patients dosing themselves with other drugs on the quiet, or even sharing the supplies of their spouses, on the basis of 'sauce for the goose and the gander'.

Age-related practical problems

One can attain to an extreme age in fine health, with intact special senses, alert in mind, positive and well-integrated. Notwithstanding, the chance of some morbid condition being present in a person of 85 and over is of the order of 65 per cent. Elderly invalids often have to contend with a variety of major and minor disabilities in addition to any illness for which they currently require drug treatment. Altered eyesight, as presbyopia, is almost universal; patients with correct glasses will see reasonably printed labels on containers; those who have mislaid their glasses or who suffer from ocular disease may very well not. Hearing may be virtually intact, but deafness is often there as a barrier, and many old people exhibit 'selective' deafness, to use a euphemism. It is thus essential when instructing them in drug matters to be sure one has their full attention and co-operation. The sense of smell and taste may be impaired also, but these days patients seldom need to identify their medicines by the taste.

The prescriber may not always appreciate that a very aged patient has become quite small in bulk and stature. Old people are indeed no larger than some children, and it might be logical to prescribe for them according to their weight rather than to the 'standard' dosages for young adults.

The very fact that having lived a long time with perhaps several illnesses encountered for which drugs were used, increases the probability of drug allergies having been established. These are notoriously common, especially in old women.

Aged hands may be fully functional, if tremulous, but arthritic or parkinsonian hands may be quite unable to open a simple screw-capped container or press a tablet out of a foil or bubble pack, while some child-proof containers defeat the elderly patient more than their grandchildren. Few old people have the dexterity to break in half a small scored tablet, and it must be unrealistic to talk in terms of 'half a tablet' of anything. 'Strokes' and their residual disabilities are common; a hemiplegic patient can seldom administer his own drugs.

Forgetfulness is a major problem. To be just a little forgetful can be counted as normal if it does not result in abnormal behaviour, but amnesia may be severe enough to cause non-compliance in a patient who is not basically unco-operative. Severe amnesia tending towards dementia, even if it is mild, makes self-medication impossible and frankly hazardous. About 20 per cent of people over the age of 80 show some clearly detectable signs of dementia, of which severe amnesia is likely to be an early sign. In such people the administration of the drugs must be put in the hands of relatives, friends or neighbours – and often there are none, or none within range, or none willing. Periodic absences of such supporters also create immediate difficulty. It is commonplace to find a mentally unreliable old person contemplating a collection of six to a dozen different drugs in various containers, muddled about how much of which to take next. Then technical 'non-compliance' is a certainty, and the patient really at risk.

It may be necessary, too, for a solitary elderly diabetic on oral or insulin treatment, active but with problems of eyesight or peripheral neuropathy, to have to be

kept in hospital indefinitely because of insuperable difficulties about diet, medication and control.

Many old men have prostatic disease and many elderly women have hanging over them at least a risk, if not the fact, of incontinence. These things, which are part of the geriatric life, do not of course mean that heart failure when it appears should not be treated energetically with diuretics – but one has to be on the watch for retention or loss of control. One can, however, suggest first, that postural oedema (which is so common) is not treated long-term with powerful diuretics on empirical grounds, and, secondly, that once an attack of congestive heart failure is overcome, diuretics might be stopped, to give the patient the best chance of remaining continent.

In general, older people have strong likes and dislikes, and their refusal to take certain preparations may not be easy to explain. One of their most usual dislikes is swallowing tablets, and to have to take a dozen or two tablets every day may be intolerable to them. For this reason they often take more kindly to suspensions and syrup formulations, but these require some dexterity also. Effervescent tablets taken in water are a good formulation for older people, when they are available.

MULTIPLE PATHOLOGY AND MULTIPLE DRUGS

When ill, old people seldom present with just one disease. Indeed, multiple pathology is the rule not the exception. Some pathological conditions may be recent and acute, others long-standing – but still under long-term drug treatment. For example, painful arthropathy, parkinsonism or diabetes are perhaps already present, underlying more acute conditions. Instinct, perhaps, suggests that one should prescribe immediately for the latter when insufficient thought may have been given to a conflict of indications, or actual incompatibility of the various drugs intended for subsequent use. Sometimes these combinations nullify each other's effects; often they potentiate them alarmingly. Further, memories being short and old patients being uncertain history-givers, significant past events which might contra-indicate a new line of treatment are often never admitted to. Examples are previous drug allergies, or peptic ulceration or the earlier finding of a hiatus hernia, either of which could make anticoagulant treatment questionable. This is particularly so when very long-term treatment has been in use, for the prescriber may literally have forgotten the fact, or a colleague is called first to a new incident and is not aware of the long-term use, for example, of corticosteroids or gastric-irritant analgesics for arthritis, or whatever.

Multiple pathology means multiple symptoms, and often intractable symptoms at that. This, undoubtedly, tempts a busy doctor to prescribe a new specific for each new symptom; it is a temptation which must be resisted, and if a fresh drug be contemplated one should try to discontinue one earlier drug to make room for it in the regimen. The habit of giving extra drugs for new symptoms can lead to prescribing for the side-effects of a drug already in use, when the correct line is probably to discontinue the latter. An extreme but not unique example was when a patient was found to be having nine drugs; three had been specifically indicated but the rest had been instituted *seriatim*, each to treat a new symptom of intolerance to a previous drug!

It is a well-established pharmacological truth that the greater the number of drugs being used, the greater by far the risk of unwanted reactions. These have to be discreetly watched for. It is not sufficient to wait for an elderly patient to report a drug intolerance, for he will probably not recognise it as such. It is an equally well-established fact that geriatric patients cannot be relied upon to report symptoms of any kind for themselves. They assume that their condition will be something inevitable, just because they are aged.

The undoubted risk of using several potent drugs simultaneously does not, however, mean that significant new disorders must be left untreated. Rather, it means that a full drug review is necessary. One might then decide that a long-term condition should be left untreated for a time while the complication is being dealt with. Thus, gastric irritants like phenylbutazone or aspirin for arthropathy might best be omitted while a threatening deep venous thrombosis was receiving immediate treatment.

RATIONAL PRESCRIBING AND DRUG MANAGEMENT FOR ELDERLY SUBJECTS

The reader will see by now that there is an almost endless number of factors to be taken into account when prescribing for old people. At this point it is appropriate to summarise the requirements of good, safe, long-term drug management. These criteria apply equally to practice in hospital and outside it, but hospital staff must, of course, be sure that the regimen they have selected can be put into effect when the patient goes home – which pre-supposes some knowledge of the personalities and the conditions at home. If it cannot, the chance of relapse and readmission may be high.

1. Determination of which pathological states actually require treatment

The supposition here is that perhaps not all can be safely treated at one time. Certain states, like established epilepsy, hypothyroidism or megaloblastic anaemias, must of course be treated continuously. Diabetes, too, must be treated appropriately – though it is often mild in old people – but treatment should be subject to periodic reviews to see if diet alone might suffice. But does arthritis always have to be treated, since the usual drugs are notorious for producing intolerance? Much rheumatoid arthritis in old people is disfiguring but has reached an inactive phase. With activity and pain present, treatment is certainly needed; without them, probably not. Does the hypertension for which the patient has had years of treatment still need continuous treatment now? Similarly, does long-term therapy for depression have to go on regardless of the patient's current mood? The policy must be to put first things first – not first in time but first in importance. There is a tendency for therapy to be over-simplistic. People say 'the up-to-date treatment for X is Y', and simply use it. With elderly patients it is often more appropriate to use Z if it is less potent, and sometimes to eschew specific treatment altogether on grounds of a conflict of indications. Geriatric prescribing is always a matter for fine judgement, and usually calls for compromises. There is absolutely no point in causing the treatment to be more unpleasant than the disorder, when therapeutic aims are limited anyway.

2. Decision as to which symptoms need treatment on their own account

First, of course, one must try to relate all the symptoms to a single cause and treat the cause itself; but things are seldom as simple with older patients. The appearance of a fresh symptom demands consideration of whether it is caused by the current therapy. If so, it is seldom right to use yet another 'corrective' drug to treat it, although occasionally the rule must be broken to get maximum response.

Failure to offer relief for real distress when drugs will help is, of course, not excusable. But old people's symptoms can be numerous yet fairly trivial, because they are more introverted and egocentric, less optimistic than they were when younger. Some have become querulous by nature. Pain and its evaluation is a recurrent problem, but many of the aches and pains of old people do respond to simple, well-tolerated minor analgesics like Distalgesic or the safer forms of aspirin. The pain of malignancy, and the fear of that pain, are a different matter entirely, and there need be no limit to the properly conducted use of drugs in terminal care.

Chronic insomnia, or alleged insomnia, is another cause of difficulty. It is a common enough complaint, but often grossly exaggerated in the event. There are many 'social' remedies to be tried before hypnotics, and the patient is often trying to organise for himself several hours more sleep per twenty-four hours than the body needs in old age – which may be as little as six or seven hours. Hypnotics have a bad reputation in geriatric work because they cause stupor, inertia, 'hangover', falls, and preventable complications like pressure sores or pneumonia. Hypnotics and analgesics also have much increased potency for old people who have anaemia or hypothyroidism. To establish chronic dependence on a hypnotic drug, especially a barbiturate, by inadvertence or by taking the easy option is to sow the seeds of a geriatric disaster.

3. Consideration if any drugs can be stopped
In view of the risks of interaction, which multiply with the number of drugs simultaneously in use, any rational reduction is to be welcomed. Compliance is sure to be better the simpler the regimen. It has been suggested that the average elderly person is not capable of reliably managing more than four preparations for himself, and some would say three is the limit. Hence the suggestion that if one is to be added, an earlier drug should be withdrawn if possible. Hospital inpatient prescribing forms almost force regular reviews of the regimen upon medical staff, since they must re-write the sheet every few weeks. Yet it remains easy with longer-term drug usage, unthinkingly, to repeat them all. The problem is magnified in general practice where face-to-face review of patients' progress is less common but prescribing goes on, and where drugs are often demanded as of right (or habit). A tendency also exists for drugs to be continued just in case of relapse, and occasionally as a calculated preventive manoeuvre where fresh problems are anticipated. This would be praiseworthy if the drugs were as well tolerated and excreted as they are in young people. Patients, once treated for cardiac failure, are so often allowed to remain for months or years on digoxin and diuretics even though their hearts are in sinus rhythm and not showing one classical sign of failure. Others are given psychotropic drugs or antihypertensives indefinitely when no clear indication for them remains. In some circles a theory persists that, once started, corticosteroids will be needed *sine die* (see below), regardless of side-effects. Whatever may be the proper policy with young patients, therefore, safety and good sense require the question to be asked – how soon could this be stopped? With most long-term treatments one should be able safely to withdraw the drug and observe,

reinstating it if need be later. For this policy to be safe, regular and critical follow-up is necessary. In hospital outpatient departments proper continuity of follow-up is often lacking; in family practice likewise, though perhaps for different reasons.

4. Consideration of the correct choice of drugs, dosage and timing
Appropriate choice of drug naturally depends on accuracy of diagnosis. It is not justifiable to place old people potentially at risk from drugs simply on unconfirmed suspicion of a diagnosis, particularly with insidious maladies for which treatment might, once started, be maintained endlessly. There are serious hazards in inappropriately treating anaemias which have not been fully investigated; likewise in treating supposed hypothyroidism on clinical suspicion alone; similarly in using potent new drugs for parkinsonism when this is not substantiated – for several conditions mimic parkinsonism, as does great age itself (see below).

Confusion, the commonest of all symptoms of physical disorder in old people, does not immediately call for drugs, but evaluation. The possibility of diagnostic error is great unless elderly people have been assessed properly in a place where all investigations are available and some are done as a routine, such as blood counts, renal function, electrocardiography, and chest x-rays.

Where the choice of drugs is concerned it is a matter of knowing which are likely to cause fewest adverse effects in old people. For example, benzhexol has a thoroughly bad reputation in elderly parkinsonism, but orphenadrine is less liable to cause confusion. Of the many drugs used for their central nervous system effects, several (notably phenothiazines) are especially prone to cause hypothermia or postural hypotension – two scourges of the elderly which are so often iatrogenically induced. With diuretics it is not always best to use the most powerful or quickest-acting. With diabetes, social factors may limit the choice of treatment, and tight control with drugs often has to be sacrificed because of the patient's fickle dietary habits or total lack of understanding of the principles of treatment.

With regard to dosage – this should generally be smaller than for younger people, especially when the drug is excreted by the kidneys. The reasons have already been examined, and so has the matter of trying to relate dose to body size. When treating acute disorders it is a mistake to be too cautious, for time is seldom on the side of the prescriber. However, with long-term drug treatment the possibility of cumulative effects with high plasma levels must always be kept in mind. In very long-term treatment extending over a large part of life, dosage might have to be reduced gradually in keeping with the reduced metabolic and excretory capacity. It is regrettable that standard adult doses of some drugs in tablets are simply too large for many old people, e.g. nitrazepam and digoxin, and a paediatric dose of the latter (0.0625mg) often has to be used. The dose level to get optimal results without unwanted side-effects can in older people be highly critical. Sedatives are a case in point, and so is levodopa. Such drugs have in effect to be titrated against symptoms and signs, and occasionally a hint of overdose has to be watchfully accepted in the interests of getting maximum general advantage. Besides those just mentioned, a list of other drugs for which it is advisable to give reduced dosage in the elderly includes at least the following: chlormethiazole, chlorpropamide, other benzodiazepines besides nitrazepam, haloperidol, thyroxine, warfarin, metoclopramide, pethidine and morphine – and many who practise geriatric medicine would think this list too short.

Timing of drug administration presents few problems in hospital, but at home they loom large. The more difficult the regimen, the more timing errors there will be. If there are several drugs, some ordered for once, some twice, some three times a day, the old person will simply make mistakes. Many drugs should be taken after food, but old people in a house alone may be capricious about eating and in their other habits. It might be best that all the patient's drugs should be arranged to be taken once or twice a day. There are not many preparations, except for potent analgesics, levodopa etc, where timing is critical. In long-term drug therapy where compliance is a problem, it might be more realistic (if heretical) to suggest that provided the day's drug 'ration' is ingested at *some* time in that 24-hour period, little harm will result. This system simply has to be used by some hard-pressed relatives, who can only pay a supervisory visit once a day. It is habit that has made many of us prescribe doses of drugs three or four times daily when once would be quite satisfactory. Since the elderly have high blood levels and slow excretion, frequent divided doses are often quite pointless.

5. Awareness of likely adverse reactions

These are legion, and likely to be met often in old people because of their changed physiology and the likelihood of being given several drugs simultaneously and on a continuing basis. All the known adverse reactions might be met, but the finding of the following fresh symptoms should raise suspicion that it is not the disease so much as the therapy which is to blame: nausea, vomiting, anorexia, drowsiness, stupor or increased confusion, skin rashes and photosensitivity, lowered blood pressure, hypothermia or extra-pyramidal disorders. The latter are well-known side-effects of phenothiazines and other drugs. Yet it is astonishing how often one finds a patient with parkinsonian signs having his aggression or restlessness treated persistently with chlorpromazine. In one note-worthy case the treatment had been maintained twice daily for 15 long years, yet no untoward behaviour had ever been reported by his wife, and not one of several doctors had suggested it should be stopped!

The 'treatment' of adverse reactions is of course to omit the suspected drugs. Only in a few well-known cases (e.g. corticosteroids and levodopa) need this be done slowly. With drug-induced skin rashes, however, immediate stopping is essential, for serious complications like exfoliative dermatitis can follow.

6. Formulation and packaging

It has already been hinted that old people dislike swallowing tablets and capsules. More research on acceptability of drugs is needed from the manufacturers. Where other considerations allow, syrups or thick creamy suspensions with a reasonable taste are well accepted. So are effervescent tablets and tasteless drugs in granule form dispensed in single-dose packages to be stirred up in a little milk or water. Benoral (benorylate) granules are a good example. Compliance is sometimes entirely dependent on an attractive formulation, or on tablets being large enough to see and pick up but small enough to swallow comfortably.

Packaging has usually to be in a medium-sized container with a simple push-on or screw-cap of manageable size. From early in 1981 most containers have been child-proof unless otherwise specified; often it will be necessary so to specify, because old people will not be able to open them. Attempts have been made to provide multiple-compartment labelled containers with a day's or a week's drugs apportioned in advance, with administration times specified. More experiments are needed. The problem is always that someone has regularly and accurately to fill up these *aide memoire* packs. Labelling must be in bold script or typewritten, clear, specific and understandable, and the name and dose of the drug should be given if only for the guidance of the professional visitor. Frequently drug doses or timings are changed after a visit, and this must be indicated by a fresh label, otherwise confusion will be total. It is also helpful for the patient to be told, as well as to have it on the label, which drug is for which condition. The use simultaneously of several drugs of indistinguishable size and colour is bound to cause confusion. Problems arise even if different brands of the *same* drug are of different sizes or colours, and if the patient has more than one source of supply, i.e. the hospital and the family doctor. This really is best avoided.

7. Instructions

A patient needs to be told about his drugs and their purposes, as well as being handed properly labelled containers. With old people the telling will usually have to be repeated, perhaps many times. This is often left to the nurse, receptionist or counter staff at the pharmacist's; it is done more or less clearly, but most patients really need it written down as well. There is a trend in hospitals to have ward pharmacists who will give specific instruction before the patient's discharge. In this way any problems of suitability of containers and their labelling, and of general comprehension, can be corrected at once. Perhaps, for weeks, the nurses have been handing the patient the drugs from the dispensing trolley at standard times, leaving nothing to chance, yet explaining nothing to the patient! Immediately on discharge the unfortunate patient may be on his own and expected to manage his drugs solo. The only logical course is for him to be given containers of his drugs for, say, one week *before* discharge and made responsible for keeping them and dosing himself appropriately. The nurses' job then is to check that all is well. Problems of security are said to make this undesirable. Any risks have, in the writer's view, to be accepted in the interests of the individual patient's proper instruction and the avoidance of error and the risk of relapse from iatrogenic causes.

In some cases the patient simply cannot supervise his own drugs. Then a relative or good neighbour must be recruited, or if once-a-day dosage is possible, the community nurse may have to be involved. The helper must above all be willing and reliable. Whoever it may be, this helper has to be clearly told all the details, and professional health workers advised of possible side-effects to be observed.

8. Follow up

In a word – it is essential, by one means or another. In any follow-up the responsible person must see and check the drugs and the containers, and if need be hold a 'rehearsal'. Therefore patients must be encouraged to bring their supplies to surgery or clinic. Follow-up is often difficult to organise for old people, especially in country districts. They may easily default if required to report to the surgery endlessly, and the doctor may not be able regularly to visit them. This, then, is where the community nurse and health visitor should take their part. Many geriatric patients are attending day hospitals or follow-up clinics precisely because the domicili-

ary follow-up seems uncertain and failure of compliance with drugs is anticipated – though when they do come, other benefits accrue. It really is no longer acceptable that the fate of old people on complex drug systems should be left to chance and the open-ended repeat prescription.

SOME COMMON THERAPEUTIC PROBLEMS IN AGED PATIENTS

Now it is appropriate to discuss a few specific conditions and categories of drugs used long term which present special problems or give rise to uncertainty where older patients are concerned. This is not of course a comprehensive review, but demonstrates a few practical applications of the principles already outlined.

Hypertension

The dilemma of whether to treat or not to treat hypertension in older people has been under close scrutiny recently. It has been well reviewed by Moore-Smith (1980). Geriatric physicians have been reluctant to use powerful drugs, partly because some rise of blood pressure takes place normally in many (but not all) people as they grow older, and partly because the effects of sudden depression of the blood pressure can be devastating, including as they do syncope, falls, fractures, loss of confidence and cerebral vascular catastrophes. Many argue that hypertension should only be treated in this age-group if there are undoubted signs of myocardial stress, in particular cardiomegaly and triple rhythm, or after a bout of heart failure when hypertension still persists. Intolerable headache, giddiness or retinopathy as a consequence of hypertension in this age-group are rare, and malignant hypertension does not occur. It might anyway be said that treating established hypertension in old age is like shutting the stable door after the horse has bolted. Or, that by the time there is established cerebral arterial disease, the patient positively needs the high pressure to maintain a reasonable cerebral blood flow. The time to start treatment should perhaps have been one or two decades earlier.

It now appears that later in life high pressure continues to carry a risk of cardiovascular morbidity and death, and that systolic readings are of more significance than diastolic values, for both are distorted by changes in the pressure waves in an ageing arterial system, the systolic moving upwards but the diastolic marginally downwards. It cannot be justifiable to treat a symptomless patient of great seniority on one or two chance findings of a high blood pressure; for one thing, old people show lability of pressure just as many young people do; for another, treatment often causes unpleasant side-effects, and the business of regular drugs and blood pressure recordings may make old people highly apprehensive. In later life this could be an example of a treatment being less acceptable to the patient than the disease.

Sizeable multi-centre studies have lately suggested that if in old people the blood pressure is consistently in excess of 180/110mmHg this should be treated, with caution, provided that there are no contra-indications – and therein lie many difficult questions. One should not be treating blood pressure figures, but a patient with a complex mixture of hopes, fears, capabilities and disabilities, and a statistically much reduced further expectation of life, regardless of the hypertension. Old women in particular have a reputation for long survival with a raised blood pressure, of which they may be quite unaware and might be better left in ignorance.

There should be no striving to reduce the blood pressure to the 'normal' for young people, for at that level many elderly hypertensive subjects feel downright ill. The choice of treatment should not be what is most immediately effective, but what is reasonably good without doing harm. Reducing the diastolic level below 105mmHg probably does not further diminish the future cardiovascular risk. The question of trying to reduce the blood pressure after a stroke incident is likewise a vexed one. Its advocates remind us of the known high risk of recurrence; its opponents point to the fact that blood pressure usually falls spontaneously without drugs after a stroke and they ask why, if the cerebral vascular accident was a thrombotic incident, it might not recur as a result of blood pressure reduction. Indeed, most geriatric physicians can recall many cases of strokes occurring in patients receiving powerful anti-hypertensive drugs.

When extended treatment for hypertension in old age is finally decided upon, it must be done circumspectly. Weight reduction would help but, unfortunately, is usually doomed to failure in this age-group. Salt restriction is advisable at any stage. The best initial drug is probably a benzothiadiazine diuretic like cyclopenthiazide with a potassium supplement, or hydrochlorothiazide, either alone or in combination with amiloride (Moduretic). The relatively slow action of these diuretics is advantageous to the elderly in many ways. Even used alone these drugs may be enough to reduce blood pressure, and with it the mortality. If they are not effective, then a more powerful preparation should be added, α-methyldopa probably being the drug of choice for old people despite the fact that its

side-effects include sleepiness, mental slowing, depression, dry mouth, salt and fluid retention etc. The dose of so potent an agent must be small at first and built up, being matched against regular blood pressure readings, and always used in association with a diuretic. Methyldopa would be hard to justify in a patient with brain damage or a history of depressive episodes – and there are many such. Beta-adrenergic blockers are sometimes used in place of methyldopa, with perhaps less certainty of effect but certain disadvantages, notably those of causing confusion, dreams and hallucinosis, broncho-constriction and the chance of precipitating heart failure. Previous obstructive airways disease and heart failure are in fact contra-indications, but if angina of effort was part of the picture a beta-blocking drug might be the one of choice.

Seldom can it be necessary to use more powerful vasodilator-type anti-hypertensive drugs like hydrallazine in old people. Whatever method is finally worked out for long-term use, regular and frequent follow-up is essential and a watch must be kept for any hint of hypotensive episodes, which the elderly are not able to endure as young people may do. In practice it is important to take the blood pressure with the patient standing. Such drugs as bethanidine and guanethidine are not advised precisely because they cause postural hypotension, and the rauwolfia series cause depression.

Cardiac failure

Apart from stroke illness and confusion (which is a warning symptom rather than a specifically treatable entity), heart failure is the commonest major disorder of later life. Mostly it can be treated quickly and efficiently, and drugs, well used, save and prolong patients' lives so that they can live independently and in fair comfort, other disorders permitting. There is seldom an argument as to whether treatment for cardiac failure is 'worthwhile'. Nevertheless, so 'standard' has heart failure treatment become that failure tends to be diagnosed in old people and treatment started upon the merest suspicion of breathlessness or even a decline in general performance. No one should suppose that just because a heart is old it must be 'weak' and on the verge of failure. Leg oedema by itself is not enough to justify treatment as if for heart failure. In old age, isolated left ventricular failure is not very common and diagnostic requirements are the presence of dyspnoea (usually nocturnal), a cardiac triple rhythm in most cases, and some consistent evidence as to cause, before treatment is used. Cardiac ischaemia may be present, but it should not be assumed. The chance finding of basal râles alone is not enough to establish this diagnosis.

Cardiac failure responds well to hospital nursing, but seldom requires prolonged rest in bed. One octogenarian patient rested in bed for 40 years, having once been told she must rest because she had a 'weak heart'; the doctor happened not to call again. Rest at night is important, however, and morphine (not more than 10mg per dose) is helpful in the early stages except in the presence of pulmonary heart disease. The value of a salt-poor diet should not be so overlooked as it has been in recent years, but a severely salt-restricted diet would be impracticable in old age, even if desirable. Otherwise, treatment largely resolves round digoxin and diuretics. This chapter is not of course the place to examine all the variants of drug treatment for heart failure from the outset to the later stages.

Digoxin is one of the most consistently over-prescribed drugs for old people, in spite of being so often positively indicated. As has been said, old people are very sensitive to it especially at low levels of serum potassium. They excrete the drug poorly, for renal function is relatively impaired in old age though the kidneys may not be diseased; therefore, maintenance dosage should be much smaller than in young adults and higher loading doses used with care. It is common to find that a dose of 0.125mg twice daily, or 0.0625mg twice or even in a single daily dose is adequate to maintain digitalisation in the long term. In reality once-a-day dosage for older patients is entirely logical. Excessive dosage often causes nausea or vomiting, or even profound anorexia without nausea or vomiting; but there are other signs of intolerance – confusion, occasionally xanthopsia, even a high-rate arrhythmia such as paroxysmal atrial tachycardia, as well as the more usual bradycardia, which however may not appear at all and throws everyone off scent. Old people who are apparently ill, eating nothing and losing weight, are often admitted for investigation of a suspected gastro-intestinal cancer when all they require is to be released from their digoxin.

To use or not to use digoxin requires sober thought. It is a most valuable drug, almost obligatory in atrial fibrillation at a medium or high rate, provided there is confirmation by ECG. It is also required as the first 'covering' drug in conjunction with other medication in most other arrhythmias – apart from those due to conduction defects involving a likelihood of bradycardia. Yet some old people with undoubted atrial fibrillation maintain a low rate without drugs (the so-called 'senile type' of fibrillation) and they do not need to be put on digoxin. Others have intermittent or paroxysmal atrial fibrillation, perhaps only detected for certain with 24-hour tape ECG monitoring, and doubt arises about using digoxin during the phases of sinus rhythm

to prevent these periodic 'escapes' into atrial fibrillation. In the treatment of cardiac failure with a regular normal pulse rate digoxin should probably be included for its inotropic effect. Since we are considering long-term drug treatment, an appropriate question to be posed is; should digoxin be in use on a long-term basis? There was a time-honoured saying, 'once digitalis, always digitalis'. In older people this dictum would not often apply, for stability of the drug level on a regular dose can seldom be relied upon, toxic effects are widespread, upsetting and serious, and the limits of therapeutic tolerance correspondingly narrow. It is necessary in the view of most geriatric physicians to use the drug when any positive indication appears, but to try withdrawing it when that indication has passed. This policy demands regular follow-up, particularly since other incidents like chest infections can quickly precipitate further cardiac failure and episodes of arrhythmia.

The number of diuretics available for the early treatment of cardiac failure is large. Most of them require the use of potassium supplements; but combinations which include potassium in the same tablet sometimes do not provide enough, though they make the patient's drug schedule simpler. Frusemide for example is widely used, effective and fairly well tolerated by old people, even in initial doses of 80 or 120mg daily. After this dramatic and life-saving stage, during which the disadvantages of a sharp diuresis in an old person can be accepted, the problem is how long to continue diuretics. Certainly until all the current signs of heart failure have gone and the patient has regained a reasonable effort tolerance. This may take several weeks in refractory heart failure in old age. Thereafter though, it is surely reasonable to stop and observe, twice-weekly weighing being a good guide to progress. The open-ended prescription of frusemide in the absence of overt cardiac failure cannot be justified, for there is a risk of potassium depletion, and old people are particularly prone to dehydration which similarly creeps up unobserved. As always, follow-up of such a potentially relapsing condition as heart failure is necessary. To continue the full drug treatment as an alternative to follow-up cannot be justified. Supposing that a longer-term diuretic does prove necessary, there is a good case for using something slower and smoother-acting, like a thiazide. The argument runs that old people would like to get the diuresis over and done with early in the day; but with them this is not always achieved by using a loop diuretic, and even if it is, the precipitant micturition may be too much for their speed of movement and the awkward layout of their houses. Older patients' compliance with potassium supplements is always suspect because of the size and number of tablets needed, though effervescent potassium tablets (e.g. Sandoz-K) may prove more acceptable. Difficulties about potassium are a further reason for questioning long-term diuretic usage, but they can be countered by using a potassium-sparing drug such as amiloride or spironolactone in combination with a thiazide.

Parkinsonism

This widespread disease provides a good example of the need for careful long-term prescribing and management, and most of its victims are quite elderly. Old age is nevertheless heir to many tremors of the 'senile', habit or other types; furthermore there are various akinetic, depressive, negativistic or slow-moving states, including pseudo-bulbar palsy, which are *not* parkinsonism though they look like it superficially. It is not appropriate to treat any of these conditions with anti-parkinsonian drugs, putting the patient at risk of distressing side-effects. Nor is it logical to treat thus the extrapyramidal side-effects of various drugs like chlorpromazine and haloperidol. The diagnosis of parkinsonism must first be clearly established, but this may not be easy at first with such an insidious disease carrying a very variable prognosis. This variability also raises a question of when powerful but effective remedies should be started, if they might, as they often do, lose their effectiveness after a time. Nevertheless it would not be logical to withhold the levodopa types of drug simply because the patient is old unless the risks were unacceptable – and generally speaking they are not.

Amantadine is useful at an initial dose of 100mg rising to 200mg daily, but its action is often not maintained more than a few weeks or months. It has few side-effects but it can cause mental symptoms. Amantadine is now used mostly when levodopa is poorly tolerated, and sometimes simultaneously when circumstances require doses of the latter to be kept to a low level.

The L-dopa drugs are remarkably effective in older patients, some 80 per cent of whom appear to benefit. The newer formulations, combining it with the dopa-carboxylase inhibitors, carbidopa (Sinemet) or benserazide (Madopar), are obviously preferable because they allow reduction of the dose of the potent, yet toxic, principal agent. This dose usually has to be rather less than for younger people as we have seen, starting perhaps at 50–100mg daily and working up gradually with increments every three to five days. The average maintenance dose may run at 500–600mg daily in this age-group. However, courage is needed, and the dose

should be raised to give optimal therapeutic effect just as in younger people. In many cases there comes a point at which side-effects appear and the balance has to be struck. These side-effects are well-known – nausea, vomiting, dystonic movements, unexpected mental changes and cardiac problems. Some care must be taken when using L-dopa drugs in people with a recent history of cardiac or mental problems, but in the writer's view these are not absolute contra-indications. It is not necessary to abandon treatment on the appearance of side-effects; there are many patients who are on the verge of postural hypotensive attacks and dystonic facial, trunk and arm movements just when the therapeutic effect is greatest. Many particularly ask to be kept at a dose level which gives some side-effects because it is a price they will gladly pay for the improvement they experience. Thus, instead of stopping, one should titrate the dose against symptoms, to fine limits; likewise arrange the timing not at 'standard' drug times but specifically to cover those times of the day when the drug seems most needed – for the variability of performance in older people, day by day, almost hour by hour, is remarkable, and often predictable after a few days' observation. Sometimes, small doses at very frequent intervals suit them best, especially later when the duration of therapeutic effect of each dose seems to be shortening. A disadvantage of early treatment and high dosage could be the earlier development of these and other manifestations of the 'on–off' phenomenon. L-dopa therapy therefore has to be well planned, purposefully but flexibly pursued, and reviewed frequently by the same person. It is effective for the akinesia and hypertonicity, but does little for the tremor, which for many old people is highly embarrassing and makes them shun the public gaze.

The other group, the synthetic anticholinergic drugs, have only a limited place. They assist with hypersalivation, may relieve the rigidity a little, but do not significantly influence the tremor. They are second-best to the foregoing drugs, and in old people are not well tolerated. Gastro-intestinal and ocular side-effects are common, and these drugs often cause drowsiness, hallucinations and mental confusion, particularly the latter. Benzhexol has already been particularly mentioned in this respect, orphenadrine being less likely to cause toxic confusion. Since these drugs are only marginally effective and have side-effects particularly detrimental to geriatric patients, there can be no brief for using them and them alone in old people while denying them the advantages of the newer drugs; of the latter bromocriptine must not be forgotten, for it is of use when the on–off phenomenon following

L-dopa therapy has become troublesome. Rather, the question may be at which point to use the newer drugs. Clearly this must be, other factors allowing, when akinesia and hypertonicity are causing the patient distress and making him dependent on others and limiting his self-confidence and his pleasures. It remains to be seen whether the prolongation of life which modern treatment gives will allow time for more elderly parkinsonian patients to develop symptoms of dementia. There is already a hint of this.

Corticosteroid drugs

A number of conditions which are common in later life require the use of steroid drugs, often quickly and with full dosage at first. Examples are pemphigus vulgaris, some urgent respiratory conditions like asthma, giant-cell arteritis and polymyalgia rheumatica; the latter are probably linked on a pathological basis. Giant-cell arteritis is the cause of dramatic blindness as well as other cranial arteritic phenomena. Whether it could be held responsible for a significant number of cases of stroke or cardiac infarction, as a few suggest, is open to much doubt, so the use of steroids for such cardiovascular and cerebral vascular episodes is very hard to justify. This is not the place for such an argument. Undeniably though, giant-cell arteritis involving the retina is a frequent geriatric occurrence and requires immediate steroid therapy. In this and the other conditions listed above, the question must soon arise – for how long does one continue? Where the diagnosis is reasonably certain and there are signs of activity, such as fresh skin lesions in pemphigus or a grossly elevated ESR in arteritis, steroid treatment should continue. However, dosage should be at the lowest level to keep the symptoms and signs in abeyance. In steroid-dependent skin disorders, with visible evidence to go on, it is easy to titrate the level of drug against the signs, but the treatment can seldom be stopped altogether. With persistent bronchial asthma it may also be possible – but less easy – to titrate or stop, and the drug can be promptly used again in a crisis. Some of the other conditions like polymyalgia are self-limiting, so it is surely unjustifiable to use these potent drugs indefinitely. Arthritis is one of old age's commonest afflictions, and the word arthritis still tempts some to use corticosteroids when the type of arthropathy is not clearly delineated. Yet, even with rheumatoid arthritis, their use, except for widespread active disease in an acute stage, can be seriously questioned. Many old women have rheumatoid-like arthritis of the hands, but should not need steroids. In rheumatoid disease and a number of other fairly acute disorders in old age these drugs are of immense benefit in the short term.

Nevertheless, whenever they are exhibited the prescriber must ask himself how quickly the dose can be reduced and how soon finally stopped. The plight of old people after years of steroid therapy, for which there so seldom seems good justification and occasionally not even a definite diagnosis, is truly pathetic. They are bloated and distorted in facial appearance, weak of muscle, bent of back, fragile of skin, so heavy and oedematous as to be usually chair-bound, dependent, diabetic, hypertensive, habituated to the drug, and at grave risk from infections and fractured bones. Whatever the original disorder, this state must be worse – and it has been iatrogenically induced. The writer was once present when two careful nurses were lifting an elderly rheumatoid patient, who was on permanent steroids, from a commode to her bed: this simple act of lifting caused bilateral mid-shaft fractures of her femurs.

Anticoagulant drugs

The use of anticoagulant regimens for old people is possible but full of hazards. Frequently they have to be stopped and counter-measures instantly used, for any significant bleeding in old people is likely to be dangerous. It is hard to justify even starting when a former bleeding tendency is on record, or if the patient has hypertension and evidence of cerebral vascular disease. For elderly sufferers from transient ischaemic attacks (when there are no such contra-indications), or for repeated arterial embolisation from a known cause, anticoagulants may be justifiable. One is frequently faced with a quite aged patient developing a deep vein thrombosis, yet having a reputation for independence, alertness and previous good health. Thus it becomes a matter of balancing risks, and in the light of a limited expectation of life in any event. Assuming that the decision to use anticoagulants in an old person has been made, how long should they continue? It cannot be acceptable to keep a patient in hospital indefinitely for this reason alone, and the hazards of using these weapons without initial hospital assessment and establishment of a stable state with an oral drug are barely acceptable. Then, to continue the treatment at home requires this stable state, good motivation, total compliance, and the willingness perhaps to attend a haematology clinic as required. Such a combination of favourable factors is not easily found among elderly patients. Even then it would be exceptional to continue beyond, say, three months, and often four or six weeks may be the limit, though a high and continuing risk of arterial embolisation could be an indication for longer treatment. Geriatric physicians, having seen so many complications of anticoagulants even when conditions are favourable, tend to be conservative in this respect. They would also encourage their patients to remain actively ambulant, since there is little advantage to anyone in ending with a bed- or chair-fast dependent invalid after such a course of drug treatment.

Long-term therapy and the central nervous system

With the exception of the suppression of epilepsy, which presents few new problems in old age, and the treatment of parkinsonism (see above), together with a few exceptional and rare diseases, it is hard to visualise when drugs acting on the central nervous system can be justified on a regular and continuing basis, particularly when their potency and toxic potentialities are remembered.

The drug treatment of depression is effective, but it should surely be tailored to the fluctuating episodes of mood change. MAO inhibitors do not suit old people well and are not advised.

As has been mentioned, a complaint of sleeplessness is often heard but is seldom fully justified, and when it is, as likely as not the patient sleeps most of the day instead – often the result of having an undesirable type, dose or timing of an all-too-regular hypnotic. The habit of demanding hypnotics is widespread, but it is best resisted, or the patient weaned as far as possible, because the eventual consequences are so often morning confusion or stupor, incontinence, falling and fractures through getting up at night, pressure sores etc. In a case of acute illness or terminal care management, the need for hypnotics may be unmistakeable. So, when an *ad hoc* drug is required it may be best to use chlormethiazole or dichloralphenazone in a moderate dose, carefully timed to fit the circumstances. Fortunately, we have passed through the era when barbiturates were the rule. It is alarming to see how easily a normal adult dose of one of the latter drugs, or of nitrazepam, can 'flatten' a frail old person and put her seriously at risk. A nightcap consisting of a hot milk drink or a regular measure of something alcoholic is a time-honoured habit. For old people it certainly has its place in preference to most drugs. The prevalence of amnesia suggests old people should not personally have control of powerful hypnotics.

Mental confusion and restlessness is a frequent problem. The writer, though acknowledging the social disturbance so often caused and the pressures put upon the doctor by people other than the patient, believes that sedation with drugs should be kept to a minimum, and on an *ad hoc* not a regular basis. The malign effects of over-sedation have been mentioned already, and must surely be well known. Clarity of mind in the patient never follows from sedation, and happiness seldom. If it has to be used from time to time in old people it is better to keep to moderate doses of chlormethiazole, haloperidol or thioridazine, for example, in a liquid or syrup form for preference. Phenothiazines can be held in reserve for crises. The concept of long-term sedation, though very occasionally necessary, is anathema to geriatric physicians. Save in extreme circumstances the sight of a stuporose, slow, unsteady, disorientated, incontinent, spoon-fed individual, rendered thus by long-term drugs for the sake of peace and quiet is not acceptable. Intelligent, sympathetic professional handling can usually achieve far more, at far less risk.

There remains the possibility of using the so-called cerebral activating drugs, whether they are held to possess neuronal, vasodilatory, metabolic or other actions, such as reducing blood viscosity or increasing red cell flexibility to improve capillary transit. Much research into this subject has been done by pharmaceutical firms in recent years in the search for drugs to combat the largest geriatric problem of all, i.e. progressive, chronic brain failure. Not all of the latter of course is attributable to reduced cerebral blood flow. If the several underlying causes of dementia were fully understood and it could later be eradicated, that would be an immense therapeutic triumph. In the meantime any drug able to increase cerebral blood flow would be worth an extended trial, and if its value were proven it would certainly be used long-term. Supposing its cost were to be very high ethical problems might arise, for the numbers of patients who could be treated would be immense. Fully-controlled trials of such drugs are often lacking and are anyway very difficult, because of the problems of evaluating cerebral performance within fine limits. Clinically, the use of so-called cerebral activators has unfortunately been very disappointing to date, but the problem is so large that we should, even in our scepticism, remain receptive to any genuine attempt to halt the march of dementia, by drugs or by any other means.

CONCLUSION

The foregoing is an attempt to put longer-term drug treatment for older patients into perspective, having regard to their altered physiology, multiple and conflicting pathologies and their response to and need for powerful modern drugs. In many cases that need is more apparent than real and it is urgently necessary to limit dosage and the numbers of drugs simultaneously in use, and to be prepared to stop as willingly as to start, for the sake of safety and good sense. This view does not mark the writer down as a therapeutic nihilist, but perhaps as a realist who sometimes sees as much harm done by drugs inappropriately used as good by their proper use. A question for debate is whether, with a few special exceptions, the concept of long-term, uninterrupted drug treatment for old people is acceptable at all. Meanwhile a good maxim might be: 'When in doubt, stop it, wait, and see'.

REFERENCES

Blackwell, B. (1972). The drug defaulter. *Clinical Pharmacology and Therapeutics*, **13**, 841.

Caranasos, G. J., Stewart, R. B. and Cluff, E. (1974). Drug-induced illness leading to hospitalisation. *Journal of the American Medical Association*, **228**, 713.

Hurwitz, N. (1969). Predisposing factors in adverse reactions to drugs. *British Medical Journal*, **1**, 536.

Moore-Smith, B. (1980). *The Management of Hypertension in the Elderly*. In *The Treatment of Medical Problems in the Elderly* (ed Denham, M. J.). M. T. P. Press Limited, Lancaster.

O'Malley, K., Judge, T. G. and Cross, J. (1980). *Geriatric Clinical Pharmacology and Therapeutics*. In *Drug Treatment*, 2nd edition (ed Avery, G. S.). Churchill Livingstone, Edinburgh.

Sackett, D. L. (1976). *The Magnitude of Compliance and Non-compliance*. In *Compliance with Therapeutic Regimens* (eds Sackett, D. L. and Haynes, R. B.). Johns Hopkins University Press, Baltimore.

Williamson, J. and Chopin, J. M. (1979). *Adverse reactions to prescribed drugs in the elderly – a multicentre investigation*. Quoted in *Drugs in the Elderly* (eds Crooks, J. and Stevenson, I. H.). Macmillan Publishers, London.

Woodford-Williams, E., Alvarez, A. S., Webster, D., Landless, B. and Dixon, M. P. (1968). Serum protein patterns in normal and pathological ageing. *Gerontologia*, **10**, 86.

Chapter 18 Prescribing during pregnancy and breast-feeding

SHEILA L. B. DUNCAN MD, FRCOG

INTRODUCTION

Throughout the ages, anxiety that a woman may be safely delivered and her child be normal has been well founded since there were many hazards. The science of embryology swept away mediaeval beliefs that adverse sights might result in structural abnormalities in the unborn child only to be replaced by the realisation that environmental factors or ingestion of apparently harmless drugs could have disastrous effects.

This chapter will deal mainly with drugs liable to be prescribed by the general practitioner for prophylactic or therapeutic reasons. There are, in addition, important environmental influences such as irradiation, industrial pollutants and chemical contamination of food, such as mercury contamination of fish which occurred in Japan (Minimata disease). Many such factors are recognised to cause adverse fetal effects but these are outside the scope of this chapter which will deal rather with prescribing for individuals. Drugs used solely for short-term effects in pregnancy or labour such as uterine inhibition or stimulation, fetal lung maturation or pain relief in labour will not be considered in detail. Rather, the problem for the family doctor is to steer a course between adequate therapeutic endeavour in the woman of childbearing age and safe prescribing before and during pregnancy and breast-feeding. Drugs given during pregnancy and lactation are usually primarily for the benefit of mother and any fetal effects are unintended or undesirable. It is, however, in the interests of the fetus that the mother remains healthy. There are a few occasions when therapy is given primarily for fetal benefit and any undesirable effects on the mother must be considered.

DRUG EFFECTS ON THE FETUS

Timing is crucial. An adverse effect around conception may result in failure of implantation or development. In the early weeks there may be disruption of orderly organogenesis while later, formed systems may suffer impairment of growth or maturation. After birth any effect is likely to be on function. For many substances the effect cannot be predicted. Experimental studies are indirect and animal studies may prove not to be relevant. Thus, thalidomide is relatively harmless in rodents while salicylates, long used in pregnancy without obvious harmful effect, cause a variety of congenital malformations in pregnant rats. It is for this reason that most new drugs carry an explicit warning about use in pregnancy since unexpected effects are always possible.

Table 1 Possible factors influencing drug action in pregnancy

Increased maternal blood volume and protein binding
Ingested drug may be altered by maternal liver before reaching placental circulation
Placental blood flow may vary
Variability in lipid solubility, molecular weight and ionisation influence transfer
Placenta contains enzymes for most known drug disposal mechanisms
Substances received into the fetal circulation are effectively 'intravenous'
The fetal umbilical vein bypasses the liver and a relatively large proportion of any drug in the circulation goes directly to the brain
Transfer into liquor and/or fetal excretion lead to recirculation by swallowing and possible alteration by fetal liver

Distribution of a drug may be altered in a woman in pregnancy and variations in placental transfer, metabolism and fetal circulation add to the possible complexities. Not only may developing tissues, e.g. limbs/teeth/bone be vulnerable in a different manner to formed tissues but the fetus may be exposed to a different metabolite. Table 1 summarises some of the variables. Many a mother is aware that ingestion of alcohol has an effect on the breast-fed infant and laxatives intended solely for herself may have a distinctly anti-social effect on her baby. Nevertheless, milk is a relatively unimportant route for drug excretion so far as the mother is concerned. Maternal absorption, renal excretion, protein binding in plasma and milk and lipid solubility vary not only between drugs but also between women so that the amount excreted may bear little relationship to the administered dosage. Studies of milk excretion are particularly complicated by difficulties in the collection of representative samples since even within a feed, concentration may vary. The actual amount received by an infant will be a function of both concentration and volume and the time from drug ingestion will affect individual feeds. The baby may digest some drugs (e.g. insulin) which therefore lose pharmacological effects while absorbed drugs may have a prolonged effect since gut motility may be slow and excretion mechanisms poor. (For a useful background review see Berlin, 1980.) Thus, the presence of a drug in milk may or may not lead to an effect in the baby. Important effects will be referred to in discussion of the relevant drug groups.

KNOWLEDGE OF DRUG EFFECTS

A good deal of present knowledge has been built up by anecdotal observation, retrospective study and only occasionally by planned observation. Anecdotal observations, for example the increased occurrence of cleft palate in women taking anticonvulsant drugs (Meadow, 1968), have been the basis for more definitive confirmatory studies. Other possibilities based on preliminary observations such as potato avoidance for prevention of neural tube defects have not proved effective on prospective study. Where a drug is a potent teratogen (e.g. thalidomide) a cause and effect relationship can be established fairly quickly once suspicion has been aroused but when a very low incidence of teratogenicity occurs (as with anticonvulsant drugs) it is much more difficult to establish an association. For many substances after years of study the most that can be said is that the drug is possibly harmful in susceptible subjects.

Drug prescribing in pregnancy may relate to:

1. Women who conceive while on long-term therapy for medical disorders.
2. Women where conception and short-term drug therapy happen to co-exist.
3. Possibilities for therapy on account of pregnancy.
4. Incidental disorders arising during pregnancy or breast-feeding.

MEDICAL DISORDERS REQUIRING PRE-PREGNANCY CONSIDERATION

Most women in the reproductive age-group are healthy and have little need for long-term drug therapy. However, several medical disorders involving drug therapy have important consequences for pregnancy and decisions concerning management are best resolved before pregnancy. The concept of pre-pregnancy counselling where there are medical disorders requires wider recognition and opportunities should not be lost for advice concerning the implications for pregnancy. Suitable occasions often arise when discussing possible changes in drug therapy or advising about contraception.

Epilepsy

The young woman requiring drug therapy for epilepsy carries additional difficulties in relation to reproduction. In some, control of fits may be less effective when using oral contraception and more specifically the taking of anti-epileptic drugs may be associated with an increased risk of failure of oral contraception (John, 1976). It becomes important therefore to ensure optimal anti-epileptic drug management at all times in girls liable to become pregnant. It is better to review the need for drugs prior to pregnancy than risk the disadvantages of stopping therapy in the early weeks of pregnancy. There can be few firm rules in this area but it is common practice to review the need for therapy if fits have been totally controlled for about two years. Any attempts to withdraw drugs should precede pregnancy since the occurrence of fits or, especially, status epilepticus could itself be damaging to the developing fetus. The effect of pregnancy on the frequency of fits is variable and certainly difficult to predict but since there is in general a tendency for fits to increase it becomes a particularly undesirable time to experiment with withdrawal of therapy. A possible factor for the increased tendency to fits is that serum concentrations of anti-epileptic drugs tend to fall possibly due to increased blood volume and increased renal excretion. An increase in drug dosage may therefore be required in pregnancy.

There have been many reports in recent years of an increased association between the use of anticonvulsants during pregnancy and an increase in incidence of congenital malformations, mainly cleft lip or palate and congenital heart defects. Attention was drawn to this possibility by Meadow in 1968 and a summary of the available studies (Smithells, 1976) suggests an incidence of about two per cent for both congenital heart lesions and for cleft lip and palate. These incidencies are about twice the background in the general population. What remains less certain is whether this increased incidence in congenital malformations, small though it is, is causally related to the drugs and, if so, whether any specific drugs are responsible. There is little doubt in animal studies that anti-epileptic drugs such as phenytoin and barbiturates are associated with developmental defects. There is some evidence that trimethadone is especially harmful. In the past there has been greater enthusiasm for combined preparations or the use of several drugs and this has complicated the analysis of specific drug effects. Most mothers on anti-epileptic treatment have normal children and the small teratogenic risk of drugs certainly does not justify withdrawal of therapy from a woman who needs treatment even if her epilepsy is well controlled. The harm likely to result from uncontrolled fits to both the fetus and the mother is a greater risk. In recent years there has been a greater tendency to use only a single drug provided this controls the fits and, if it does not, to change the drug rather than add a second or third drug. Hopefully, single drug therapy will enable better evaluation of specific drug risks. There is substantial advantage in surveillance of serum concentrations of drugs and there should be readiness to increase the dosage of drug should fits occur. (For a review of this topic see Editorial, *BMJ*, 1980.)

Women on anticonvulsant drugs are especially prone to folate deficiency and supplements should be given. Phenobarbitone, primidone and phenytoin have all been associated with a deficiency of vitamin K-dependent clotting factors and vitamin K should therefore be given to the neonate.

Anticonvulsant drugs are excreted in milk and tend to depress the infant. However, this effect is not necessarily of clinical significance in most instances and the advantages of breast-feeding may be considerable. Usually lactation should be encouraged unless the mother is on exceptionally high doses or the baby is especially sleepy. Breast-feeding should be discontinued if there is any suspicion of clotting deficiency.

There is a dearth of information on long-term evaluation of the children of mothers taking anticonvulsant drugs during pregnancy. Epilepsy is not a single entity with predictable genetic effects and the relative effect of drugs in pregnancy and later environmental influences would be singularly difficult to discriminate.

Diabetes

The outlook for pregnancy in women with diabetes has improved steadily and dramatically over recent decades at the expense of good compliance of the patient and meticulous control of the blood sugar. The main problems affect the juvenile-onset type of diabetes and such women are usually established on insulin. Prior to pregnancy diabetic women should be educated in the importance of adequate control of blood sugar during pregnancy and should have some knowledge of the additional time and trouble that will be required of them for safe management of their pregnancy. In the early weeks the main relevant event is that the increase in glomerular filtration results in increased excretion of sugar in urine and unreliability of urine testing to control the dose of insulin. Unless the girl is warned of this in advance she may increase her dose of insulin because of glycosuria and this, especially if accompanied by some degree of nausea associated with early pregnancy, may result in hypoglycaemia. While there is no certainty at present that maternal hypoglycaemia is associated with an increased risk of congenital anomalies nevertheless one of the most disappointing features in the management of diabetic pregnancy has been that there has been no decrease in the incidence of infants born with significant congenital abnormalities. At present this rate is approximately three times that of the general population. It remains to be seen whether optimal blood sugar control during the early weeks of development contributes to a reduction in this high congenital anomaly rate.

Most of the problems later in pregnancy so far as insulin dosage is concerned relate to the appropriate increase in insulin dosage as pregnancy proceeds. It is often necessary to change to shorter-acting types given more frequently and the general aim should be to keep the blood sugar as normal as possible throughout the 24-hour period. There is no alternative at present to frequent blood sugar measurements and the use of home monitoring has been a significant advance. Although the metabolic disturbance in diabetes and the effect on pregnancy is complex and poorly understood, nevertheless the improved outlook for normal growth of the fetus and optimal condition at birth relates very closely to blood sugar control and this is where the main therapeutic efforts should be directed. It is, of course, also important to identify disorders of pregnancy such as pre-eclampsia. Optimal management of the insulin-taking diabetic woman in pregnancy hinges closely on a team approach between diabetic physician and obstetrician and should only be undertaken in a centre with adequate facilities for monitoring of blood glucose and facilities for the care of the ill newborn.

The role of drugs in the milder diabetic is more controversial. Problems relate both to the woman with abnormal glucose tolerance only in pregnancy (gestational diabetic) and the older woman with maturity-onset diabetes. Outside pregnancy such women may be treated with diet only or with one of the sulphonylurea group of drugs. Oral hypoglycaemic agents have certainly been associated with successful outcome of pregnancy and there is no evidence of any increase in congenital abnormalities but, in general, control of the diabetes may be poor; some women require insulin in late pregnancy, and the perinatal outcome both in terms of survival and of avoiding macrosomia is not so good as the outcome with good insulin control (Sutherland et al, 1974). In addition there have been particular problems with hypoglycaemia in the baby after birth. The drugs are certainly found in the baby, they metabolise slowly and it may be very difficult to maintain glucose levels. Very profound symptoms have occurred in carefully studied cases and there have been occasions when exchange transfusion of the infant has been required to reduce the drug level. On the whole, oral hypoglycaemic agents are a poor alternative to insulin in pregnancy.

Even the group of women with no symptoms and only abnormal glucose tolerance have a higher perinatal mortality compared with the normal population. Although it is at present uncertain how much this can be reduced by drug therapy, it seems rational to use the blood sugars as a guide and to try to achieve normal glycaemia during the entire pregnancy. If insulin would help to achieve this then it seems the appropriate treatment.

Thyroid disorders

Since disorders of the thyroid gland particularly affect women in the childbearing age-group the association in pregnancy is quite common. Untreated hypothyroidism is an exception to this since infertility is common and it would be more usual for pregnancy to occur in women already having replacement therapy. However, a mild degree of hypothyroidism may co-exist with pregnancy and diagnosis may be difficult. Increased protein binding of thyroxine renders many of the usual thyroid function tests unsatisfactory and an important feature of the diagnosis of hypothyroidism is an elevated TSH level in a patient with features that are clinically suspicious. Treatment would normally be with thyroxine to a replacement level sufficient to ensure adequate suppression of TSH to normal levels. The therapeutic aim, therefore, is to provide a sufficient dose of thyroxine so that the mother is euthyroid. Provided treatment of the mother is adequate the outcome of the pregnancy should not be prejudiced.

Hyperthyroidism complicates pregnancy in approximately 1 in 500 pregnancies. The most common situation is that the patient is already on anti-thyroid treatment since untreated hyperthyroidism is likely to result in amenorrhoea. However, the onset of hyperthyroidism in pregnancy is attended with particular difficulties in diagnosis since many of the features are closely mimicked by the physiological changes in pregnancy. Radioactive iodine tests should not be used in pregnancy as iodine readily passes to the fetus. The increase in protein binding in pregnancy also confuses the interpretation of tests of thyroid function. Under-treatment with anti-thyroid drugs carries a risk of cardiac failure, thyroid crisis, abortion or preterm labour in the course of pregnancy while overtreatment carries a risk of suppression of the fetal thyroid. Thus the objective of drug therapy is to steer a suitable course between these risks. While there may be occasions where thyroidectomy is preferable, drug treatment with anti-thyroid drugs is usually satisfactory. Propylthiouracil up to 100mg eight-hourly is a satisfactory drug to use in pregnancy and as pregnancy proceeds it may well be possible to reduce the dosage. As the increased metabolic rate in pregnancy 'absorbs' some of the increased thyroid output, the need for drugs may well reduce. Anti-thyroid drugs cross the placenta and there is, therefore, a risk of suppression of the fetal thyroid. This is an important argument for the reduction of the dosage as the pregnancy proceeds. In certain women, particularly where the cardiac effects of hyperthyroidism are predominant, the addition of propranolol may aid control. The aim of management should be to maintain the mother as euthyroid as possible assessing the matter clinically and by serum thyroxine and TSH levels. It is usually possible to reduce the drug dosage substantially towards the end of pregnancy even at the expense of slight hyperthyroidism and thus reduce the risk of suppression of the fetal thyroid. There has been uncertainty in recent years as to the value of adding thyroxine to the regimen to try to avoid hypothyroidism in the infant. However, thyroxine crosses the placenta poorly and the net effect of combined therapy is that a greater dose of anti-thyroid drug is necessary. This seems a conflicting objective and there is no evidence that the management with the combined regimen is in any way superior to the minimum dosage of anti-thyroid drug used alone.

Particular difficulties occur in a minority of patients with hypothyroidism who have high levels of maternal long-acting thyroid stimulator (LATS) and/or LATS protector – immunoglobulins associated with some cases of toxic goitre. These immunoglobulins remain in the mother even after thyroidectomy and when she is euthyroid. Babies born to such mothers may suffer from neonatal thyrotoxicosis even if the mother has required no therapy during her pregnancy. When a high level of immunoglobulin can be detected in the mother during pregnancy the management for the protection of the baby becomes complex but essentially depends on anti-thyroid treatment for the infant given via the mother and thyroxine therapy for the mother to maintain her in a euthyroid state (Munro et al, 1978).

Both iodides and thiouracil drugs pass readily into milk. Radioactive iodine tests should not therefore be used in breast-feeding women since even tracer doses can suppress the fetal thyroid. Lactating women can produce enough thyroxine normally in milk after the first week that the infant with congenital hypothyroidism may have the features obscured. For this reason screening tests for hypothyroidism should be done in the first week of life. Thiouracil is actually concentrated in milk so that levels may be higher than in maternal plasma. As it is then absorbed by the baby after ingestion, mothers who require anti-thyroid drugs after delivery should not breast-feed.

Cardiovascular disorders

Hypertension, valvular and congenital heart defects and thrombo-embolism all have important implications for pregnancy. Drug therapy is, however, only a relatively small component of total management in such women.

HYPERTENSION

Between one and two per cent of women in pregnancy have hypertension pre-dating their pregnancy. Although there are especial risks in pregnancy there is no need to advise against pregnancy except in a few very severe cases or a few with underlying auto-immune disease. Where hypotensive drugs are required these should be continued during pregnancy although in a few women dosage can be reduced in mid-pregnancy. Choice of drug from the wide variety of hypotensive agents available may be a problem. In general, adrenergic-blocking drugs such as guanethidine and debrisoquine have the disadvantage of depending largely on postural effects and are not the optimal drug in late pregnancy. Ganglion-blocking drugs are not much used now for long-term therapy but have no place in pregnancy because of their parasympathetic effects of gut and urinary inhibition (already sluggish in pregnancy) and the occurrence of ileus in the fetus. Methyldopa, which has both central and peripheral adrenergic-blocking effects, is a preferred drug which has stood the test of time in pregnancy. Vasodilators, such as hydralazine are usually reserved for acute episodes. In general, there is no necessity to alter whatever regimen a woman is satisfactorily stabilised on, at least during the early weeks. From mid-pregnancy onwards the regimen should be carefully evaluated and change to methyldopa may be feasible. Drowsiness, depression and bradycardia in the mother and, very rarely, haemolysis in the newborn have been reported but the incidence of drug complications is very low.

HEART DISEASE

Women with significant heart disease carry very definite additional risks in pregnancy and require close supervision and access to cardiac care facilities. If digitilisation is required before pregnancy because of heart failure or fibrillation then it will certainly be required during pregnancy and the dosage for effective blood levels may need to be increased. Diuretic therapy may assist the prevention of pulmonary oedema.

The fetus shares digoxin given during pregnancy but in practice this appears to have no harmful effect. There is substantial transfer of digoxin into milk so that levels of the drug in milk are just below those in maternal plasma. Nevertheless, levels found in infant plasma are low and the baby receives only a small proportion of a daily maintenance dose. The decision about whether a woman requiring long-term digoxin treatment should breast-feed or not depends more on other factors than transfer of digoxin to the baby. There is no contra-indication to breast-feeding but if the father will cope with night feeds by bottle this may be in the mother's best interests.

THROMBO-EMBOLISM

There are few indications for long-term anticoagulant treatment in women likely to conceive but the insertion of artificial heart valves is one. Stopping anticoagulant therapy may be disastrous and if pregnancy is to be risked, the disadvantages of anticoagulation must be accepted. In other situations when anticoagulation is advised for some months, such as after venous thrombosis or pulmonary embolism, perhaps following surgery or oral contraception usage, postponement of pregnancy until after therapy is finished should be strongly advised. This will usually mean the use of alternative contraception and women should be warned that anticoagulant therapy carries risks in early pregnancy. Further discussion will be included under occurrence of thrombo-embolism during pregnancy and the puerperium.

Respiratory diseases

The important long-term respiratory disorders influencing management in pregnancy include asthma, bronchiectasis and tuberculosis.

ASTHMA

The outcome for pregnancy depends mainly on the severity of the disease. In general, pregnancy is an acceptable risk and medical management of asthma should proceed. There is a slight increase in the incidence of cleft palate in women on corticosteroids in early pregnancy but if they are already required for a woman with asthma the increased risk is justified and therapy should continue. Status asthmaticus could be a greater risk. Long-term use of adrenergic-stimulant drugs such as salbutamol does not appear to inhibit uterine activity at term.

BRONCHIECTASIS

Drug management with antibiotics and antispasmodics, if necessary, should proceed in pregnancy.

TUBERCULOSIS

Every effort should be made to complete the therapy for tuberculosis before pregnancy. However, it may be diagnosed *de novo* during or just after pregnancy. As the therapeutic considerations overlap these situations will be discussed together. Many women on active therapy have had successful pregnancies and problems relate more to the loss of functioning tissue in diseased organs (e.g. lung or kidney) rather than drug ingestion. Before and during pregnancy the general principle of drug therapy for tuberculosis obtains, that chemotherapy should involve at least two drugs and be prolonged and uninterrupted. Streptomycin, isoniazid and para-aminosalicylate (PAS) have been used for many years with few demonstrable harmful effects. There is, however, a low incidence of ototoxicity with streptomycin, and isoniazid causes increased excretion of pyridoxine (B_6) (supplement should therefore be given). Rifampicin and ethambutol are newer drugs which may be preferred to streptomycin or PAS but there is less documentation of their effects in pregnancy. Sensitivity of the organism will determine drug choice. Sputum conversion occurs quite quickly in pregnancy and unless the diagnosis has first been made in late pregnancy there should be little need nowadays to separate the infant.

Psychiatric disorders

Women requiring psychotropic drugs pre-dating pregnancy have problems and decisions to make well beyond drug therapy *per se*. If pregnancy is going to be embarked upon, the drug regimen should be reviewed. For most drugs in common use there is no certain teratogenic effect and any effect on growth and development or increased perinatal mortality would be hard to identify as due to drug effects alone. It is difficult to separate these from other adverse factors not least of which is compliance and uptake of services. A particular exception is lithium carbonate, much used at present in manic-depressive disorders. There is a substantial increase in perinatal loss in pregnancies where mothers have taken lithium (often together with other drugs) and for some forms of heart disorders the risk is increased tenfold. Information is accumulating in this area by virtue of an International Register of Lithium Babies (Weinstein, 1976) and more data should become available. At present there is justification to consider termination of pregnancy in women who must continue lithium in early pregnancy. When pregnancy continues there is substantial excretion of lithium in breast milk resulting in therapeutic levels in the infant. Breast-feeding is not, therefore, advised.

Other medical disorders

There are many other medical disorders such as ulcerative colitis, Crohn's disease, auto-immune disorders and rheumatoid arthritis requiring specific therapy for their control. Some involve the use of new drugs relatively untested in pregnancy. Generally, review of the need for therapy, discussion among the medical staff involved and ascertainment of present knowledge of the drug (often from the manufacturers) should enable an informed plan to be made for the management in pregnancy.

INADVERTENT DRUG USAGE AROUND THE TIME OF CONCEPTION

Drugs may be used to aid conception or women may chance to conceive while on therapy. Diagnostic x-rays are relevant in this context and enquiry should always be made concerning the likelihood of conception and the date of the last period before x-ray involving the chest, abdomen or pelvis.

Rubella vaccination

While not quite a 'drug', rubella vaccination may be given to women of child-bearing age. The vaccine is a live, attenuated virus and there is a risk of viraemia in an existing or soon to be conceived fetus. The exact risk of fetal damage is uncertain and is almost certainly less than after infection with wild virus. When vaccination has occurred during or soon before pregnancy many pregnancies have been terminated but many healthy children have been born without any evidence of the known abnormalities. A problem in risk estimates is that the immune status of the woman before vaccination has often not been known and where she was already immune the risk is minimal. Rubella vaccine virus has, however, definitely been found in the fetal tissues after pregnancy termination and it has been estimated that where the woman is known to have been sero-negative before vaccination the risk of viraemia, but not necessarily congenital defect, is about 25 per cent (Modlin et al, 1975). Where immune status is unknown the risk would be much less. Thus, contraception is advised for three months after vaccination.

Drugs to promote fertility

When drugs to assist fertility are used a concomitant problem is often irregular menstrual cycles and recognition of pregnancy may be problematical. This is not likely to arise with pituitary drug stimulation since each cycle is followed through. With clomiphene, however, there may be failure to distinguish between anovulatory or conception amenorrhoea but there is no evidence that clomiphene intake after conception has any specific adverse effect. Bromocriptine may be used in women with or without hyperprolactinaemia and diagnosis of pregnancy confounded by co-existing amenorrhoea. Again, there is no present recognition of adverse effects and in women known to have enlargement of the pituitary gland there may be positive advantage in continuing bromocriptine during pregnancy.

Tetracycline

This is popular current therapy for young women with acne and is discussed later with other antibiotics. Discontinuation should be advised as soon as pregnancy is planned but should conception occur while on therapy there is no evidence of immediate harm.

Oral contraception

Use of oestrogen and progestogen hormones in early pregnancy is suspected of carrying adverse effects (discussed later) and even the inadvertent use of oral contraceptive doses around the time of conception has been reported to be associated with an increased incidence of cardiovascular malformations. Precise information in this area is especially difficult although the clinical association is a common one in view of the prevalence of the use of oral contraception. The failure rate due to the method is low but usage is under the direct control of the woman and, in circumstances of failure, there is frequently poor motivation, missing of tablets, intercurrent gastro-intestinal upsets and failure to anticipate temporary exhaustion of supply. Some of these features, which may result in the continuation of usage after conception, are also associated with poor 'recall' of precise events. Clarification of the exact relationship of oral contraceptive usage to the time of conception (not usually known with accuracy anyway) may be impossible. Most of the studies arousing anxiety about hormone use have not identified inadvertent oral contraception use after conception separate from diagnostic or therapeutic use. In a study on the outcome of pregnancy in former oral contraceptive users conducted by the Royal College of General Practitioners an interim report (1976) identified 136 pregnancies associated with inadvertent use. The abortion rate was no greater than in controls and of the 102 pregnancies that went to term there was only one infant with significant structural abnormalities. None had cardiovascular anomalies. There is, therefore, at present no basis to arouse anxiety in girls who conceive while taking oral contraception.

DRUG THERAPY INITIATED DURING PREGNANCY

Drugs taken during pregnancy may be either because of incidental medical reasons and despite the existence of the pregnancy or specifically to help the safety or welfare of the pregnancy.

Both self-medication and prescribing of drugs in pregnancy occurs to a very high extent. Forfar and Nelson (1973) found that about 80 per cent of women had an average of four drugs prescribed in pregnancy (excluding iron) and 65 per cent used self-medication of drugs. Despite increasing concern with the use of drugs in recent years there is evidence that a high level of prescribing, often for relatively trivial conditions, is maintained (Lewis, Boylan and Bulpitt, 1980). Analgesics, antacids and anti-emetic drugs contribute heavily to this drug usage.

Drugs in early pregnancy used because of pregnancy

The vulnerability of the developing fetus makes early pregnancy a time of especial concern in drug prescribing. The time of greatest risk may be associated with uncertainty or failure of recognition of the pregnancy and, except in the medical conditions requiring therapy discussed previously, the use of any drugs in women who may be pregnant must be critically considered. Some of the more common situations will be discussed.

ANTI-EMETICS

Since the dramatic decrease in the use of drugs for nausea and vomiting in pregnancy during the 1960s as a result of thalidomide their place in therapy continues to be questioned. Severe vomiting associated with acetonuria is best treated in hospital; the change in environment and intravenous fluids, if necessary, usually obviates the need for drugs. Women with milder symptoms can usually adapt their eating habits or life style to minimise their discomfort. Where nausea remains a significant problem then drugs may help some women so substantially that their use may be reasonable. For drugs such as prochloperazine maleate (Stemetil) 10mg at night, firm risk estimates simply cannot be given. If any teratogenic risk is associated it is so low as to be indistinguishable from the background risk. Nevertheless, the current concern with Debendox raises difficulties. If a child is born with a congenital deformity and any such drug has been given it could be impossible to exclude an adverse drug effect. At the very least women should be made aware of the theoretical risk before prescribing anti-emetics but there seems no reason to withhold therapy where nausea and/or vomiting is distressing, and especially if weight loss is occurring. Continued vomiting or failure of food intake may itself be a greater threat to the pregnancy.

The position at present in relation to Debendox is unclear. This preparation is a mixture of drugs containing doxylamine succinate and dicyclomine hydrochloride together with pyridoxine hydrochloride in a timed-release capsule. The Committee on Safety of Medicines at present advise that they can find no scientific evidence that this preparation is the cause of congenital abnormalities and no indication to suspend its use.

HORMONE PREGNANCY TESTS

Suspicions that oestrogen/progestogen preparations used for diagnosis might be teratogenic were first raised more than 10 years ago. While none of the studies reported can be regarded as conclusive, suspicion has increased with the accumulation of publications on the topic. The argument at present against their use rests not so much on firm evidence that they are harmful but recognition that there are other much better methods for diagnosing pregnancy and that the practical problems resulting from their use are avoidable. Thus, if the woman is not pregnant and bleeding occurs, the cause of amenorrhoea is not clear and diagnosis is still required. If the object of the diagnostic test is the diagnosis of pregnancy, then concern with awareness of the possible risk may become a significant problem. If the couple learn of this afterwards they may seek termination of pregnancy (even if the pregnancy was planned) and although the risk of abnormality of the

fetus cannot be regarded as substantial, nevertheless the woman's mental anxiety may justify termination. Despite the low risk, difficulties may ensue if a child should be born with a congenital abnormality and attention had not been drawn to the point. Discussion of the risk in the first instance would preclude use. This is therefore an example where the benefit of a drug is so minimal that no increased risk can be contemplated. Tablets for this express indication have been withdrawn from the market but oestrogen/progestogen mixtures in other forms are available and this iatrogenic problem is mentioned only to be condemned.

HORMONE THERAPY FOR HABITUAL THREATENED ABORTION

In comparison with the above situation high doses of oestrogen and/or progestogen have been used for several weeks or even months in pregnancy and certain adverse effects have been observed. These cover a range including masculinisation of the female fetus (Grumbach and Ducharne, 1960), hypospadias in the male fetus (Aarskog, 1979) and the long-term risk of vaginal adenocarcinoma in adolescent girls (Herbst, Ulfelder and Poskanzer, 1971). The latter situation is an example of effects arising many years after exposure and arouses anxiety that no new therapy can be regarded as safe for many years.

A dismal aspect of hormone use in pregnancy to prevent abortion is that such therapeutic endeavours continued long after the regimens in use were shown to be without effect (Dieckmann et al, 1953). There is, therefore, no place for the use of such hormone therapy in pregnancy.

IRON AND VITAMINS

Iron is perhaps the drug most commonly prescribed in pregnancy and together with folic acid and other vitamin preparations may be regarded as dietary supplements rather than drugs. Iron, however, is not entirely without risk: not only is over-dosage toxic to the pregnant woman but the ready availability of brightly coloured tablets is a well-recognised risk for children in the house. No adverse effects on the fetus can be specifically attributed to iron taken throughout pregnancy, although individual studies have shown a higher proportion of mothers of infants with major abnormalities taking iron in early pregnancy compared with controls (Nelson and Forfar, 1971). Such therapy is not usually the only drug used and a causal relationship is certainly not established.

Controversy centres more around the need for supplemental iron and whether this can be regarded as physiological. Iron requirements have long been established in pregnancy and amount approximately to:

Baby and placenta	350mg
Expansion of red cell mass	200mg
Blood loss at delivery	200mg
Lactation	150mg
	900mg

This increased requirement is offset by a saving of about 150mg due to pregnancy amenorrhoea and the iron going towards increased red cell volume is retrieved after delivery. Thus a pregnant woman requires to absorb about 600mg of iron during pregnancy in addition to the normal 'wear and tear' requirement of about 1mg/day. Although a good diet will contain at least 10mg, absorption is less and variable, and many older studies (e.g. Magee and Milligan, 1951) have shown convincingly that, in a population, a decline in haemoglobin level is not fully retrieved even one year after delivery. Supplemental iron will not only tend to maintain a higher Hb level in a higher proportion of the population but will result in faster recovery to pre-pregnancy levels and is the basis for recommending supplementation. The assessment of iron deficiency during pregnancy is complicated by wide variations in the increase in blood volume, and levels of Hb are arbitrary. The more meaningful event is the oxygen-carrying capacity of the blood which is impractical to measure but is usually increased even with a modest reduction in Hb levels. Unless a woman is anaemic before her pregnancy, or has already depleted her stores, then her increased requirements can usually be readily met for the first few months of pregnancy. Iron supplements started about mid-pregnancy will suffice for the majority of the population. Starting later avoids the prejudice which may arise if the woman attempts to take supplemental iron when she has nausea of early pregnancy. In healthy women taking a good diet and with only one or two spaced out pregnancies the incidence of iron deficiency in pregnancy may be extremely low even if iron supplements are not taken. Women in poorer socio-economic groups and with poorer dietary intake obviously have greater need, especially if pregnancies occur in quick succession. The practice of an individual practitioner, therefore, will depend very much on the population served.

FOLIC ACID

The additional haemopoesis in pregnancy makes demands on folic acid, the intake of which depends enormously on the type of diet and mode of food preparation. The incidence of frank megaloblastic anaemia

in the UK is low – usually less than one per cent, but varies greatly with the population. Biochemical or bone-marrow deficiency is commoner and suggests that in many women folate requirements are often not fulfilled. Where folate absorption is just adequate to maintain peripheral blood but not stores, then an additional demand such as occurs with haemorrhage or even treatment of iron deficiency may convert the latent folic acid deficiency into overt anaemia. These considerations have led to the popularity of a small prophylactic dose (e.g. 300 micrograms a day) of folic acid conveniently combined with iron. As with iron supplementation it is impossible to demonstrate any benefit in the healthy woman taking a good diet but at least in some populations the incidence of anaemia will be increased if supplements are not given or taken.

The precise formulation of supplements used owes more to individual preference by patient and doctor rather than pharmacological superiority. A 200mg tablet of ferrous sulphate contains 65mg of elemental iron and one tablet daily should suffice. There is obvious advantage in combining folic acid into a single tablet to be taken daily. If more elegant preparations improve acceptability and, therefore, compliance their use should be accepted.

VITAMINS

Vitamins are intimately involved in basic metabolic processes and cellular growth and requirements increase in pregnancy. Their precise role in human reproduction is not, however, clearly established. The increased requirement can be met by a good diet. Nevertheless, additional intake of vitamin preparations may be taken currently by about 80 per cent of pregnant women. Clear evidence to support the need is not available since it is hard to demonstrate specific deficiency and prescribing is often irrational. In animals, deficiency of vitamins can produce resorption of fetuses, congenital abnormalities and/or growth retardation. Observations in the human that folate deficiency was commoner among women who had infants with neural tube defects and with an increased incidence of placental abruption opened up the notion that additional vitamins around the time of conception and placentation might contribute to a reduction in these problems. This is a tempting concept encouraged by the apparent relevance of environmental factors such as social class and seasonal variations to these conditions. Current interest in this area has been heightened by the report of a reduction in neural tube defects in a group of women given peri-conceptional vitamin supplementation for at least 28 days before conception (Smithells et al, 1980). There are, however, some problems in interpretation of this study since the supplemented and non-supplemented groups may not have shared the same recurrence risk. Vitamins in high dosage are not harmless and excess vitamin A is itself a teratogen in animals.

In summary, therefore, the addition to the diet of small doses of vitamins is probably harmless though often unnecessary but advice to use substantial doses before conception is not, as yet, soundly based. (For an account of adverse reaction to vitamins see Lewis, 1980.)

PARASITE INFESTATION

Moderate or severe anaemia (e.g. Hb 7g or less) in women in pregnancy, may be the alerting indication of a parasitic infestation especially in women recently arrived from countries with endemic infestation. While not exclusive to pregnancy the urgency for treatment is greater and there is often accompanying poor diet in such women. Therapy will depend on the infestation. Hookworm which is often associated with anaemia will usually respond to one dose of 2.5g bephenium (Alcopar) and the anaemia can be rectified by oral supplementation.

ACCOMPANYING OR INCIDENTAL DRUG THERAPY IN PREGNANCY

Antacids

Reflux oesophagitis is a frequent problem, especially in late pregnancy. Delayed gastric emptying may contribute to the reflux but also tends to prolong the effect of ingested antacids. If postural adjustments, especially after meals, do not help sufficiently then antacids should be offered. There is no likely harmful effect in small or occasional doses. Some preparations contain a lot of sodium and this may be a disadvantage to some women in late pregnancy but this would be clinically significant only with very large doses. Alginate preparations produce a more mechanical than pharmacological effect but tend to be more expensive.

Laxatives

Constipation is such a common accompaniment of pregnancy that advice about this is frequently sought. Although not of itself very important, passage of a hard stool may be painful or damaging if haemorrhoids are present. The first aim should be to try to improve bowel function by increased bulk in the diet and dependence on purgatives should be avoided. Bulk purgatives such as methylcellulose or agar seem more physiological than irritants such as senna or bisacodyl

but as they are not specifically harmful in moderate doses, personal preference should prevail.

Analgesic drugs

The use of salicylates is hallowed more by tradition than by therapeutic approval. High doses in rodents have undoubted teratogenic effects but no such effect has been convincingly demonstrated in the human. Retrospective studies on infants with congenital abnormalities have demonstrated an increased intake of salicylates in early pregnancy compared with control mothers (Richards, 1969) but as in all such studies when the outcome of the pregnancy is known the significance of retrospective questioning is uncertain. Subsequent studies have not shown a teratogenic effect (Slone et al, 1976). Salicylates also have antiprostaglandin effects and therefore there is the theoretical risk of premature closure of the ductus arteriosus and adverse effects on blood clotting. The clinical significance of these actions in pregnancy is not certain but in Australia, where self-medication with salicylates is commoner, an increased incidence of prolonged gestation and obstetric haemorrhage has been found in regular salicylate takers (Collins and Turner, 1975). Such an association cannot be assumed to be causal, however, since there may be other factors distinguishing these populations. An effect on haemostasis in the neonate has been shown (Bleyer and Breckenridge, 1970). Even in present-day studies the use of salicylates in pregnancy is high (Lewis et al, 1980) and it would seem reasonable to advise restriction of their use in the last month or so of pregnancy. There is, however, no basis for withholding occasional doses when symptoms warrant it. Salicylates and other analgesic drugs, e.g. phenacetin are excreted into milk but cause little harm. Methaemoglobinaemia with phenacetin has, however, been described.

Antibiotics and chemotherapy

Most antibiotics cross the placenta into the fetus and liquor, although to a varying extent. In general, greater protein binding limits passage. This variability may be utilised depending on whether the therapeutic intention includes the fetus as well. For example, if the intention is to treat maternal urinary tract infection or pneumonia there is no positive advantage in fetal treatment as well. For maternal syphilis or uterine infection the chief aim of therapy may be fetal and good therapeutic levels in the fetal compartment are essential.

Where drugs pass rapidly across the placenta the initial equilibrium between mother and fetus yields to higher levels in the fetus, as maternal but not fetal excretion proceeds. Frequent doses may lead to accumulation of drugs in the fetus.

As with all antibiotics, identification of the organism and recognition of sensitivity are desirable where possible before selecting the appropriate antibiotic.

Penicillin and ampicillin (where a broader spectrum of effect is required) have been widely used in pregnancy and there seem no specific adverse effects. Tetracycline is nowadays avoided because of its affinity for developing bone and teeth with consequent interference with bone growth and discolouration of teeth. These effects are important from the fourth month onwards and it is not certain whether there is a critical time earlier in pregnancy. Although definite limb deformities have occurred in rodents there is no proven teratogenicity in the human. This point is important because of the use in acne and girls given tetracycline should therefore simply be warned to stop its use if pregnancy occurs or is suspected. Apart from the fetal effects there have been reports of fatty degeneration of the liver and even liver failure and altogether this group of antibiotics should be avoided in pregnancy.

Chloramphenicol has not been shown to be harmful to the developing embryo but if used in late pregnancy may cause the 'grey syndrome' in the neonate. Streptomycin was widely used in former times in tuberculosis in pregnancy and although VIIIth nerve deafness has been described the incidence is low. There seems no specific contra-indication to the cephalosporin groups of drugs.

Chemotherapeutic agents

Sulphonamides have been used for a long time particularly in urinary tract infections. They tend to be highly protein bound and when given in late pregnancy may compete for bilirubin binding sites so that where bilirubin is high as in neonatal jaundice, kernicterus becomes a greater risk.

Trimethoprin, often used in conjunction, has an anti-folate effect but the clinical relevance of this is doubtful. It is not certain at present whether trimethoprin or sulphamethoxazole alone might be as effective as the combination (Septrin) which, at least *in vitro*, is synergistic. However, there are other chemotherapeutic agents for urinary tract infections without specific disadvantages and which are preferred at present.

In essence, antibiotic therapy should not be withheld in pregnancy if it is otherwise desirable but the timing, choice of antibiotic and effect on the pregnancy should be considered.

Specific common disorders requiring antibiotic or chemotherapy

URINARY TRACT INFECTION

The treatment of asymptomatic bacteriuria has been consistently shown to reduce the incidence of acute pyelo-nephritis in pregnancy although the long-term effects have been disappointing. Screening the urine in all antenatal women therefore generates a need for therapy which is selected according to bacterial sensitivity. Nitrofurantoin 100mg q.d.s. for 7 to 10 days is commonly chosen because of its safety. Alternatives are nalidixic acid or ampicillin. Unusual organisms or sensitivities may demand other choices.

SEXUALLY TRANSMITTED DISEASE

There are additional considerations in pregnancy. Untreated gonorrhoea carries a hazard of ophthalmia for the newborn while treatment of the syphilitic mother was one of the first instances of therapy given to the mother specifically for its fetal effect. Thus, treatment of a woman in the latent stages of syphilis when not actively requiring treatment herself may prevent either a stillborn infant or one with congenital syphilis.

Penicillin remains the basic therapy for gonorrhoea. Precise regimens vary but ampillicin 3g orally or procaine penicillin-G 4.8 mega units intramuscularly (IM) are currently used.

If the organism produces β-lactamase or the patient is sensitive to penicillin then erythromycin 3g followed by 750mg q.d.s. for four days may be used. Experience in pregnancy with spectinomycin as an alternative for erythromycin is too limited yet for confidence in its safety in pregnancy.

Most antibiotics pass into milk but in small concentrations and clinical effects are, in general unimportant.

SYPHILIS

Treatment requires to be more prolonged than for gonorrhoea and should be given both to those with a new diagnosis in pregnancy and also to women with a diagnosis made within recent years. A possible regimen is procaine penicillin-G 600 000 units IM daily for about 14 days. If the patient is sensitive to penicillin then erythromycin would be alternative therapy.

TRICHOMONAS VAGINALIS

Metronidazole 200mg for seven days is effective treatment for this condition. Systemic therapy is, however, best avoided in the first three months of pregnancy since the anti-protozoal effect carries at least theoretical risks to the embryo. Although specific teratogenic effects have not been established, clotrimazole (Canesten) or hydrargaphen (Penotrane) pessaries may be effective alternatives in early pregnancy. After the fourth month there is no basis for withholding systemic treatment.

Candida, while not usually sexually transmitted, may conveniently be considered here. It is especially common in pregnancy and although local treatment with nystatin or clotrimazole may be effective, recurrence is common. Newer more elegant pharmaceutical preparations and shorter duration of therapy as with econazole (Ecostatin) may be more acceptable but there are no certain advantages.

GENITAL WARTS

Drug therapy with podophyllin applied locally may be acceptable for small lesions but the drug is toxic and anti-mitotic. Absorption is enhanced with the increased blood supply in pregnancy and serious neuropathy has occurred when use has been extensive. Small areas may be carefully treated with podophyllin but extensive areas are better treated by excision, cryosurgery, cautery, or laser therapy.

Corticosteroids

There is relatively little place for long-term use of corticosteroid drugs in pregnancy apart from conditions such as severe rheumatoid arthritis or asthma where their use has pre-dated pregnancy. Because of the increased output of placental hormones in pregnancy it is often possible to reduce the dosage. Adverse effects include a slight increase in the incidence of cleft palate when used in early pregnancy, a greater susceptibility to infection and at least a theoretical risk of pre-term labour and adrenal hypoplasia in the neonate. The incidence of these problems is very low and corticosteroid drugs should not be avoided if there is likely therapeutic benefit. However, when benefit is unproven as in Bell's palsy occurring in pregnancy there seems little point in adding even a small extra risk. Betamethasone 12mg for two consecutive days given IM to the mother for the express effect on maturing the fetal lung if delivery is planned before 34 weeks of gestation has little effect on the mother except for a risk of fluid retention in severe pre-eclampsia. Possible long-term effects on the baby have not been demonstrated as yet.

Anti-mitotic drugs

Indications for the use of potent anti-mitotic drugs are very infrequent in pregnancy. There is only a narrow range between toxicity to mitotic and to normal cells.

Aminopterin is recognised to have a teratogenic effect and may cause abortion. Used later in pregnancy there is a high likelihood of low birth-weight. In situations of malignancy before pregnancy it would always be preferable to complete therapy before embarking on pregnancy. When an indication for anti-mitotic chemotherapy arises up to mid-pregnancy the circumstances may warrant termination of the pregnancy. Later in pregnancy treatment of the mother should not be delayed although diagnosis in the last few weeks may be better dealt with by delivery first. The nature of disease, choice of chemotherapy and individual circumstances make it difficult to generalise but where a variety of malignant conditions have been observed there is a high incidence of spontaneous abortion and malformations but also a large number of apparently healthy live infants (Nicholson, 1968).

Anticoagulants

Thrombo-embolism ranks as one of the commonest causes of maternal mortality. Although there has been improvement in recent years this has occurred mainly in the puerperium, and thrombo-embolism during pregnancy remains a significant problem in diagnosis and management.

Effective anticoagulation in pregnancy carries the additional risks of uterine or fetal haemorrhage. In addition, oral anticoagulant therapy in the first trimester is associated with specific embryopathy involving sunken nose, eye defects and sometimes mental retardation. The incidence of this teratogenic effect is about four per cent where the mother is given oral anticoagulation in the first trimester with the highest incidence between the sixth and ninth weeks of gestation (Hall et al, 1980). Given later in pregnancy there is a further incidence of a variety of CNS abnormalities believed to be due to scarring from fetal haemorrhage. These considerations lead to a reluctance to provide anticoagulation in pregnancy since overall, only about 70 per cent of pregnancies thus treated have a normal outcome. There is evidence that women treated with heparin to achieve effective anticoagulation fare no better. It is probable that prophylactic treatment with subcutaneous heparin is completely safe so far as haemorrhage and the fetus are concerned but it is doubtful if this is adequate therapy in certain high risk groups (Duncan, 1978). What, then, is the best advice? Whenever possible it is better to avoid oral anticoagulation in the first trimester. An exception to this is the patient with artificial heart valves already stabilised on oral anticoagulation. Discontinuation may be disastrous. The price may include not only clotting in the valves but also cerebral embolism, and the risk of embryopathy should be accepted in preference. A new episode of thrombo-embolism in early pregnancy should be treated with intravenous (IV) heparin until about 14 weeks then warfarin or sub-cutaneous (s.c.) heparin given. The choice would depend not only on the presence of other risk factors, e.g. obesity, but also on patient preference. Prior to delivery heparin only should be used. Where the indication for therapy is a previous thrombo-embolic episode then the choice between prophylactic anticoagulants and the risk of recurrence (about 15 per cent) should be discussed.

The condition is commoner in the puerperium and the management simpler. Where the diagnosis is even suspected heparin should be commenced and if it is confirmed a choice made between oral anticoagulation or s.c. heparin. There is no effective passage of warfarin into milk and no adverse effect on the infant (Orme et al, 1977) so that breast-feeding should be normally encouraged.

Tranquillisers

Apart from patients with established psychiatric disorders requiring therapy before pregnancy there is some need for psychotropic or sedative drugs as pregnancy proceeds. In later pregnancy, discomforts may be sufficient to interfere with adequate sleep; late pregnancy hypertension may be benefited in some women by sedation and significant psychiatric disturbance may arise *de novo*. The choice of drugs is wide and there are few firm facts in pregnancy on which to base therapy.

BENZODIAZEPINES

Diazepam (Valium) and chlordiazepoxide (Librium) are useful drugs in some women during disturbed periods and there is no specific contra-indication to their use, although final assurances cannot be given concerning teratogenicity. High doses given in later pregnancy may have a significantly depressant effect on the newborn and this action tends to be prolonged. With moderate doses especially only at night the effect is slight. In severe pre-eclampsia delivery is usually preferable to heavy sedation but there may be occasions when sedation is the lesser risk than eclamptic fits.

Barbiturates

Use of barbiturates during as well as outside pregnancy has been much reduced in recent years. Their use in early pregnancy is mainly in anticonvulsant therapy and often in conjunction with other drugs as previously discussed. Used alone in non-epileptic women there is no convincing teratogenic effect although restriction of use is recommended. Later in pregnancy, concern is more for maternal addiction and prolonged usage is undesirable. Neonatal sedation and even withdrawal effects (Desmond et al, 1972) have been described. There may still be a need for barbiturates for short-term use in severe pre-eclampsia especially after delivery.

Phenothiazines

Chlorpromazine is useful in psychiatric disorders occurring in pregnancy, although drug therapy would be only one aspect of comprehensive psychiatric care.

Tricyclic antidepressants

While useful in depression, drugs such as imipramine carry definite disadvantages. There are important anti-cholinergic and cardio-toxic effects with urinary retention and feeding problems in the newborn. Although the safety of this group of drugs has not been fully evaluated in pregnancy and lactation, there is no convincing evidence of teratogenic effects and if the benefit derived from the drug is substantial there is no basis for withholding it. In general if a woman requires such therapy before pregnancy her need will not diminish and withdrawal could be more harmful.

PUERPERIUM

The borderline between normal reaction and puerperium depression is hard to define. Most sedative drugs appear in milk and may cause sleepiness in the baby but this may be preferable to interfering with bonding by stopping breast-feeding or to a wakeful baby in a depressed mother. The effect of any sedation should be carefully observed in both mother and infant.

Psychosis in the puerperium may be sudden and extremely distressing for the relatives. Drug therapy is only one part of total care but chlorpromazine may prove valuable. In high doses the baby may certainly be depressed. ECT may be preferable treatment. Lithium passses readily into milk. As the toxic and therapeutic levels are close, either lactation should be avoided or, at the very least, lithium levels should be checked in the baby.

DRUGS USED FOR SPECIFIC EFFECTS ON THE PREGNANCY

Most of the therapeutic situations already discussed involve intercurrent disorders in pregnancy or common incidental problems. Drugs used specifically to influence the course of events in pregnancy or the outcome are mainly the responsibility of the obstetrician but a few common situations will be discussed.

Diuretics

Oedema is a problem in late pregnancy but it is now recognised that retention of water and sodium is largely a physiological adjustment. The increase in glomerular filtration in pregnancy leads to constant loss of sodium which is further aggravated by the antagonism of aldosterone by increased progesterone. There are adjustments in the renin-angiotensin system to compensate for this. Formerly, low-salt diets and diuretics were used in a misguided belief that they would prevent fluid retention but instead, these measures may just interfere with a normal, physiological process. Although there have been many studies to try to establish whether diuretic drugs prevent pre-eclampsia there is no evidence that they influence the pathophysiology in any useful way and their use may be positively harmful. Thus, there may be significant electrolyte loss, and blood volume, already reduced in pre-eclampsia, may be further depleted. For the mother their use may result in an increase in uric acid (which prevents this being used as an index of renal function), impaired glucose tolerance or acute haemorrhagic pancreatitis. Hyponatraemia and thrombocytopaenia have been described in infants after maternal use.

The main problem in severe oedema in pregnancy, especially if associated with pre-eclampsia, is a reduced plasma protein level. Increase of the osmotic properties within the circulation by administration of albumin or other protein seems more logical. This risk of hypovolaemia in severe pre-eclampsia was recognised early in the evaluation of diuretic agents in pregnancy (Brewer, 1962) and there seems no more recent observations to alter this evaluation. The value of diuretic agents in reducing blood volume can be usefully exploited in valvular heart disease in pregnancy when a failing heart may temporarily be unable to cope with rapid haemodynamic changes. By diminishing venous return and, hence, cardiac filling, pulmonary oedema may be avoided or relieved.

Drugs influencing uterine activity

Although the precise mechanisms controlling uterine activity and the onset of labour in the human are unclear many drugs affect uterine activity and some have important clinical applications. To induce or accelerate labour both oxytocin and prostaglandins are in current use and ergometrine enjoys world-wide use to aid efficient contraction of the uterus after delivery. Although these drugs are important in obstetric practice the short-term nature of their therapeutic effect puts them largely outside the scope of this chapter. Ergot is, however, excreted in milk and high doses given to the mother in the puerperium have caused ergotism in the infant.

Important among the wide variety of drugs used to inhibit uterine activity are the beta-adrenergic-receptor stimulators such as isoxsuprine, ritodrine, orciprenaline and salbutamol. Although acting mainly on β_2-receptors where the inhibition of uterine activity lies, these drugs also act on β_1-and α-receptors. All this group of drugs therefore, tend to cause tachycardia (both maternal and fetal) and peripheral dilatation. Lipolysis is an important side-effect causing a significant rise, at least initially, in blood glucose. It is usually unwise to use any of this group of drugs in the diabetic woman. Evaluation of these drugs in threatened pre-term labour is confounded by the uncertainty of whether or not labour will really proceed anyway. There is no doubt of their pharmacological effect *in vivo* and many studies testify to prolongation of the pregnancy with their use. A blind, controlled trial is not possible because of the side-effects and a disappointing feature is that in countries in Western Europe where their use is high there has been no reduction in the incidence of low birth-weight. Nevertheless, when it seems desirable to inhibit suspected pre-term labour their use intravenously is at least an option. If uterine activity subsides conversion to oral maintenance dosage is usual although proof that oral use is effective is lacking. It is hard to find reasons to prefer one drug to another in this group although side-effects will dictate the choice in individual women. Other drugs with inhibitory effects on uterine activity include indomethacin and ethanol but the side-effects of premature closure of the ductus arteriosus and intoxication effects respectively, limit their use.

Analgesic drugs in labour

The short-term use of analgesic drugs in labour, including pethidine and morphine used in appropriate dosage have few consequences for the mother. Their use requires considerable judgement, luck and guess-work in order to steer between adequate pain relief yet participation in the birth without distressing amnesia. The effect on the infant may be cumulative if several doses are given and sleepiness in the infant and neuro-behavioural depression may occur. Where substantial doses are used after delivery, e.g. after caesarean section there may be significant excretion in milk. Local or regional analgesia may help to minimise systemic intake but in this area a compromise must be sought in the individual case.

HORMONES, ORAL CONTRACEPTION AND LACTATION

If lactation is not commenced, milk production is usually very temporary and enthusiasm for the use of oestrogens to suppress lactation was much dampened by recognition of their role in thrombo-embolism. Nowadays, if drug assistance to suppress lactation is desired (e.g. after perinatal loss) it is preferable to use bromocriptine 2.5mg b.d. for 14 days.

Advice is frequently sought concerning the advisability of oral contraceptive use during lactation. The contraceptive effect of breast-feeding is variable and unreliable so that anytime from six weeks onwards from a term delivery conception may occur. Contraceptive precautions should therefore be in effect by then. The doses of oestrogen used to suppress lactation are large and there is little evidence that the low dose used in a combined-contraceptive pill inhibits lactation and certainly not after it is well established. However, there is wide individual variation on this point. Although oestrogen has certainly been found in milk, the level after contraceptive doses has usually been below detectable levels. There have been reports of gynaecomastia in infants during maternal oral contraceptive use while lactating and this, together with the increased risk of thrombo-embolism after delivery, make other contraceptive methods preferable. Even these small objections do not apply to progestogens. Lactation once established is not diminished and there are no specific adverse effects in the baby. The benefits of family spacing are so great especially in underprivileged groups or nations that no impediment should be put in the way of women wishing to breast-feed and yet avoid another pregnancy.

SMOKING, ALCOHOL AND DRUG ABUSE

These often inter-related problems have important consequences on pregnancy and involve medical advice if not, usually, drug prescribing.

Smoking

Women who smoke in pregnancy have a higher risk of a low birth-weight baby and of perinatal loss. The association is clear but the mechanism is not and there is not even certainty that the relationship is causal. There are so many other factors influencing pregnancy outcome that it is hard to isolate the specific contribution that smoking makes. However, there are other long-term health hazards associated with smoking and motivation in pregnancy may be sufficient to enable some women to give up. Medical and other health care support may be crucial in aiding this and no such opportunity should be lost. Substitution for smoking should be neither by drugs nor additional food. (For a useful review of this topic see Witter and King, 1980.)

Alcohol

Until recently, society (including the medical profession) has been reluctant to acknowledge that alcohol intake has had any specific adverse effect in pregnancy. However, in 1973 Jones and his colleagues in Seattle described a syndrome in infants of 'heavy' alcohol-taking mothers sufficiently characteristic to be called the *fetal alcohol syndrome*. The main features include growth deficiency *in utero*, facial dysmorphism, short nose with low nasal bridge and short palpebral fissures. These physical features may be accompanied by mental deficiency. The efforts of this group have aroused extensive interest in the USA and Europe and subsequent studies suggest in addition an increased rate of abortion and of perinatal loss. Major difficulties in this area include assessment of the actual amount of alcohol intake and the specific effect of alcohol apart from concomitant nutritional and other social deficiencies. Other studies have failed to identify a specific fetal alcohol syndrome but have confirmed a high perinatal loss and incidence of congenital abnormalities, including microcephaly and cardiac defects, among 'heavy drinkers' (Ouellette et al, 1977). Longer-term follow-up of children born to such mothers includes especial difficulties because of poor environmental factors and level of maternal care, so that the drug effect *in utero* would be very hard to identify. Alcohol is definitely passed to the baby in milk and, in heavy drinking mothers, carries adverse effects for the baby. The group in Seattle have the greatest experience in this area and the best advice they can offer at present is that there is no identifiable harm in pregnant women having less than two 'drinks' daily. Problems have been identifiable in women having four or more and increase with intake (Smith, 1980).

Drug addiction

Pregnancy occurs in women addicted to narcotic drugs although fertility may be impaired in the more severe degrees. Most of the systematic studies derive from the USA where the association is both commoner and well-documented. Pregnancy in women addicted to heroin and methadone has a high complication rate of pre-eclampsia, low birth-weight and perinatal mortality. It is unclear how much of this increased morbidity is due to background social factors, poor nutrition, lack of antenatal care and associated infection, including hepatitis and sexually transmitted disease. It is clear that the neonate can suffer from withdrawal features and it is possible that withdrawal of the drug in late pregnancy can adversely affect the fetus.

The therapeutic management must be comprehensive in terms of psychiatric and social support and further drug therapy may play little part. If drug dependency cannot be controlled by mid-pregnancy it is probably better to continue with a small, maintenance dose through the later weeks of pregnancy, maintaining the nutrition and co-operation of the mother, than to try to enforce abstinence and probably lose co-operation. The birth may be a stimulus to rehabilitation although relapse rate is high (Connaughton et al, 1977).

CONCLUSION

This chapter perhaps owes more to a discussion of why individual drugs should not be used during pregnancy and breast-feeding. This seems a good premise from which to start, and drugs should be prescribed only for positive reasons. Where the maternal need is clear, then treatment should proceed taking due account of the safest drug where there is a choice. Where the primary objective of treatment is fetal, then due explanation to the mother will usually permit her to be a willing 'carrier'. In these situations the risks of failure to treat must be considered. When the disorder to be treated carries a relatively low risk then the advisability of treatment may be more problematical and the safest drug for the shortest possible time should be chosen. If there is doubt, drug avoidance is usually preferable. There is no place during pregnancy or lactation for the use of active drugs for a marginal or placebo effect – where two are joined together by an umbilical cord one man's meat may indeed be another's poison!

REFERENCES

Aarskog, D. (1979). Current concepts in cancer. Maternal progestins as a possible cause of hypospadias. *New England Journal of Medicine*, **300**, 75–8.

Berlin, C. M. (1980). *The Excretion of Drugs in Milk*. In *Progress in Clinical and Biological Research*, Vol 36, pp 115–28 (eds Schwarz, R. H. and Yaffe, S. J.). Alan R. Liss Inc, New York.

Bleyer, W. A. and Breckenridge, R. T. (1970). Studies on the detection of adverse drug reactions in the newborn. II. The effects of prenatal aspirin on newborn haemostasis. *Journal of the American Medical Association*, **213**, 2049–53.

Brewer, T. H. (1962). The limitations of diuretic

therapy in the management of severe toxaemia: the significance of hypoalbuminaemia. *American Journal of Obstetrics and Gynecology*, **83**, 1352–9.

Collins, E. and Turner, G. (1975). Maternal effects of regular salicylate ingestion in pregnancy. *Lancet*, **2**, 335–8.

Connaughton, J. F., Reeser, D. and Finnegan, L. P. (1977). *Pregnancy Complicated by Drug Addiction*. In *Perinatal Medicine*, pp 265–76 (eds Bolognese, R. J. and Schwarz, R. H.). Williams and Wilkins Co, Baltimore.

Desmond, M. M., Schwanelcke, R. P., Wilson, G. S., Yasumage, S. and Burgdorff, I. (1972). Maternal barbiturate utilization and neonatal withdrawal symptomatology. *Journal of Pediatrics*, **80**, 190–7.

Dieckmann, W. J., Davis, M. E., Rynkiewicz, L. M. and Pottinger, R. E. (1953). Does the administration of diethylstilboestrol during pregnancy have therapeutic value? *American Journal of Obstetrics and Gynecology*, **66**, 1062–81.

Duncan, S. L. B. (1978). Long-term self-administered subcutaneous heparin in pregnancy. *British Medical Journal*, **2**, 125.

Editorial (1980). Epilepsy and pregnancy. *British Medical Journal*, **2**, 1087–8.

Forfar, J. O. and Nelson, M. M. (1973). Epidemiology of drugs taken by pregnant women: Drugs that may affect the fetus adversely. *Clinical Pharmacology and Therapeutics*, **14**, 632–42.

Grumbach, M. M. and Ducharne, J. R. (1960). The effect of androgens on fetal sexual development. Androgen-induced female pseudohermaphroditism. *Fertility and Sterility*, **11**, 157–80.

Hall, J. G., Pauli, R. M. and Wilson, K. M. (1980). Maternal and fetal sequelae of anti-coagulation during pregnancy. *American Journal of Medicine*, **68**, 122–39.

Herbst, A. L., Ulfelder, H. and Poskanzer, D. C. (1971). Adenocarcinoma of the vagina. Association of maternal stilboestrol therapy with tumour appearance in young women. *New England Journal of Medicine*, **284**, 878–81.

John, A. (1976). Epilepsy and the pill. *British Medical Journal*, **2**, 528.

Jones, K. L., Smith, D. W. and Ulleland, N. (1973). Pattern of malformation in offspring of chronic alcoholic mothers. *Lancet*, **1**, 1267–71.

Lewis, J. G. (1980). Adverse reactions to vitamins. *Adverse Drug Reaction Bulletin*, **82**, 292–9.

Lewis, P. J., Boylan, P. and Bulpitt, C. J. (1980). An audit of prescribing in an obstetric service. *British Journal of Obstetrics and Gynaecology*, **87**, 1043–6.

Magee, H. E. and Milligan, E. H. M. (1951). Haemoglobin levels before and after labour. *British Medical Journal*, 2, 1307–10.

Meadow, S. R. (1968). Anticonvulsant drugs and congenital abnormalities. *Lancet*, 2, 1296.

Modlin, J. F., Brandling-Bennett, A. D., Wittee, J. J., Campbell, C. C. and Meyers, J. D. (1975). A review of five-years experience with rubella vaccine in the United States. *Pediatrics*, 55, 20–29.

Munro, D. S., Dirmikis, S. M., Humphries, H., Smith, T. and Broadhead, G. D. (1978). The role of thyroid stimulating immunoglobulins of Graves' disease in neonatal thyrotoxicosis. *British Journal of Obstetrics and Gynaecology*, 85, 837–43.

Nelson, M. M. and Forfar, J. O. (1971). Associations between drugs administered during pregnancy and congenital abnormalities of the fetus. *British Medical Journal*, 1, 523–7.

Nicholson, H. O. (1968). Cytotoxic drugs in pregnancy. *Journal of Obstetrics and Gynaecology of the British Commonwealth*, 75, 307–12.

Orme, M. L'E, Lewis, P. J., de Swieet, M., Serlin, M. J., Sibeon, R., Baty, J. B. and Breckenridge, A. M. (1977). May mothers given warfarin breast-feed their infants? *British Medical Journal*, 1, 1564–5.

Ouellette, Eileen M., Rosett, H. L., Rosman, N. P. and Weiner, L. (1977). Adverse effects on offspring of maternal alcohol abuse during pregnancy. *New England Journal of Medicine*, 297, 528–30.

Richards, I. D. G. (1969). Congenital malformations and environmental influences in pregnancy. *British Journal of Preventive and Social Medicine*, 23, 218–25.

Royal College of General Practitioners' Study (1976). The outcome of pregnancy in former oral contraceptive users. *British Journal of Obstetrics and Gynaecology*, 83, 608–16.

Slone, D., Heinonen, O. P., Kaufman, D. W., Siskind, V., Monson, R. R., and Shapiro, S. (1976). Aspirin and congenital malformations. *Lancet*, 1, 1373–5.

Smith, D. W. (1980). *Alcohol Effects on the Fetus*. In *Drug and Chemical Risks to the Fetus and Newborn*, pp 73–82 (eds Schwarz, R. H. and Yaffe, S. J.). Alan R. Liss Inc, New York.

Smithells, R. W. (1976). Environmental teratogens of man. *British Medical Bulletin*, 32, 27–33.

Smithells, R. W., Sheppard, S., Schorah, C. J., Seller, M. J., Nevin, N. C., Harris, R., Read, A. P. and Fielding, D. W. (1980). Possible prevention of neural-tube defects by periconception vitamin supplementation. *Lancet*, 1, 339–40.

Sutherland, H. W., Bewsher, P. D., Cormack, J. D., Hughes, C. R. T., Reid, A., Russell, G. and Stowers, J. M. (1974). Effect of moderate dosage of chlorpropamide in pregnancy on fetal outcome. *Archives of Disease in Childhood*, 49, 283–91.

Thiersch, J. B. (1952). Therapeutic abortions with a folic acid antagonist 4-aminopteroylglutamic acid (4-amino PGA) administered by the oral route. *American Journal of Obstetrics and Gynecology*, 63, 1298–304.

Weinstein, M. R. (1976). The International Register of Lithium Babies. *Drug Information Journal*, 10, 94–100.

Witter, F. and King, T. M. (1980). *Cigarettes and Pregnancy*. In *Progress in Clinical and Biological Research*, Vol 36, pp 83–92 (eds Schwarz, R. H. and Yaffe, S. J.). Alan R. Liss Inc, New York.

Chapter 19 Chronic gynaecological problems

ANTHONY JOHNSON MD, MRCOG

and ALBERT SINGER DPhil (Oxon), PhD, FRCOG

PELVIC INFLAMMATORY DISEASE

Pelvic inflammatory disease (PID) affects the uterus, the Fallopian tubes, the ovaries and the adjacent structures. It may be acute or chronic. It is caused by ascending infection of pyogenic organisms after childbirth or abortion, by gonorrhoea (which is nearly symptomless in a quarter of female cases), by tuberculosis, or by pyogenic infection of the pelvic peritoneum from a primary cause in the alimentary duct (e.g. appendicitis or diverticulitis).

Pelvic infections may also be present as a pyometra when the cervix is obstructed. The cause of the obstruction is usually a carcinoma.

Puerperal and post-abortal pelvic infections

The organisms involved are usually *staphylococci*, *E. coli* or *streptococci*. Rarely *Clostridium welchii* may be the causative organism. Acute PID is an acute surgical emergency and may present with an acute abdomen and the condition must be distinguished from the other causes of the acute abdomen. The patient must be admitted to hospital. Her general condition is improved by intravenous fluids and analgesics. Swabs from the cervix, the vagina and the urethra are taken for bacteriological examination; antibiotics are administered. Ampicillin lg by intramuscular injection followed by 500mg IM six-hourly and metronidazole 400mg usually are given. In cases where there is evidence of a spreading peritonitis or where the diagnosis is in doubt, it may be necessary to perform a laparotomy.

Chronic pelvic inflammatory disease

Chronic PID is often asymptomatic and may be discovered during investigation for infertility. It may, however, cause dysmenorrhoea, menorrhagia and dyspareunia. There is usually a past history of acute PID. The patient will often have a chronic pelvic ache, which is worst in the week or so preceding menstruation. On vaginal examination the pelvic organs will be found to be fixed and tender. The uterus is commonly retroverted. The diagnosis is confirmed by laparoscopy and the extent of the disease can be delineated. There will usually be adhesions and bilateral hydrosalpinges.

It is worth treating the patient with a prolonged course of antibiotics and the most useful are ampillicin and metronidazole. Often, however, a cure can only be effected by carrying out a hysterectomy and bilateral salpingo-oophorectomy. In relatively young women efforts are made to conserve some ovarian tissue and it is sometimes possible to carry out a conservative procedure in a nulliparous woman, with a view to attempting an operation to restore tubal patency at a later date.

Tuberculosis of the pelvis

This disease is becoming more common and it occurs particularly in immigrant women. It is most usually caused by the human tubercle bacillus with a small minority of cases being due to bovine tubercle bacillus. The infection is almost always secondary to a primary focus somewhere else in the body, which has spread to the pelvis by the blood supply.

The infection is commonly silent and may only be detected during investigations for infertility. There are usually bilateral hydrosalpinges with calcification in the walls and this is demonstrated by hysterosalpingography, or by laparoscopy. The diagnosis is confirmed by bacteriological examination of the endometrial curettings, which can be notoriously unreliable, or preferably by guinea-pig innoculation with an emulsion made from endometrial curettings. Repeated curettage may have to be carried out to establish a positive diagnosis.

Treatment is carried out by antibiotic therapy. Combinations of streptomycin, para-aminosalicylic acid and isoniazid are most commonly used. Treatment is carried out for at least two years and the patient must be kept under observation for many years subsequently, to be certain that she is cured. It is unusual for a woman with pelvic tuberculosis to conceive and if she does so, there is a possibility of miscarriage and of ectopic pregnancy. In cases where the disease has demonstrably caused tubal occlusion, the chances of subsequent fertility are extremely remote and hysterectomy and bilateral salpingo-oophorectomy is considered in these cases.

Actinomycosis

This disease is caused by *Actinomycoses israeli* and is unusual. It is, however, becoming more common and may be associated with the use of intra-uterine contraceptive devices. The diagnosis is confirmed by bacteriological examination of material obtained by curettage or biopsied from suspicious areas in the pelvis via laparoscopy or laparotomy. Treatment is by penicillin in large doses given pre-menstrually over a long period of time. It is sometimes possible to achieve therapeutic blood levels by giving massive doses of penicillin orally in conjunction with probenecid.

HORMONE THERAPY IN GYNAECOLOGY

Dysfunctional uterine haemorrhage

Dysfunctional uterine haemorrhage (DUH) is a common abnormality accounting for 10 to 15 per cent of patients seen at gynaecological outpatient clinics. It is a result of ovarian dysfunction which is expressed by irregular, scanty or prolonged bleeding from the uterus. The diagnosis can only be made after any anatomical lesion of the genital tract has been excluded and this will require a rigorous history and physical examination of the patient, a blood picture and a curettage. It may also be necessary to exclude other endocrine disturbances, e.g. thyroid and adrenal pathology.

DUH has the following patterns:

POLYMENORRHOEA

Bleeding occurring at regular intervals which are of less than 18 days. It is more common in post-menarchal girls and pre-menopausal women than in the established reproductive years.

OLIGIMENORRHOEA

Bleeding at regular intervals of more than 45 days.

MENORRHAGIA

Bleeding which is profuse and is often prolonged but which is basically regular.

METRORRHAGIA

Bleeding which is characterised by being irregular and prolonged but which is not heavy.

Treatment of DUH is either surgical or medical. All patients must have a curettage in order to exclude a carcinoma. The curettings will also allow a histological diagnosis to be made and, in addition, curettage is the quickest way of controlling excessive uterine bleeding. Curettage is best avoided, however, in the young adolescent. The place of wedge resection of the ovaries and hysterectomy is outside the scope of this chapter.

The drug treatment of DUH is in the main hormonal, although claims have been made for haemostatic preparations such as tranexamic acid (Cyklokapron), aminocaproic acid (Epsikapron) and ethamsylate (Dicynene). Haematinic preparations are used to correct any iron deficiency resulting from heavy and prolonged uterine bleeding.

DUH may be suppressed by the use of progestogens, either alone or in conjunction with oestrogens. Clomiphene citrate (Clomid) is used to induce ovulation and hence a normal menstrual cycle. This form of treatment is particularly applicable to those patients who are complaining of infertility in association with DUH. It should only be given with appropriate warning to patients who do not wish to conceive.

Menorrhagia due to hypothyroidism can be controlled by thyroid preparations. Where normal ovarian periodicity is inhibited by cortical dysfunction due to adrenal hyperplasis, control can be effected with glucocorticoids.

Releasing factors may soon be used to achieve appropriate secretion of follicle stimulating hormone and lutenising hormone in patients in whom it is deranged due to hypothalamic-pituitary malfunction.

Progestogen suppressive therapy

Prompt control of dysfunctional bleeding can be achieved with progestogen therapy. Norethisterone (Primolut N) 5mg three times a day for five days will usually stop the bleeding. Thereafter 5mg twice a day from day 19 to day 26 of the menstrual cycle is prescribed for four months. A normal menstrual cycle will often ensue following this regimen. Medroxy-progesterone acetate (Provera) is an alternative preparation which may be used in a similar fashion.

The pituitary-ovarian axis may also be suppressed and dysfunctional bleeding controlled by the use of the combined contraceptive pill, e.g. ethinyloestradiol 50 micrograms and norethisterone acetate 1mg (Minovlar) in a dosage of one tablet daily for 21 days followed by seven tablet-free days. These preparations are particularly useful in young women who also need contraception. They should be used with caution in women with oligomenorrhoea lest post-pill amenorrhoea results.

Dysfunctional bleeding and infertility

Patients who wish to conceive and who have DUH can be treated by progestogens followed by clomiphene citrate. The bleeding can be controlled by medroxy-progesterone acetate 5mg three times a day for five days. A withdrawal bleed occurs within one week and clomiphene citrate 50mg daily for five days, commencing on the first or second day of bleeding, is then prescribed. An assessment of whether ovulation has occurred is made by reviewing the patient's temperature chart and measuring the progesterone level in plasma on the 21st day of the cycle. The dose of clomiphene citrate is adjusted up to 200mg a day for five days until an appropriate response has occurred. Treatment is maintained until conception occurs or up to six months.

Patients who do not respond to clomiphene may have to be treated with human menopausal gonadotrophins followed by human chorionic gonadotrophins. This therapy requires laboratory control and the dosage is individually assessed.

Progestogens have superseded androgens for the control of DUH. Recently, however, a new androgenic preparation danazol (Danol) which does not have virilising side-effects has been shown to be effective in controlling menorrhagia. The dose is 200mg daily; and treatment is maintained for four months (Chimbera et al, 1979).

Hyperprolactinaemia

Hyperprolactinaemia may be either physiological as in post-partum conditions or it may be inappropriate hyperprolactinaemia. It may occur when women take dopamine-antagonist drugs and also in association with prolactinomas of the pituitary.

Post-partum lactation may be suppressed by bromocriptine 2.5mg twice daily for two weeks. Rebound lactation rarely occurs and responds to another course of treatment. Bromocriptine is now the treatment of choice for the suppression of lactation in patients for whom it is considered necessary to use drugs for this purpose. Oestrogens are contraindicated for this purpose because of the risks of thrombo-embolic phenomena.

INAPPROPRIATE HYPERPROLACTINAEMIA

Drug-induced hyperprolactinaemia and hyperprolactinaemia due to pituitary tumours must be excluded, and in patients who have raised plasma prolactin in association with primary hypothyroidism, the treatment depends upon replacement therapy with thyroxine.

The patient has secondary amenorrhoea and some-times, but not always, galactorrhoea. Bromocriptine is started in small doses of 1.25mg daily, gradually increasing to 2.5mg three times a day, in order to minimise the side-effects of vomiting and nausea. The treatment may be monitored by reviewing the patient's temperature chart, by observing a fall in plasma prolactin into the normal range, and by observing a serum progesterone concentration of greater than 25nmol/litre, indicating a normal luteal phase.

There is usually little point in treating patients with hyperprolactinaemia if they do not wish to conceive, except in cases where galactorrhoea is troublesome. In such patients, a mechanical form of contraception should be advised and bromocriptine prescribed as indicated above.

Polycystic ovarian syndrome

This syndrome consists of sclerocystic ovaries associated with secondary amenorrhoea. The classical syndrome described by Stein and Leventhal also included obesity and male distribution of hair.

The diagnosis is confirmed by laparoscopy when the enlarged pearly-white ovary may be visualised. Treatment may be either surgical or by means of drugs. Ovarian biopsy at the time of laparoscopy is easy and besides being helpful diagnostically, it is sometimes therapeutic in promoting normal ovarian steroidogenesis. Formal laparotomy and wedge resection of the ovaries may be undertaken and this may be followed by drug therapy or drug therapy alone may be used.

Clomiphene citrate is the treatment of choice for patients with this syndrome and is successful in inducing ovulation in up to 75 per cent of these patients, although only half of these women succeed in conceiving.

The polycystic ovary is often hyper-responsive to clomiphene and treatment should be commenced cautiously. Small doses of the drug such as 25mg daily for five days is an appropriate regimen to commence with. Patients who fail to ovulate with anti-oestrogen treatment will sometimes do so when exogenous gonadotrophin therapy is used. Great care and meticulous laboratory control is needed to avoid the risks of hyperstimulation in these patients.

Women who have evidence of excessive adrenal activity will often respond to suppression of androgen secretion to a level which allows an increased gonadotrophin secretion from the pituitary. This may be achieved by prescribing dexamethasone 2mg daily.

A number of patients with polycystic ovarian syndrome have dysfunctional bleeding due to unopposed action of oestrogens on the endometrium. This may result in hyperplasia of the endometrium which may be pre-malignant.

In patients who do not wish to conceive, cyclical bleeding can be achieved by prescribing the combined oral contraceptive pill. Where contra-indications to exogenous oestrogen therapy exist, then cyclical bleeding can still be achieved by using norethisterone 5mg twice a day for the last two weeks of the cycle.

HIRSUTISM

The surgical and drug regimens outlined above will often lower androgen secretion but have no effect on excessive hair growth. Treatment with the anti-androgen, cyproterone acetate suppresses the secretion of the anterior pituitary hormones. Regression in abnormal hair growth is seen in the majority of patients within nine months. Cyproterone acetate has a contraceptive effect because of the pituitary suppression it induces. It is, however, a powerful anti-androgen and if conception did occur a male fetus would be feminised. In view of this risk, and also to achieve reasonable cyclical control, it is usual to prescribe ethinyloestradiol in conjunction with the cyproterone acetate. Cyproterone acetate 50mg twice a day from day five to day 15 of the cycle is given and ethinyloestradiol 50mg daily is given from day five to day 25.

Hormone therapy for endometriosis

Endometriosis may be treated surgically or medically or by a combination of both. It is important to confirm the diagnosis and assess the severity of the disease by laparoscopy or laparotomy, and to monitor the treatment by repeated laparoscopy in selected cases. Patients who have severe endometriosis with large cysts and extensive adhesions will usually require surgery. Drug treatment of this condition is only applicable to patients who have mild to moderate endometriosis or as a suppressive adjunct to surgery, postoperatively. Pregnancy is usually curative in this condition but 40 per cent of patients with endometriosis are infertile and indeed the diagnosis may be made during infertility investigations.

OESTROGENS

Oestrogens in large doses have been used in the treatment of this disease. They act by pituitary suppression, but they are a direct stimulus to endometriosis and should only be used in conjunction with progestogens.

PROGESTOGENS

Progestogens are given in large doses in order to mimic the beneficial effects of pregnancy on this disease. Their effect is to decidualise the stroma. Treatment is carried out for at least six months in the hope that the glands will be permanently destroyed and the endometriosis cured. A suitable preparation is norethisterone (Primolut N), and a dose of up to 20mg a day is given. Purely progestogen preparations, however, have problems especially when used for prolonged periods. Breakthrough bleeding and post-treatment amenorrhoea are relatively common. For these reasons combination treatment with oestrogen and progesterone preparations, e.g. mestranol 75 micrograms and norethynodrel 5mg (Enavid), is much used. The risks of thrombo-embolic phenomena and hypertension must be remembered when these drugs are prescribed.

DANAZOL

Danazol is a derivative of 17α-ethinyl testosterone; it has weak androgenic effects and its main action is thought to be suppression of gonadotrophin release. Danazol is the most effective hormone treatment for relieving the symptoms of endometriosis (Noble and Letchworth, 1979). The same authors report a pregnancy rate of 58 per cent following completion of a course of treatment of danazol. This drug has been used in the treatment of severe endometriosis with good results but the disease tends to return in the months following cessation of therapy.

Dysmenorrhoea

Primary spasmodic dysmenorrhoea is a common problem in girls and young women; it must be distinguished from secondary dysmenorrhoea which occurs later in life and is due to pelvic pathology, e.g. endometriosis.

There is still much folklore associated with menstruation, and psychological conditioning of a young girl by an over-anxious mother who accentuates the child's perception of the discomfort, is common. In the present day there is a more open and sensible attitude to sexuality and as a result it is probably becoming less common to see young women suffering from incapacitating dysmenorrhoea.

The pain is due to myometrial contractions producing uterine spasm. It is colicky in nature but is usually perceived by the patient as an ache in the lower abdomen, the vulva and the inside of the thighs. Low backache is also common. An excessive amount of prostaglandins has been suggested as a causative factor for dysmenorrhoea (Baker et al, 1962).

Treatment of dysmenorrhoea is medical rather than surgical. Careful explanation and reassurance are necessary; in the majority of cases this will suffice with perhaps the use of simple analgesics such as aspirin.

Prostaglandin synthatase inhibitors are potent and

effective drugs for the treatment of dysmenorrhoea. Mefenamic acid (Ponstan) is the most widely-used drug and is prescribed in a dose of 50mg to 500mg six-hourly on the first and second day of menstruation.

HORMONE THERAPY

The most effective method of curing dysmenorrhoea is by the suppression of ovulation, and this is most easily achieved by prescribing the combined oral contraceptive pill. This therapy is particularly indicated for patients who require contraception. It is widely known that doctors commonly prescribe oral contraception therapy for the treatment of dysmenorrhoea and it is common for young women to present with this complaint when their real desire is for oral contraception. It is necessary for the physician to be sensitive to this need, as in a particular patient the combined pill may be contra-indicated. In such cases the dysmenorrhoea should be treated by alternative therapy and appropriate contraceptive advice tendered.

The low-dose combined preparations are the most appropriate for young women. A suitable preparation would contain 30 micrograms of ethinyloestradiol and 250 micrograms of levonorgestrel (Eugynon 30).

PROGESTOGEN THERAPY

In patients in whom hormone preparations containing oestrogen are contra-indicated, dysmenorrhoea may be treated using only progestogenic compounds. The most commonly used is dydrogesterone (Duphaston) in a dose of 10mg twice daily from day five to day 25 of the menstrual cycle. Dydrogesterone has no oestrogenic, androgenic or corticoid activity and does not inhibit ovulation.

All patients with dysmenorrhoea can be very effectively helped by these regimens. Surgical treatment by cervical dilatation is contra-indicated, and treatment by pre-sacral neurectomy is carried out extremely rarely and only with expert assessment after suppression of ovulation has failed to relieve symptoms.

Pre-menstrual syndrome

This syndrome is the occurrence of symptoms in the pre-menstrual phase which usually occur in a group with one or two symptoms predominating. The symptoms not only vary from one patient to the next but may vary from one month to the next.

Physical symptoms include weight increase, enlarged and tender breasts, abdominal distension, headaches and peripheral oedema. Psychological symptoms of mood change, inability to cope and a difference in libido are also common. Assessment of these symptoms is necessarily subjective but there is no doubt that the patient's and the families' lives can be difficult during this period. The aetiology is not clearly understood but it is probably multi-hormonal.

Differing forms of treatment are available and in assessing a patient's response, it must be remembered that there is a large placebo effect.

NON-HORMONAL TREATMENT

Diuretics are commonly prescribed and are effective in relieving oedema and increased weight due to fluid retention. Bendrofluazide 5mg daily or frusemide 40mg daily, starting two days before the symptoms are expected and continuing until the onset of menstruation, are suitable preparations.

Tranquillising drugs are indicated in patients who experience particularly severe aggressive tendencies during the pre-menstrual phase. Diazepam up to 30mg a day in divided doses may be effective in the short-term.

HORMONAL TREATMENT

Progestogen therapy is widely used. Progesterone suppositories (Cyclogest) 400mg daily from the 14th day of the cycle until the onset of menstruation are sometimes effective. Dydrogesterone (Duphaston) 10mg orally twice a day throughout the menstrual cycle is also effective and is more acceptable to most patients. Suppression of ovulation with the combined oral contraceptive preparations is perhaps the most effective therapy. The use of danazol and bromocriptine have also been advocated, but experience with these drugs in this syndrome is limited and as yet there is no scientific evidence to justify their use.

EPITHELIAL DYSTROPHIES OF THE VULVA

Vulval skin is often affected by chronic changes and the aetiology of these changes is frequently obscure. Pruritus is a common symptom and constant scratching results in chronic inflammation, abrasions of the skin can occur and secondary infection may result. The common fungal and protozoal infections must be excluded.

Atrophic vulvovaginitis

This condition is found in post-menopausal women, or those women who have been subjected to bilateral oophorectomy without oestrogen replacement.

The patient complains of dryness, pruritus and dyspareunia. On examination, atrophy of the vulva is apparent. The vaginal mucosa is thin and pale and petechial haemorrhages readily appear on minimal trauma. Secondary infection is common and should be treated before hormone replacement therapy is initiated. Oestrogen replacement can be administered both systemically, or by the local application of dienoestrol cream through a vaginal applicator nightly for a few weeks' course, which may be repeated when symptoms recur. Occasionally this may cause mild symptoms (e.g. gynaecomastia) in the male partner through local skin absorption of oestrogen during intercourse.

Lichen sclerosis planus et atrophicus
The skin is thin with white glistening areas and red areas. The condition may affect the labia, perineum and perianal regions and may spread to the buttocks and inside of the thighs.

Leucoplakia
The skin is white and thickened due to hyperkeratinisation and cracks in the affected areas are common.

Carcinoma in situ (Bowen's disease)
The patient will usually have pruritus vulvae but the skin can sometimes appear normal. The classical appearance however is bright red with a clear serpiginous edge. The diagnosis can only be made on histological examination of a biopsy.

Paget's disease
The clinical picture of this unusual dystrophy is identical to that seen in Bowen's disease. There is often an underlying adenocarcinoma. The diagnosis is made on histology.

Squamous cell carcinoma of the vulva
This carcinoma shows the same clinical features as any skin cancer. It is usually seen as an ulcer with a necrotic base and raised edges. The lesion can occur anywhere in the vulva but is found most commonly on the labia and clitoris, and 'kiss ulcers' are common.

Treatment
Treatment depends upon an accurate diagnosis. Fungal infections and vulvitis due to *Trichomonas* can be diagnosed by swabs and culture or hanging-drop preparation even when the clinical features are obscured by excoriation and secondary infection from excess scratching.

General skin disorders such as psoriasis are excluded by a careful physical examination, when the general manifestation of the disorder will be observed. Pruritus, scratching and a chronic vulvitis can sometimes be caused by skin sensitivities to perfumes, deodorants and antiseptic preparations. The chronic epithelial dystrophies of the vulva are sometimes found in association with one or other of these factors, and a diagnosis can only be made by the histological examination of an adequate biopsy of the vulval skin.

SURGICAL TREATMENT
Patients with squamous cell carcinoma are treated by radical vulvectomy. Patients with a vulval dystrophy in which it is thought that there is a risk of invasive disease developing are considered for local vulvectomy. These dystrophies include Bowen's disease, Paget's disease and those conditions where very atypical epithelial activity is demonstrated on histological examination. Following simple vulvectomy the patient is kept under prolonged observation as the dystrophy commonly recurs in skin adjacent to the excised area and repeated excisions are often necessary. Vulvectomy is avoided in those cases in whom it is thought that there is a minimal risk of invasive disease. The operation is mutilating and the dystrophy very frequently returns.

GENERAL TREATMENT
Attempts are made to stop the patient scratching, hypnotics are prescribed to ensure sleep and systemic antihistamines may be given. Soothing and cooling local applications of cold cream and calamine lotion may be helpful. Hydrocortisone ½% or 1% cream is often used and is sometimes effective in relieving the pruritus and hence stopping the patient scratching. The inflammation in the skin is relieved but the effect is usually only temporary and the pruritus returns when the patient stops applying the cream.

A cream containing clobetasone butyrate, nystatin and oxytetracycline 3% (Trimovate) is particularly effective. Patients with pruritus which cannot be relieved by these measures may need admission. In intractable cases injection of the vulva with absolute alcohol in order to destroy the cutaneous nerves is usually effective.

It is important that all patients with chronic vulval dystrophies are followed up carefully for many years. Repeated biopsy of the vulva may need to be undertaken in patients in whom the lesion persists or recurs, in order to be quite certain that the atypical activity or even cancer is not developing.

GYNAECOLOGICAL MALIGNANCY

Cancers of the vulva and vagina are treated by surgery, and cervical cancer is treated by surgery or radiotherapy or a combination of the two. There is as yet no chemotherapeutic agent or hormonal compound which is effective against these cancers, and their use is, in general, contra-indicated because of their unpleasant side-effects. Palliation of recurrent disease of these organs is best effected by other means.

Adenocarcinoma of the endometrium

The primary treatment of this disease is surgical, a modified radical hysterectomy being the operation of choice. Pre-operative irradiation from radio-active isotopes is of value in 'sterilising' the surface of the tumour and hence preventing spread through implantation of neoplastic cells dropping from the lesion during surgery.

Progestogens are useful in this disease. They are sometimes employed over the operative period in an attempt to suppress any metastatic foci of tumour; but their main use is for palliation of recurrent disease especially where this is metastatic.

The most commonly used preparation is medroxyprogesterone acetate (Provera) up to 400mg daily being given in divided doses.

Ovarian cancer

The primary treatment of malignant conditions of the ovary is by laparotomy and hysterectomy and bilateral salpingo-oophorectomy in patients in whom this is technically feasible. Ascites due to peritoneal or omental spread of ovarian cancer can sometimes be temporarily controlled by the instillation of alkylating agents such as thiotepa into the effusion. Spironolactone is often helpful in delaying the re-accumulation of fluid. Cisplatin (Neoplatin) is useful in obtaining temporary remission in patients with ovarian cancer who have recurrent masses of tumour, and recurrent excision to reduce tumour bulk may be helpful. Vomiting may be a difficult and severe problem in these cases.

Choriocarcinoma

There are three centres in Great Britain where all cases of choriocarcinoma are referred for treatment and follow-up. Chemotherapeutic measures employed in this disease are often curative rather than palliative, and are based on the antimetabolic drugs methotrexate, a folic acid antagonist, and 6-mercaptopurine, a purine antagonist.

General and symptomatic treatment of inoperable and recurrent pelvic cancer is effected by the measures applicable to recurrent malignant disease anywhere in the body.

REFERENCES

Baker, J. C., Clitheroe, H. J. and Pickles, V. R. (1962). The menstrual stimulant in primary dysmenorrhoea. *Journal of Endocrinology*, **25**, 1.

Chimbera, T. H., Anderson, A. B. M., Cope, E. and Turnbull, A. C. (1979). Preliminary results on clinical and endocrine studies in the treatment of menorrhagia with danazol. *Postgraduate Medical Journal*, **55** (suppl 5), 90–4.

Noble, A. D. and Letchworth, A. T. (1979). Medical treatment of endometriosis: a comparative trial. *Postgraduate Medical Journal*, **55** (suppl 5), 37–9.

Chapter 20 Pelvic inflammatory disease from the viewpoint of the genito-urinary physician

GEORGE R. KINGHORN MB, MRCP

Whereas tuberculous salpingitis has become a comparative rarity in most western countries, accounting for less than five per cent of all cases, the incidence of non-tuberculous salpingitis has risen at a rapid rate in association with the pandemic of gonorrhoea and other sexually transmitted diseases in the past two decades. The size and economic consequences of the pelvic inflammatory disease (PID) problem in the USA, and the cost effectiveness of health care strategies designed to reduce the incidence of sexually transmitted diseases (STD), have recently been put into perspective. It is estimated that in the USA each year one million women suffer from PID and its sequelae of infertility, recurrent salpingitis, ectopic pregnancy and chronic pelvic pain. The direct costs of spending for health services and indirect costs of loss of industrial output due to disease and premature death together amounted to 1.3 billion dollars each year. Moreover, this estimate did not take into account the intangible costs to sufferers caused by deprivation of parenthood, school absenteeism or marital discord.

Certain epidemiological features are noteworthy. The age distribution of acute PID mirrors that of uncomplicated lower genital tract infections, for two-thirds of cases occur in women aged less than 25 years, and one-third in women who have not yet started their reproductive life. It has been calculated that one in eight sexually active 15-year-old girls will develop PID each year, which represents 10 times the risk to sexually active 24-year-olds. The use of intra-uterine contraceptive devices also holds a four times increased risk to young nulliparous compared to multiparous women, whereas the 'pill' may have some preventive effect against PID. Assessment of PID risk factors should be made when contraceptive advice is sought. Effective action to prevent acute PID will also prevent the need for the long-term management of the physical and psychological conditions associated with its sequelae.

MICROBIOLOGICAL CAUSES OF PID

During acute salpingitis caused by ascending spread of sexually transmitted pathogens, damage occurs to the tubal mucosa which thereby facilitates secondary infection with facultative pathogens that are usually present in low numbers in the lower genital tract. Although there is evidence of a different tubal and endocervical flora in sub-acute, recurrent and chronic PID from that in acute salpingitis, a consideration of these initiating causes is relevant to their appropriate management and understanding, not least because it is the experience of genito-urinary physicians that many cases of so-called chronic salpingitis are in reality recurrent acute or sub-acute attacks resulting from further exposure to the same initiating sexually transmitted pathogens.

Gonococcal PID

It is estimated that PID complicates 10 to 15 per cent of all gonococcal infections in women. There is a considerable geographic variation in the relative prevalences of cases due to gonococcal disease, being of the order of 40 to 60 per cent in the USA but of a lower order in most European studies. Different strains of gonococci have a variable propensity to cause PID. It is commoner in the young and in negroes; the onset of symptoms frequently occurs with menstruation; and has a better prognosis for future fertility. Cervical, urethral and rectal swabs directly plated on to selective Gc culture media is the most reliable means of diagnosing the infection, although placing swabs in Amies transport medium is an acceptable alternative. Single-dose treatment with either aqueous procaine penicillin IM 2.4 to 4.8 mega units or ampicillin 2 to 3g plus 1g probenecid by mouth is preferred for uncomplicated gonorrhoea. Gonococcal PID is normally managed in hospital with systemic penicillin G but in less acute cases oral ampicillin 2g daily for 7 to 10 days can be given.

Investigation for accompanying genital pathogens,

contact tracing and tests of cure following treatment are mandatory in all cases. The increasing prevalence of gonococcal strains which are relatively resistant to penicillin or which produce a β-lactamase, especially in infections acquired abroad, suggests that gonococcal infections are still best referred for specialist management.

Non-gonococcal PID

Long-term clinical and microbiological studies in Sweden showed that the prevalence of gonococcal PID fell from 50 per cent of all cases in 1960 to 10 per cent of all cases in 1975. A similar trend is to be anticipated in the UK, for lower genital tract infections in both men and women have shown a similar change in favour of non-gonococcal rather than gonococcal causation, during the past 10 years. Non-gonococcal PID is more prevalent in older women and IUCD users; although symptoms are more often sub-acute and patients frequently apyrexial, there is a worse prognosis for future fertility and other sequelae than after gonococcal PID. Improved microbiological techniques in recent years have lead to a clearer understanding of the causative organisms of non-gonococcal PID and their management.

1. CHLAMYDIA TRACHOMATIS (*C. trachomatis*)

In recent Scandinavian studies, *C. trachomatis* was isolated from the endocervix and Fallopian tubes of women with PID more often than any other pathogen and is implicated in the causation of up to 60 per cent of all PID cases. The organisms are obligate intracellular pathogens with a unique growth cycle and cannot be grown in artificial media. They are the commonest cause of non-specific urethritis, and cause a very wide spectrum of disorders in the male and female genital. tracts. Transmission to the fetus during passage through the birth canal results in chlamydia conjunctivitis, which in the UK is now four times as common as gonococcal ophthalmia, and a distinctive pneumonitis. Early infections in women are often without symptoms or signs. The association of muco-pus with ectopy, oedema and contact bleeding of the cervix (so-called 'hypertrophic erosion') may give a clue to the diagnosis. Lower genital tract complications, such as bartholinitis, peri-urethral abscess and frequency/dysuria syndrome, and the upper genital tract complications of endometritis causing abnormal uterine bleeding, salpingitis and peri-hepatitis which may mimic acute cholecystitis, are increasingly being recognised in women infected with *C. trachomatis*.

Diagnosis is most reliably made by inoculating tissue cultures with swabs obtained from infected mucous membranes and placed in specific chlamydia transport medium. Unfortunately a chlamydia culture service is restricted to relatively few centres and is not available to general practitioners.

C. trachomatis infections do not respond to penicillin and its derivatives, and single-dose treatment even in uncomplicated cases is ineffective. The drugs of choice are the tetracyclines given in courses lasting 14 to 21 days. Alternatives are erythromycin or sulphonamides but resistance to the latter does occur.

2. UREAPLASMA UREALYTICUM AND MYCOPLASMA HOMINIS (*U. urealyticum: M. hominis*)

Although these organisms frequently colonise the lower genital tract of sexually active persons, most often as commensal flora, they have been implicated in the causation of non-specific urethritis and cervicitis. *M. hominis* has been isolated as the sole agent directly from Fallopian tubes of women with salpingitis and from blood of women with post-abortal and post-partum fever. Both agents can be grown in agar media to which horse serum has been added. Specimens for inoculation can be sent to the laboratory in Amies transport medium. Treatment with penicillin and its derivatives, sulphonamides alone or in combination with trimethoprim, are ineffective. Tetracyclines again are the drugs of choice.

3. FACULTATIVE PATHOGENS

E. coli, H. influenzae, Group A and *B streptococci* and anaerobic bacteria play an important causative role in salpingitis which follows uterine instrumentation or childbirth. Anaerobes such as Bacteroides and Clostridial species are important in clinically severe infections, particularly where a tubo-ovarian abscess has formed, and in recurrent chronic PID. Bacteroides can be cultured from swabs sent in Amies transport media, and are best treated with metronidazole 400mg b.d. for 7 to 14 days.

Management of PID

The investigation and management of PID sequelae such as infertility, abnormalities of menstruation, and end-stage disease manifested by chronic pelvic pain and fixed fibrotic pelvic organs lies principally within the province of the gynaecologist. The role of the genito-urinary physician lies in investigating acute, sub-acute and recurrent attacks of PID for the microbiological cause and in investigating male consorts for infection. Studies of consorts in women with acute salpingitis have shown up to 50 per cent to have asymptomatic gonococcal or *C. trachomatis* infections.

Any drug therapy should be preceded by attempts

to diagnose the microbiological cause of PID by taking swabs from the cervix, urethra and rectum. Polymicrobial PID is the rule rather than the exception. It is worth remembering that 40 per cent of women with gonorrhoea have concomitant *C. trachomatis* infection. In unspecified PID combined therapy with tetracyclines 2g daily and metronidazole 400mg b.d. for 14 days is recommended as it will cover the widest spectrum of potential pathogens. Compliance with tetracycline therapy, particularly advice to avoid ingestion of milk products and antacids may be a major problem for some patients and doxycycline 100mg b.d., although more expensive, is a useful alternative. Erythromycin 2g daily can be substituted for tetracyclines.

Patients should also be warned about the possible 'Antabuse'-like reaction if alcohol is taken during metronidazole therapy.

Chronic pelvic pain which is often worse before menstruation, may benefit from continuous progestogen suppressive therapy, and danazol has also been used with some success. However, the increasing ingestion of simple analgesics or resort to potentially addictive drugs are an indication for gynaecological referral with a view to surgery.

The high incidence of STD, the importance of making an aetiological diagnosis in PID, following up patients after treatment to ensure a microbiological as well as a clinical cure, and the need to investigate and treat consorts, cannot be over emphasised. Prevention and control of sexually transmitted diseases must therefore be seen as being an important part of PID management. To be effective it requires close co-operation between the general practitioner, genito-urinary physician, microbiologist and gynaecologist. The incidence of chronic and painful disease may require co-operation between these colleagues over a period of many years.

BIBLIOGRAPHY

Report of a WHO Scientific Group. (1981). *Non-gonococcal urethritis and other selected sexually transmitted diseases of public health importance.* Technical Report Series 660. World Health Organisation, Geneva.

Harris, J. R. W. (ed) (1981). *Recent Advances in Sexually Transmitted Diseases*, No. 2. Churchill Livingstone, Edinburgh.

Pelvic Inflammatory Disease Symposium. (1980). *American Journal of Obstetrics and Gynecology*, **138**, 845–1112.

Chapter 21 Oral contraceptives

PAMELA BUCK MB, BS, MRCOG

INTRODUCTION

Oral contraceptives have been in use for over 20 years and it is estimated that some 40 to 50 million women throughout the world are using this method. It is a safe, effective method and, being separate from the act of coitus, has no aesthetic drawbacks.

Few other drugs have received such scrutiny from the medical profession and public alike. Such attention is hardly surprising since the drugs are not being used to treat disease but to prevent the physiological state of pregnancy. Serious side-effects, however uncommon, receive much publicity, being promptly reported in the popular press. It is important to put this problem into perspective by comparing the risks of drug usage with the risks of pregnancy. Both morbidity and mortality are greater in pregnancy than in oral contraceptive users, and this difference is even more marked in countries where maternal mortality rates are high.

The combined oral contraceptive is the most effective reversible method of contraception available. The failure rate is of the order of 0.1 to 0.4 pregnancies per 100 women-years, when taken correctly.

TYPES OF ORAL CONTRACEPTIVE

There are three basic forms of oral contraceptive, the fixed dose combined oestrogen/progestogen, the sequential oestrogen/progestogen and the progestogen-only preparation. Each type will be considered separately since there are important differences between them.

Combined oral contraceptive

These preparations consist of constant proportions of an oestrogen and a progestogen, usually administered over 21 days followed by a period of seven days when no tablet is taken, allowing withdrawal bleeding to occur. Some preparations are taken continuously but seven of the tablets are inert. Combined pills are usually classified according to the dose of oestrogen which they contain. Preparations in current use in Britain contain either 50, 30 or 20 micrograms of oes-

trogen. It is no longer recommended that doses of more than 50 micrograms of oestrogen be used for contraception since serious side-effects are more likely to occur. Effective contraception can be assured when the preparation contains 50 or 30 micrograms of oestrogen but there is a higher failure rate when only 20 micrograms is present in each tablet.

Sequential preparations

Older sequential preparations contained large (by current standards) doses of an oestrogen administered for 14 days followed by a combined oestrogen and progestogen tablet for seven days. This preparation was designed to mimic more closely the normal menstrual cycle where oestrogen is present in the first half and oestrogen and progesterone are secreted together following ovulation. Unfortunately, some cycles were even more physiological than intended, when ovulation took place and pregnancies resulted. Sequential preparations of this type should no longer be used because of their high oestrogen content and the higher failure rate.

The recent introduction of two triphasic sequential preparations has been heralded by the manufacturers as a major breakthrough in the development of oral contraceptives. Tablets in each of the three phases contain a combination of oestrogen and a progestogen, levonorgestrel, and this proportion is varied through the phases to achieve a step-wise increase in progestogen with an oestrogen boost at the time when ovulation would normally occur. In this way a lower total dose of progestogen but a slightly higher total dose of oestrogen is taken each cycle. The efficacy and side-effects are similar to those of 30 microgram combined preparations though the incidence of break-through bleeding is less. They cost nearly twice as much as a fixed dose combined 30 microgram preparation containing the same hormones.

Progestogen-only pills

Sometimes called the 'mini-pill' – a term to be avoided since the patient confuses this with low-dose pills, or erroneously, the progesterone-only pill. The

COMBINED ORAL CONTRACEPTIVES

	OESTROGEN	PROGESTOGEN
A. *Containing 50 micrograms oestrogen*		
Anovlar 21	Ethinyloestradiol	Norethisterone acetate 4mg
Demulen 50	Ethinyloestradiol	Ethynodiol diacetate 500 micrograms
Eugynon 50	Ethinyloestradiol	Norgestrel 500 micrograms
Gynovlar 21	Ethinyloestradiol	Norethisterone acetate 3mg
Minilyn	Ethinyloestradiol	Lynoestrenol 2.5mg
Minovlar	Ethinyloestradiol	Norethisterone acetate 1mg
Minovlar ED	As Minovlar + 7 inert tablets	
Norinyl-1	Mestranol	Norethisterone 1mg
Norinyl-1/28	As Norinyl-1 + 7 inert tablets	
Norlestrin	Ethinyloestradiol	Norethisterone acetate 2.5mg
Orlest 21	Ethinyloestradiol	Norethisterone acetate 1mg
Ortho-Novin 1/50	Mestranol	Norethisterone 1mg
Ovran	Ethinyloestradiol	Levonorgestrel 250 micrograms
Ovulen 50	Ethinyloestradiol	Ethinodiol diacetate 1mg
B. *Containing 35 micrograms oestrogen*		
Brevinor	Ethinyloestradiol	Norethisterone 0.5mg
Norimin	Ethinyloestradiol	Norethisterone 1mg
Ovysmen	Ethinyloestradiol	Norethisterone 0.5mg
C. *Containing 30 micrograms oestrogen*		
Conova 30	Ethinyloestradiol	Ethynodiol diacetate 2mg
Eugynon 30	Ethinyloestradiol	Levonorgestrel 250 micrograms
Microgynon 30	Ethinyloestradiol	Levonorgestrel 150 micrograms
Ovran 30	Ethinyloestradiol	Levonorgestrel 250 micrograms
Ovranette	Ethinyloestradiol	Levonorgestrel 150 micrograms
D. *Triphasic preparations*		
Logynon	Ethinyloestradiol 30 / 40 / 30	Levonorgestrel 50 micrograms / 75 micrograms / 125 micrograms
Logynon ED	As Logynon + 7 inert tablets	
Trinordiol	Ethinyloestradiol 30 / 40 / 30	Levonorgestrel 50 micrograms / 75 micrograms / 125 micrograms

PROGESTOGEN-ONLY PREPARATIONS

Femulen	Ethinodiol diacetate 500 micrograms
Micronor	Norethisterone 350 micrograms
Microval	Levonorgestrel 30 micrograms
Neogest	Norgestrel 75 micrograms
Norgeston	Levonorgestrel 30 micrograms
Noriday	Norethisterone 350 micrograms

preparations consist of a low dose of a synthetic progestogen administered continuously. Its mode of action differs from that of combined prepàrations and the failure rate is higher (two to three pregnancies per 100 women-years), but it is particularly useful in women in whom oestrogen administration is undesirable, e.g. women with a history of thrombo-embolism.

The hormones

All hormones used in oral contraceptives are synthetic.

Only two oestrogens are in use, ethinyloestradiol and its less potent relative mestranol. They are both suitable for use in oral contraceptives since they are (a) active when given orally, (b) have a duration of action which permits daily administration and (c) are similar to natural oestrogens in their effects on the hypothalamus and the reproductive tract.

The progestogens, five in number, are derived from the parent compound 19-nortestosterone. They vary in their potency and in androgenic and oestrogenic activity. They do not have all of the progestational effects of natural progesterone. For example, they induce secretory endometrial changes, alter cervical mucus, but will not maintain pregnancy in animals which have undergone oophorectomy. In addition to the progestational properties, all but norethynodrel have androgenic actions when given in higher doses than normally used for contraception. The racemic mixture norgestrel is only half as potent as the active compound levonorgestrel, which is the most potent of the synthetic progestogens in contraceptive usage today.

MODE OF ACTION

Oral contraceptives have more than one mode of action and it is these multiple actions which make them so effective in preventing pregnancy.

1. *Inhibition of ovulation*: Both oestrogens and progestogens can block the hypothalamic-pituitary-ovarian feedback control of ovulation. Oestrogens are more potent in this respect but in the oral contraceptive, oral oestrogen and progestogen work synergistically. Gonadotrophin secretion is not completely suppressed.

2. *Changes in the genital tract:*

(a) Cervical mucus: Progestogens induce a change in the physical state of cervical mucus. It is rendered thick, viscid and inpenetrable to sperm.

(b) Endometrium: Progestogens produce a change in endometrium which is seen histologically as oedematous stroma with atrophic glands. Such endometrium is unsuitable for implantation of a fertilised ovum.

(c) Tubal motility: Altered motility affects the speed of transport of both sperm and zygote through the Fallopian tubes. This mechanism has been suggested as the explanation for those tubal pregnancies which have been observed in patients taking progestogen-only preparations.

Combined oral contraceptives, including the triphasic preparations, act using all of the above mechanisms, while progestogen-only preparations have only the local genital tract effect in the doses used.

SYSTEMIC EFFECTS

General consideration

The actions of oral contraceptives have been investigated using laboratory techniques and using much larger numbers of women in both prospective and retrospective epidemiological studies. Difficulties arise, however, because of the very many preparations in current use. A glance at the list above reveals very many different combinations of either of two oestrogens and any one of five progestogens. Clearly, not only the actual hormone used but its dose and oestrogen/progestogen ratio will determine its pharmacological action. In terms of serious side-effects, very large numbers of women need to be studied in order to observe a small number of, say, deaths from cardiovascular causes. In the Oxford Family Planning Survey there were nine such deaths over nearly 50 000 women-years of observation. If figures such as these are further broken down and analysed for different preparations, interpretation becomes even more difficult and estimation of statistical significance may be impossible.

Until recently, oestrogen was considered to be the 'villain of the piece' but recent evidence indicates that the progestogen may also be implicated in the role of oral contraceptives in cardiovascular disease.

The genital tract

The use of oral contraceptives alters the flora and the pH of the vagina. This is considered to be the reason for the increased incidence of monilial vaginitis which is also observed in pregnancy. Each episode of candidiasis should be treated with an appropriate antifungal. It is uncommon that the infections be so intractable as to necessitate withdrawal of the oral contraceptive.

Fibroids were noted to enlarge when the high-dose oestrogen oral contraceptives were in use. The newer low-dose preparations do not seem to have such a marked effect. The presence of small, asymptomatic fibroids is *not* a contra-indication to oral contraceptive use but makes regular supervision essential.

Oral contraceptives may be associated with altered bleeding patterns and, occasionally, withdrawal bleeding fails to occur. Women do find these symptoms disturbing and require reassurance or investigation as appropriate. First, break-through bleeding is common with low-dose combined preparations and tends to occur early in treatment cycles, improving with continued use. If the spotting continues a higher dose of either oestrogen or progestogen or a changeover to one of the triphasic preparations is indicated. When break-through bleeding develops after several trouble-free cycles, the patient should be investigated for a possible gynaecological cause, as if she has intermenstrual bleeding. Irregular cycles and intermenstrual bleeding are not uncommon in women taking progestogen-only preparations and it seems that failures are more likely to occur in those women who continue to menstruate regularly. The withdrawal bleeding induced by cessation of oestrogen and progestogen administration in the 'pill-free week' is lighter and often shorter than a woman's natural menstrual loss. This beneficial effect is one of the main advantages of oral contraceptives over other contraceptive methods. Women are alarmed when withdrawal bleeding fails to occur. Pregnancy, of course, should be considered and excluded. There is evidence that, in women who fail to experience withdrawal bleeding, the hypothalamic-pituitary axis is less suppressed and the logical remedy, therefore, is to increase the dose of oestrogen. However, manufacturers recommend that should this occur for three consecutive cycles or more, the oral contraceptive be stopped until normal regular menstrual cycles are re-established. In each individual case the advantages of withdrawing this effective contraceptive method must be balanced against the risk of accidental pregnancy should the woman fail to use alternative methods of contraception.

Post-coital bleeding should always be taken seriously and a full gynaecological assessment be made.

Primary dysmenorrhoea is associated with ovulatory cycles and always improves on oral contraceptive therapy. Dysmenorrhoea secondary to endometriosis may also improve but the pain associated with pelvic inflammatory disease does not.

Should a woman be found to have abnormal cervical cytology oral contraceptives should *not* be discontinued. It is far easier to investigate and treat such patients when they are not pregnant. Oral contraceptives will not interfere with management and do not adversely effect the course of invasive cervical carcinoma. Endometrial carcinoma is less likely to be a problem with oral contraceptive users since it affects older women. There is no evidence that oral contraceptive use increases the risk of endometrial carcinoma but since the growth of this tumour is promoted by oestrogen it is wise not to prescribe oestrogens in women who have endometrial carcinoma.

The breast

Some breast cancers are hormone dependent and since it is not possible to know which tumour is promoted by oestrogens and which by progestogens, except by tissue culture techniques, it is wise not to prescribe oral contraceptives to women who have or who have had breast carcinoma. Similarly, oral contraceptives should not be prescribed to a woman with a breast mass until a firm diagnosis has been made.

Benign breast disease is quite another matter. Several studies have shown that oral contraceptives protect against benign breast disease and that their presence is no contra-indication to prescribing oral contraceptives.

That oestrogen suppresses lactation is a well-established fact. The dose of oestrogen in currently available contraceptives is unlikely to suppress well-established lactation, but the slight reduction in milk volume may be important in those women where milk production is not so copious. For this reason it is better to prescribe a progestogen-only preparation during lactation, changing to a combined form when baby is weaned.

Breast tenderness is a common complaint in the first treatment cycle and usually improves in subsequent cycles. Reassurance is all that is required.

Thrombo-embolism

In the 1960s, several isolated cases of fatal thrombo-embolic disease in oral contraceptive users were reported in the literature. These reports were substantiated by the findings of Inman and Vessey (1968) and Vessey and Doll (1968), both retrospective studies. The findings of the Oxford Family Planning and the Royal College of General Practitioners studies (both of which were prospective) confirmed these earlier reports. The increased risk in oral contraceptive users varied from study to study but was between two- and seven-fold. It is clear that the risk is greatest when the dose of oestrogen exceeds 50 micrograms, when duration of use exceeds five years, and where there are other predisposing factors such as obesity, family history of thrombo-embolism, age over 35 years and smoking. The risks are also increased at times of immobilisation and surgery. It is recommended that oral contraceptives be withdrawn six weeks before elective surgery and not recommenced until four weeks afterwards.

Progestogen-only preparations are not associated with an increased risk of thromboembolism. Varicose veins *per se* are not a contra-indication to oral contraceptive use, but if there is a history of thrombophlebitis it is wiser to select a progestogen-only preparation or an alternative method.

Myocardial infarction

Few deaths from myocardial infarction have occurred in oral contraceptive users in the absence of other risk factors and these cases have tended to be older women. All studies reported to date agree that smoking is a much more important risk factor in myocardial infarction in pre-menopausal women. There is a very strong link with smoking and other factors such as hypertension, hyperlipidaemia, obesity and diabetes. There is evidence that a reduced dose of oestrogen to 50 micrograms or less has reduced the number of these tragic deaths.

Hypertension

Some five per cent of oral contraceptive users develop hypertension. Many of these women have a positive family history or were themselves hypertensive during pregnancy. The hypertension is reversible on discontinuation of oral contraceptives and this fact would suggest that the effect is due to the preparation itself. The mechanism involved is thought to be related to a disturbance of the renin-angiotensin system which is activated by the administration of oestrogen. In addition, progestogens contribute to this hypertensive effect, for in the Royal College of General Practitioners Study there was an increasing reporting rate of hypertension with increasing doses of norethisterone acetate combined with the same dose of oestrogen (50 micrograms of ethinyloestradiol).

Cerebrovascular disease

An excess of cerebrovascular accidents has been reported in oral contraceptive users when compared with non-users. These accidents appear to be mainly of the thrombotic type and the comments made above about thrombo-embolism apply. Oral contraceptive usage is not as important an aetiological factor in haemorrhagic cerebral vascular accidents. The hypertensive oral contraceptive user who also smokes is more likely to suffer a stroke.

Endocrine system

With the exception of the effects of gonadotrophin secretion which have already been mentioned, and the effect on prolactin secretion which is described below, oral contraceptives do not appear to alter pituitary function in such a way as to be of clinical importance. Oestrogens stimulate prolactin secretion from the anterior pituitary and galactorrhoea can occur. However, a relationship between oral contraceptives and subsequent hyperprolactinaemic amenorrhoea and galactorrhoea has not been established.

Oestrogens increase levels of thyroxine binding globulin and protein binding of iodine. They are not contra-indicated in women with treated thyroid disease.

Transcortin and unconjugated cortisol levels are also increased in oral contraceptive users and these effects are similar to those seen in pregnancy.

Carbohydrate metabolism

Carbohydrate metabolism is altered by oral contraceptive administration. Glucose tolerance is reduced and in those patients who already have impaired glucose tolerance, deterioration is to be expected, such that they may become overtly diabetic. Known diabetics, when prescribed oral contraceptives, will almost certainly require alteration in insulin doses, especially in the first few cycles of administration. Close supervision of such patients is therefore essential. The effects of oral contraceptives on carbohydrate metabolism are reversible on discontinuation.

Lipid metabolism

Much attention has been paid to lipid metabolism, the development of atherosclerotic heart disease and oral contraceptive use. One important factor in the development of atherosclerosis is the level of high density lipoprotein (HDL) in the blood. A low level of HDL is associated with high incidence of atherosclerosis and vice versa. Oestrogens increase and progestogens decrease HDL levels in plasma. It has therefore been postulated that the ratio of oestrogen to progestogen is important when considering atherosclerosis in oral contraceptive users. Indeed, this is one rationale for the introduction of the triphasic preparation which has been shown to reduce HDL levels less than 20 and 30 micrograms ethinyloestradiol preparations with 150 and 250 micrograms of levonorgestrel.

Porphyria

Oral contraceptives are one of the factors known to precipitate exacerbations in the porphyrias. Oral contraceptives should not therefore be prescribed to women known to have porphyria. Pregnancy has similar adverse effects on this disorder.

Gastro-intestinal tract

Two of the commonest minor side-effects of which oral contraceptives users complain are nausea and weight gain. These two complaints are often given as reasons why women discontinue the method. Nausea is particularly apparent during the first cycle of administration and women should be reassured that this symptom is likely to improve and they should be encouraged to continue. A weight gain of 1 or 2kg due to fluid retention is to be expected and although many women blame their weight gain on the pill, clinical trials have failed to show a difference of more than 1 or 2kg weight gain between users and non users. It has been suggested that the excess weight gain is attributable to the effect of progestogens in improving appetite, to a sense of well-being and happiness when the fear of pregnancy is removed. Clearly, there are very many physical, biochemical and emotional factors involved and excessive weight gain cannot be entirely explained on the pharmacological actions of oestrogen and progestogen.

Peptic ulceration invariably improves during oral contraceptive use.

The liver

Liver function is altered in pregnancy and on oral contraceptives. It is wise to avoid oral contraceptives until liver function tests have returned to normal following viral hepatitis. Oral contraceptives are contra-indicated in women with a history of idiopathic recurrent jaundice of pregnancy and women with chronic liver disease. When jaundice occurs on the pill it tends to occur early, within the first few cycles of administration, and is reversible following cessation of the drug. There is a small, but increased risk of hepatocellular adenoma among oral contraceptive users and former users. The risk is very small indeed and is related to the dose of oestrogen as well as the duration of use, and is more common in older women.

An excess of gall bladder disease has been reported in a number of studies including the Royal College of General Practitioners prospective study. Oestrogens alter the solubility of cholesterol in bile such that the formation of gallstones is favoured. Women known to have gallstones should not therefore be prescribed oral contraceptives.

Skin

Increased pigmentation on the face similar to chloasma of pregnancy has occurred and is caused by oestrogen. The condition resolves only very slowly after withdrawal of the hormone and does not occur on the progestogen-only pill. Acne vulgaris usually improves in oral contraceptive users since sebum production is

decreased. However, a small proportion of women may experience a deterioration, and this has been explained by an androgenic effect of the progestogens in current use.

Women who have developed herpes gestationis or severe pruritus of pregnancy should not be prescribed oral contraceptives since these conditions may return.

Neurological conditions

Epilepsy is not a contra-indication to oral contraceptive administration. Some epileptics deteriorate but the majority do not; clearly, those who have a history of deterioration of their epilepsy during pregnancy should be observed very closely.

Many migraine sufferers are improved while taking oral contraceptives. However, if migraine appears for the first time during oral contraceptive use or if severe episodes are experienced, for example associated with hemiparesis or visual disturbance, then oral contraceptives should be withdrawn. This does not imply, however, that the migraine will cease, for this may take a considerable time.

Headache is not an uncommon complaint among women and this is also true of oral contraceptive users. Some experience the headache in the pill-free week, a phenomenon which has not been adequately explained. Severe or prolonged headache or headache of an unusual nature has preceded cerebral vascular accident during oral contraceptive administration and is an indication for discontinuation.

Psychiatric disorders

Subjective symptoms of depression have been reported and the literature abounds with reports that depression is either increased, decreased or remains unchanged. It seems that many of these women who complain of depression have a previous history. Depression occurring during oral contraceptive usage is ascribed to alteration of tryptophan metabolism in the brain. Oral contraceptives are unsuitable for women with severe depression and women whose depression has deteriorated during pregnancy. The pre-menstrual syndrome is related to ovulatory cycles, it follows therefore that induction of an anovulatory state will improve this condition. Oral contraceptives are useful therefore in the treatment of the pre-menstrual syndrome. However, there is a small number of women whose symptoms persist or who develop pre-menstrual syndrome-like symptoms when taking oral contraceptives. This is thought to be due to fluid retention.

Studies on the effect of oral contraceptive on libido have shown conflicting results. While sexual behaviour in animals is directly related to the activity of the sex steroids, such behaviour in women is greatly modified by social, cultural and psychological factors. One consistent finding among many studies is that coital activity is increased in women using oral contraceptives when compared with women using other methods of contraception and this has been attributed to freedom from fear of an unwanted pregnancy and does not necessarily reflect increased libido. Women who complain of decreased libido on oral contraceptives, or indeed in relation to any other family planning method, may have psychosexual problems to which they wish to draw the attention of a doctor. This possibility should therefore be borne in mind and the patient should be encouraged to identify and discuss the underlying problem.

Anaemias

Since the blood loss of withdrawal bleeding is less than that of normal menstruation, and menorrhagia is improved, patients with iron deficiency anaemia benefit from oral contraceptive administration. The situation concerning sickle cell anaemia is far from clear. An increased frequency of crises has been noted in pregnancy, and since many of these women have thrombotic tendencies it is wiser not to prescribe oral contraceptives containing oestrogens.

CONTRA-INDICATIONS

From the foregoing, a list of conditions in which oral contraceptive administration is absolutely contra-indicated or in which there are relative contra-indications can be compiled. The latter group would be considered as additional risk factors and when more than one is present it would be unwise to prescribe oral contraceptives.

Absolute	*Relative*
Thrombo-embolism	Smoking
Porphyria	Age over 35 years
Sickle cell anaemia	Hypertension
Hyperlipidaemia	Diabetes
Recurrent jaundice of	
pregnancy	Severe depression
Impaired liver function	Obesity
Myocardial infarction	
Cerebrovascular accident	
Carcinoma of breast or	
endometrium	

PRACTICAL MANAGEMENT

1. The history

At the first consultation, when oral contraceptives are requested or when a woman seeks contraceptive advice, a full personal and family history should be taken to determine the presence of contra-indications or risk factors. It is important to include her obstetric history and to enquire specifically whether she became either hypertensive or diabetic during her pregnancies. The gynaecological history should include an assessment of the quantity and duration of the menses and the cycle length. She should be asked specifically if intermenstrual or post-coital bleeding are present, for if so they require specialist gynaecological investigation. Some concept of her hormone balance can be assessed by the amount of her menstrual loss, the amount of leucorrhoea and the presence of pre-menstrual symptoms.

2. Physical examination

At the initial examination the blood pressure should be recorded, the patient weighed and the urine tested for glucose and protein. Breasts should be examined for the presence of masses, abdominal palpation should always precede pelvic examination, and any abnormal finding would require appropriate investigation and treatment; for example an enlarged liver would preclude oral contraceptive administration. Ideally, a pelvic examination should be made but one accepts that abnormalities are most unlikely to be found in young women seeking oral contraceptive in preparation for their forthcoming marriage and who are virgins. In all sexually active women a cervical smear should be taken and a pelvic examination and cervical smear are especially important if there are any abnormal gynaecological symptoms.

3. Prescribing

In the absence of contra-indications, and if the examination is satisfactory, a low-dose combined oral contraceptive should be prescribed. I would select a preparation containing 30 micrograms of oestrogen with levonorgestrel. This combination is satisfactory in the majority of women and has the advantage of excellent contraceptive efficacy and a low oestrogen content. Levonorgestrel and, of course, norgestrel have marked systemic anti-oestrogen effects which are beneficial when considering risk factors and the local genital tract effects are less marked than those of norethisterone acetate.

The patient should be instructed to start the first tablet on day one of her next menstrual cycle and she does not need to use other contraceptive methods. If a progestogen-only preparation is chosen she should also start on day one of her next menstrual cycle but requires additional contraceptive measures for the first 14 days. It should be noted that alternative contraceptive methods do not include methods based on assessment of cervical mucus or temperature.

She should be warned of side-effects which are likely to occur during the first course. They are: breast tenderness, nausea and break-through bleeding. She should be instructed not to discontinue the oral contraceptive should these side-effects occur because they will improve with continued use. I prescribe four packs initially but arrange to see her again after 12 weeks, in this way, should she be unable to keep her appointment, she will not run out of pills before she makes another appointment.

4. Review

At the next and subsequent visits the patient should be weighed, blood pressure should be checked and urine tested for glucose. Any problems having occurred during her three cycles of oral contraceptives should be noted and dealt with. It is unreasonable to assess the suitability or otherwise of any particular preparation unless it is taken for three months.

If there have been no problems she should be seen at six-monthly intervals and prescribed an appropriate number of packs so that she always has one pack in reserve.

Oral contraceptives should be discontinued should any of the following occur: pregnancy, jaundice, severe headache or migraine or visual disturbance, thrombosis or even strong suspicion of thrombosis, six weeks before elective surgery, and if the blood pressure rises above 160mmHg systolic or 105mm diastolic. Whenever oral contraceptives are stopped for reasons other than the desire for a pregnancy, alternative contraceptive advice should be given. It is highly likely that pregnancy has an adverse effect on the condition for which the oral contraceptive was discontinued (for example, hypertension). Such conditions require further investigation, if not treatment, before embarking on a pregnancy. It is not necessary to stop oral contraceptives in mid-pack on the eve of a woman's thirty-fifth birthday, it is more sensible to gradually introduce the idea of an alternative method to women in their early thirties so that they might give adequate consideration to the alternatives and therefore accept them more readily when advised to change from the pill.

There are some circumstances in which additional contraception is required:

(a) on changing from a high to a lower dose of oestrogen or on changing from a combined to a progestogen-only pill, additional contraceptive methods should be used for the first 14 days of the pack,

(b) if a tablet is omitted or if there is a gastro-intestinal disturbance, especially if these occur early in the pack, another method should be used as well until the next pack is commenced,

(c) when another drug is prescribed which is known to impair contraceptive efficacy of oral contraceptives.

DRUG INTERACTIONS

Concurrent administration of oral contraceptives with other drugs may result in an interaction whereby either contraceptive efficacy is diminished or the oral contraceptive alters the pharmacology of the other drug. It should be noted that the 30 microgram preparations allow less margin for error and even a small reduction in efficiency may result in break-through bleeding or unwanted pregnancy.

The problem of reduced contraceptive reliability came to light following the publication of reports of pregnancies occurring when other drugs were prescribed even though the oral contraceptive had been taken correctly. In recent years, sensitive radio-immuno assays for plasma levels of ethinyloestradiol, norethisterone and levonorgestrel have been developed and it has been possible to demonstrate alterations in blood hormone levels when certain drugs are administered concomitantly. This work has substantiated many of the earlier observations.

Drugs which may reduce contraceptive efficacy

(a) *Antituberculous drugs:* rifampicin.
(b) *Antibiotics:* ampicillin, chloramphenicol, neomycin, nitrofurantoin, penicillin, sulphamethoxypyridazine.
(c) *Anticonvulsants:* hydantoins, phenobarbitone, primidone, ethosuximide.
(d) *Analgesics:* phenacetin.
(e) *Anti-inflammatory agents:* phenylbutazone, oxyphenbutazone.
(f) *Sedatives and Tranquillisers:* chlordiazepoxide, chlorpromazine, diazepam, meprobamate.

It can be seen that these drugs are widely used in general practice and the possibility of reduced contraceptive efficacy must always be borne in mind when these other drugs are prescribed. This is especially important when a 30 microgram oestrogen contraceptive is being used. The appearance of break-through bleeding when one of these drugs is prescribed suggests that the level of circulating hormone is reduced.

Similarly oral contraceptives are known to reduce the antidepressant response when tricyclic antidepressants are administered. Oestrogens reduce the effect of dicoumarol anticoagulant but in my opinion if an anticoagulant is indicated then the oral contraceptive is contra-indicated.

PREGNANCY AND ORAL CONTRACEPTIVES

Women occasionally continue to take oral contraceptives inadvertently when they have conceived. Both large British surveys, the Oxford Family Planning and Royal College of General Practitioners studies have shown no excess of congenital abnormalities when oral contraceptives were taken in early pregnancy. Some abnormalities have, however, been described, the commonest of which are limb reduction deformities and cardiac lesions. The current concensus is that oral contraceptives when taken in prescribed doses in early pregnancy are not teratogenic. When larger than recommended doses are taken, for example as a means of either diagnosing pregnancy or in an attempt to induce abortion, abnormalities have certainly occurred.

There is no difference between former oral contraceptive users and users of other methods in the outcome of pregnancies conceived after discontinuation of the method.

When an oral contraceptive is stopped in order that a woman might conceive, the return of ovulatory menstrual cycles may be delayed with consequent delay in the return of her fertility. Cumulative conception rates for women stopping oral contraceptives lag behind those of IUCD and barrier method users but the difference disappears at the end of two years.

Occasionally, women stopping oral contraceptives experience periods of amenorrhoea. It is estimated that this group of women forms about two per cent of pill-users. Whether oral contraceptives cause this amenorrhoea or whether it is coincidental to oral contraceptive use is a controversial subject. The problem of amenorrhoea in women in the general population is not known accurately; but some reports suggest that it is also in the order of two per cent. Amenorrhoea of more than six months duration, whether related to pill taking or not, requires further investigation to exclude serious pathology and to select appropriate treatment.

The results of induction of ovulation with clomiphene among this amenorrhoea group are very good.

REFERENCES

Inman, W. H. W. and Vessey, M. P. (1968). Investigation of deaths from pulmonary, coronary and cerebral thrombosis and embolism in women of childbearing age. *British Medical Journal*, 2, 193.

Royal College of General Practitioners. (1974). *Oral Contraceptives and Health* – an interim report. Pitman Medical Books, London.

Royal College of General Practitioners. (1977). Effect on hypertension and benign breast disease of progestogen component in combined oral contraceptives. *Lancet*, 1, 624.

Royal College of General Practitioners Oral Contraceptive Study. (1977). Mortality among oral contraceptive users. *Lancet*, 2, 727.

Vessey, M. P. and Doll, R. (1968). Investigation of the relation between use of oral contraceptives and thromboembolic disease. *British Medical Journal*, 2, 199.

Vessey, M. P., McPherson, K. and Johnson, B. (1977). Mortality among women participating in the Oxford Family Planning Association Study. *Lancet*, 2, 731.

BIBLIOGRAPHY

Back, D. J., Breckenridge, A. M., Orme, M. and Rowe, P. H. (1980). Clinical pharmacology of oral contraceptive steroids: drug interactions. *Journal of Obstetrics and Gynaecology*, 1, 126.

Gillmer, M. D. G., Fox, E. J. and Jacobs, H. S. (1978). Failure of withdrawal bleeding during combined oral contraceptive therapy. *Contraception*, 18, 507.

Jacobs, H. S., Knuth, U. A., Hull, M. G. R. and Franks, S. (1977). Post-pill amenorrhoea – cause or coincidence. *British Medical Journal*, 2, 940.

Vessey, M. P., Doll, R., Peto, R., Johnson, B. and Wiggins, P. (1976). A long-term follow-up study of women using different methods of contraception – interim report. *Journal of Biosocial Science*, 8, 373.

Vessey, M. P., Kay, C. R., Baldwin, J. A., Clarke, J. A. and McLeod, B. (1977). Oral contraceptives and benign liver tumours. *British Medical Journal*, 1, 1066.

Vessey, M. P., Wright, N. H., McPherson, K. and Wiggins, P. (1978). Fertility after stopping different methods of contraception. *British Medical Journal*, 1, 265.

Chapter 22   Hormone replacement therapy

I. D. COOKE MB, BS, DGO, FRCOG

The term *hormone replacement therapy* has come to be used generally in relation to the treatment of post-menopausal symptoms, so this chapter will not deal with the replacement of other hormones such as cortisol, thyroxine, insulin or vasopressin which should properly be included in this term. The title is also relevant to replacement of testosterone for hypogonadal males but apart from noting the introduction of an orally active testosterone as the undecanoate (40mg tabs Restandol) this will not be discussed.

Many authors object to the term hormone replacement therapy (HRT) as the physiological state after the menopause is characterised by very low oestrogen levels and the formulations prescribed usually differ from the physiological substance oestradiol; such therapists refer to 'menopausal therapy'.

A. ASSESSMENT

TYPE OF PATIENT

(a) Spontaneous menopause

SYMPTOMS

The typical patient presents during her climacteric with vasomotor symptoms and signs of oestrogen deficiency. If more than six months has elapsed since her last episode of vaginal bleeding she is termed menopausal, if not, peri-menopausal. The hot flushes may be severe but the signs of oestrogen deficiency, vaginal dryness or dyspareunia, are not usually as obvious in the peri-menopausal era.

Many symptoms occur at this time of life but those that reliably respond to oestrogen therapy are the vasomotor component, hot flushes and the vaginal dryness which usually presents as dyspareunia but may not be volunteered and should be specifically sought. The patient of course may not have a partner but this should not be assumed – dyspareunia may be the underlying reason for the consultation. Blatt's Menopausal Index (Table 1) is a useful way of quantitating the symptoms and a score of eight suggests and of 12 signifies a clinical problem.

A recent Oxford survey found that flushing, night sweats, difficulty in making decisions and loss of confidence were closely associated with the mean age of menopause, which is 50 years in the United Kingdom. There was also a *reduction* in the incidence of irritability, low backache and aching breasts. However, anorexia, formication, headache and dyspareunia (remembering that there are also other causes for dyspareunia) were unrelated to the age of menopause, these symptoms occurring equally in males of the same age. Similarly insomnia, loss of libido and frequency and urgency of micturition were also unrelated to the age of menopause.

These symptoms must be clarified as the non-oestrogen responsive symptoms may be important in the context of some other disorder and neither patient nor doctor should expect them to respond to oestrogen. Failure to appreciate this may lead to an attempt to increase the oestrogen dose to quite high levels and out of all proportion to the need to remedy the oestrogen lack.

EXAMINATION

Physical examination may often reveal signs of oestrogen deficiency. The more gross tissue thinning and shrinkage, particularly around the vulva, are usually obvious; the diagnostic problem tends to arise when there is little obvious abnormality, the vagina is perhaps less rugose or a pinker colour. Confirmation of the symptoms may be obtained by taking a smear of the upper lateral vaginal wall using an Ayres' cervical spatula and fixing the smear in the usual way so that it can be read in the cytology laboratory. The percentage of cornified cells (Karyopyknotic Index) is likely to be 40 per cent or less and there will be increased intermediate or parabasal cells seen. Alternatively a 24-hour urinary total oestrogen excretion of less than $20\mu g$ $(70\mu mol)/24hr$ or a plasma oestradiol of less than 100pg/ml (350pmol/litre) would also support the diagnosis.

Table 1 Blatt's menopausal index

Symptoms	Factor	Severity (0–3*)	Score
Hot flushes	4		
Perspiration	2		
Paraesthesiae	2		
Insomnia	2		
Muscle, joints, bone pain	1		
Fatigue	1		
Headache	1		
Irritability	1		
Vertigo	1		
Depression	1		
Shortness of breath	1		
Palpitation	1		
Psycholability	1		
		INDEX:	

*0 – no complaint
1 – slight
2 – moderate
3 – marked or severe

The score for an individual symptom is the product of the factor and severity.
The total index is the sum of all the products.

A problem also arises in the peri-menopausal woman who may still have a cycle, albeit slightly prolonged, where symptoms such as hot flushes only occur during the follicular phase. This is because they come only when the circulating oestrogen has remained low after a period and there is a delay before some follicular activity begins in the next cycle. This late start accounts for the prolongation of the cycle. Nevertheless, the failing ovary can still ultimately achieve oestrogen levels compatible with ovulation – seemingly a contradiction where the patient has menopausal symptoms and yet ovulates and may be at risk of pregnancy. This ovarian activity in a woman who is still bleeding makes timing of samples to obtain a definitively low level quite difficult, so much so that it is hardly worth attempting. On the other hand, if the symptoms are causing significant difficulty in maintaining her lifestyle, drug therapy should be offered.

Flushes can be counted and a record kept by the patient – this serves as a useful index of response. An amenorrhoeic woman with flushes is likely to be menopausal. She is usually thin as adipose tissue by converting circulating adrenal androgens to oestrogen provides endogenous support.

(b) The younger menopausal woman
Women younger than 43 (the fifth centile) may have a spontaneous menopause but this should be carefully checked by estimating plasma follicle stimulating hormone (FSH). It is not possible, however, to make a definitive diagnosis. Until recently it was thought that in addition to an exaggerated response to luteinising hormone releasing hormone (LHRH), an absence of follicles on a very small (usually laparoscopic) ovarian biopsy provided firm evidence. However, patients have been reported who have follicles seen histologically in the biopsy and, after suppressive treatment for their 'menopause', pregnancies have been reported. It is thought that there may be a temporary functional dislocation of ovarian granulosa and theca cells such that inadequate oestrogen is produced by the follicles and this allows the plasma FSH to rise as no longer being under feedback control.

These patients should be treated and although one needs to investigate them adequately (she may be only 21 years old) to exclude other causes of secondary amenorrhoea and then give a poor prognosis, it is no longer possible to be definite if the patient still has her ovaries. Commonly the patient has had her ovaries removed surgically at total hysterectomy; bilateral oophorectomy is being done less frequently in women under 50, but a fibroid uterus may have presented technical difficulties or gross endometriosis may have warranted removal of all ovarian tissue. She may be a younger woman who has had a radical hysterectomy for carcinoma of the cervix. Ovarian removal for cystadenoma may have been complete and not simply cyst removal, or ovaries may have been consecutively removed at the time of ruptured ectopic gestations, a practice no longer recommended.

Irradiation of the pelvis in younger women is only likely to have been done for carcinoma of the cervix. Carcinoma of the breast would itself contra-indicate the use of oestrogen. Treatment of Hodgkin's disease should be able to spare the ovaries even if it means laparotomy to fix them near the midline to avoid the field of irradiation.

(c) The very young patient
Occasionally a pre-pubertal girl will have had her ovaries removed as part of a radical procedure for sarcoma botryoides, or a more general illness such as ulcerative colitis leading to ileostomy may require induction of puberty as a prelude to long-term hormone therapy. Similarly, early gonadal excision in testicular feminisation, or simply a Turner's syndrome, may need a comparable sequence. If these young girls have had no oestrogen given to them previously they will have no menopausal symptoms but rather will wish for breast development or in gonadal dysgenesis even another half-inch in height as part of the pubertal growth spurt.

GENERAL HEALTH SCREENING

A symptomatic patient who may be a candidate for long-term drug therapy must be screened for other disease. Historically one wishes to exclude breast or endometrial carcinoma. Although ovarian carcinoma is usually included in this bracket there is no evidence that ovarian malignancy is oestrogen dependent. Ischaemic heart disease, deep venous thrombosis or pulmonary embolism are contra-indications to therapy. Other factors perhaps are more reasonably risk factors that need to be taken into account, thus hypertension, diabetes, smoking and cholelithiasis may all be relative contra-indications that depend on the cumulative risk 'score' and the incapacity against which it needs to be balanced in an informed patient. There is evidence that cholelithiasis is increased by oestrogen replacement therapy but the validity of the other factors is not established and rests mainly on

extrapolation of data relative to oral contraceptive formulations in pre-menopausal women.

Pregnancy, of course, must be excluded and a pelvic examination should also exclude obvious fibroids; a cervical smear should be obtained if it has not been known to be negative within the past two years. Any undiagnosed irregular or heavy vaginal bleeding should be further investigated by curettage before HRT is contemplated. Less obvious is the problem of the patient who has suffered major side-effects on oral contraception, such as migraine.

Of major importance is the recognition of psychiatric disturbance which needs separate treatment. Established menopause clinics have a high proportion of patients resistant to therapy and these patients mostly have significant psychoneuroses.

Laboratory investigation should be directed by positive results of the specific interrogation or a strong family history; in this way we have detected abnormalities that led to a diagnosis of diabetes mellitus, hyperlipidaemia, hypothyroidism and hypertension. Urinalysis may show glycosuria but routine biochemical or coagulation screening has not, on the whole, been rewarding, although asymptomatic abnormalities in serum cholesterol or triglycerides have been detected.

COUNSELLING

Menopause therapy has been much discussed in women's magazines and by the media and unfortunately sometimes held up as a panacea. Some women will therefore be well informed and others will be anxious because of the stated 'cancer risk' and yet others simply wish to be informed reliably and with sympathy. We have been surprised at the not inconsiderable number of women who elect *not* to use any drug therapy or at least hormone therapy when the background has been explained to their satisfaction. Whether they are at long-term risk by *not* accepting treatment is as yet an open question (but see the section on osteoporosis). It seems, therefore, to be worthwhile spending time explaining the pathophysiology of the menopause, its sequelae and the effect of treatment to promote rational understanding, irrespective of whether endocrine treatment is ultimately begun. Investigations, alternative supporting therapy or hormone preparations should have their individual role delineated, so that expectations are not falsely raised. The patient must recognise that she is very likely to have regular induced bleeding (and this may ultimately become unacceptable). She will need long-term surveillance and in the light of present knowledge, an initial endometrial biopsy and probably one every two years. Treatment should probably be continued for at least ten years but the duration of treatment required for the optimum chance of reducing the risk of osteoporosis is not yet known.

OBJECTIVES AND DURATION OF TREATMENT

(a) Symptom relief

The usual reason for presenting is hot flushes which occur in nearly 50 per cent of women at 50 to 55 years of age. Population studies have shown that 10 per cent of women are so severely affected that their ability to work is sometimes impaired, whereas one-third indicate that it does not interfere with their lifestyle. Even in castrate women the number experiencing hot flushes is not higher than 50 per cent.

Double-blind cross-over studies have found that placebo decreases the flush rate although oestrogen does so to a greater extent. In those given placebo first for six months there is a continued reduction in the flushes when oestrogen is given whereas there is a rapid increase in the flush rate when changeover from oestrogen to placebo occurs.

There is little information available about the duration of treatment required for symptomatic relief and in any case it varies from patient to patient. Experience gained in a self-referral, non-hospital-based clinic suggests that if the decision is primarily made by the patient there is a progressive fall in numbers of about 20 per cent every nine months. (In that clinic the patient was treated for six months, then as part of a research protocol treatment was stopped for three months for both patient and doctor to evaluate responses and assess the need for continuing therapy.) In general, however, either a philosophical decision regarding duration of treatment is made based on the need to maintain the skeleton and hence is long term, or an arbitrary decision is made to stop after six months. If the need for further treatment becomes obvious it can be readily restarted.

Vaginal dryness as a cause of dyspareunia may occur a little later but responds equally well to oral or local therapy; each has a comparable local effect and each achieves similar blood levels – there is no exclusive or disproportionate local effect. Cessation of therapy allows a slow reversion to an atrophic vaginal mucosa and eventually would lead to some vaginal shrinkage. Intermittent therapy such as two months on and two months off would deal with this. An alternative is continuous therapy by either route but using once-daily administration of a small dose so that the plasma oestrogen concentrations are only elevated for a short time in the 24 hours gives a similar biological effect (see later).

(b) Prevention of osteoporosis

Twenty per cent of all women will suffer a fracture of the hip by the age of 90 and 80 per cent of these will have osteoporosis. As a result of complications of the hip fractures 16 per cent will die within three months. About 25 per cent of all white women over the age of 60 will develop spinal compression due to osteoporosis. Fractures are less in black women and in those societies where physical labour by these women is more common. A retrospective case control study has shown that protection against fracture by oestrogen medication started within five years of the menopause was highly significant.

Bilateral oophorectomy results in mobilisation and loss of bone, shown by a rise in plasma and urinary calcium and by rises in the urinary calcium/creatinine ratio and the hydroxyproline/creatinine ratio. This change is also evident in those experiencing a spontaneous menopause.

The best data on the effect of oestrogen treatment come from the randomised double-blind controlled trial of 120 who had undergone oophorectomy treated in Glasgow with 25 micrograms oral mestranol daily, beginning at the time of oophorectomy. Bone density has been assessed by photon absorption at the mid-point of the third metacarpal of the right hand. A nine-year follow-up showed that the metacarpal mineral content is maintained in the treated women and there is a progressive bone loss in the placebo-treated group. If there is a delay of three to six years after the menopause before treatment is begun there is even an initial increase in bone density over the first three treatment years. This is then maintained but not increased further, so that delay in initiating treatment is not a long-term handicap. However, in the placebo-treated group the rate of bone loss was greatest for the first few years and then declined. In those women who were treated for four years and then stopped therapy, the rate of bone loss was the same as for the first four years' loss in the placebo group. There was therefore no difference at eight years in bone density between those that had mestranol treatment for the first four years and those that had no oestrogen. This strongly suggests that long-term therapy is required.

Group differences in this study were similarly shown for the degree of spinal osteoporosis, but within individuals there was no correlation of the extent of the spinal osteoporosis and the metacarpal mineral content.

Short-term studies have also examined the efficacy of

calcium supplements, 1α-hydroxy vitamin D_3 or new steroids having effects only on bone and not on the genital tract, but the optimum regimen has not yet been devised and the long-term prospective data have only been obtained using oral oestrogens.

It is not yet possible to predict which patients are at risk of osteoporosis, although bone scanning using labelled diphosphonate shows some promise. The only clinical indicator at present is the asthenic woman who is not protected by sufficient endogenous oestrogens from her adipose tissue.

It seems that the fracture or spinal compression rate could be substantially reduced by deferring major bone loss for 10 to 15 years by some form of treatment. The age of the patient when she then first becomes at risk of fracture would be much greater but in view of the rapid bone loss after short-term treatment long-term reduction in morbidity must still be in doubt. On the other hand, the retrospective case control study quoted above, which showed oestrogen protection, is likely to be an *underestimate* of the likely effect of long-term therapy if there is rapid bone loss again after short-term therapy. At present, therefore, there seems to be a case for long-term treatment if this benefit outweighs the problems of surveillance for both patient and doctor. The advice to a woman must be tailored to the individual woman.

COMPLICATIONS AND MONITORING OF TREATMENT

(a) Endometrial carcinoma

The principal concern of recent years has been the association of endometrial carcinoma and the history of oestrogen treatment, noted in a series of American retrospective case control studies. They highlight the increased relative risk ratio for, or prevalence of, endometrial carcinoma after long-term, often continuous, oestrogen, with usually no, or only sporadic, progestogen. These studies are important as they have drawn attention to the theoretical need to use progestogen sequentially to induce regular withdrawal bleeding if the patient still has a uterus, and prevent unrestricted endometrial proliferation by this medical curettage. Long-term studies adequately monitored by endometrial biopsy have not yet been completed but shorter-term studies in quite large numbers (850 women) have shown that 7 to 13 days of progestogen added towards the end of a course of cyclical low-dose oestrogen does not increase the risk of endometrial hyperplasia or carcinoma. The incidence of hyperplasia fell as the duration of progestogen therapy increased and reached zero when given for 10 days.

Thus a sequential oestrogen/progestogen regimen containing 10 days' progestogen is likely to be the minimum sex hormone regimen required. In view of the above, monitoring of the endometrial response to treatment is important. To exclude pre-existing pathology a biopsy should be obtained before starting therapy if the patient is amenorrhoeic more than six months (i.e. if a diagnosis of menopause has been made) and if heavy or irregular bleeding is present in a woman still menstruating. At the menopause there is a reduction in amount, frequency or duration of periods or a sudden cessation; an increase in these is pathological.

The biopsy may be obtained by any small curette (such as a Novak, Randall or Vabra aspiration) that can be inserted without cervical dilatation. It may be necessary to apply a volsellum to the cervix to straighten out an anteverted uterus by downward traction if the fundus cannot be reached. The single-toothed volsellum causes less discomfort if closed slowly but the biopsy or aspiration usually generates quite an unpleasant dysmenorrhoea-like pain that sometimes subsequently stops the patient returning for long-term therapy. If the curette or aspiration tube cannot be inserted through the cervix without dilatation, a further attempt may be made three months later after therapy has been given as then the cervix may be softer and the endocervix more readily negotiable. If the biopsy attempt fails then one must resort to dilatation and curettage under anaesthesia, following which an office procedure can be subsequently accomplished without difficulty.

The object of biopsy is to identify hyperplasia, atypical hyperplasia and endometrial carcinoma. The first may be treated with one or two courses of norethisterone (Primolut N) 5mg for 21 days and the biopsy repeated. Atypical hyperplasia does not respond to this therapy and is best treated by hysterectomy. However, whether endometrial carcinoma or atypical hyperplasia are actually caused by the steroids has not yet been settled, the evidence rests on the epidemiological association. Pre-treatment biopsy should identify most problems. In the American studies where patients are under surveillance and endometrial carcinoma has been found incidentally at biopsy, it has been at an earlier stage than found in the controls. It could, therefore, be argued that the surveillance actually promotes the prospects of an earlier diagnosis and presumably higher survival rates in response to definitive treatment.

If no biopsy, or mucus only, is obtained, then this is acceptable as long as the technique is satisfactory, there being no endometrial proliferative response to the therapy. Present thinking suggests that a biopsy should be checked every two years provided that the induced bleeding pattern remains regular and the loss not excessive.

(b) Breast carcinoma

Data on the development of breast carcinoma are less clear-cut. Two studies suggest no increase and two others a marginal increase and a 2.5-fold increase after 12 years' oestrogen therapy respectively. Information on long-term treatment with sequential preparations is not available.

(c) Cardiovascular disease

Deaths due to coronary artery disease do not change significantly around the age of menopause. The cardiovascular system does, however, seem to be affected if oestrogen deprivation occurs early enough in life. Castration before the age of 40 has been found to result in a higher incidence of coronary atherosclerosis than in controls at autopsy more than 10 years later. Again, subjects castrated between the ages of 25 and 30 have been compared with age-matched controls 30 years later and a significant increase in the frequency of coronary vascular disease up to the age of 70 has been found in the group who had undergone oophorectomy. The Boston Collaborative Drug Surveillance Program found no association between oestrogen taking and non-fatal myocardial infarction in women aged 40 to 75. However, if the youngest cohort aged 39 to 45 was examined there *was* an increased incidence of myocardial infarction but this was virtually limited to those who were smokers. These data are reminiscent of the oral contraceptive oestrogen effect in older pre-menopausal women. The Framingham study showed that women in the 40 to 45 year age-group who had a spontaneous or surgical menopause had a substantially greater risk than *pre*-menopausal women of developing coronary vascular disease and this was doubled by oestrogen treatment. These data, of course, refer to oestrogen-only medication which, if the patient has a uterus, should no longer be given because of the potential neoplastic problem. Nevertheless, the problems seem greater in younger women and in smokers, and these aspects should be recognised in selecting patients for therapy. A clinical history or a strong family history of cardiovascular disease may, therefore, be predictive.

Serum lipids are influenced by oestrogens. Higher concentrations of serum cholesterol correlate with an increase in myocardial infarction rate, but an increase in high density lipoprotein (HDL) cholesterol is thought to be beneficial and is found in people who exercise and those who have a decreased incidence of myocardial infarction. The type of oestrogen used appears to be important as ethinyloestradiol has a worse effect on HDL cholesterol than oestradiol valerate (Progynova). Although conjugated equine oestrogens (Premarin) move HDL cholesterol levels in a 'beneficial' direction (i.e. an increase) they also increase circulating phospholipids and triglycerides. Recent work on the sequential preparations suggests that they reduce mean serum cholesterol concentrations to those of age-matched pre-menopausal controls. Different formulations however have different effects on serum triglycerides as mestranol/norethisterone (Menophase) causes an increase and oestradiol valerate/norgestrel (Cycloprogynova) a decrease. These data then suggest a preference for a sequential preparation.

No increase in thrombotic episodes in post-menopausal women taking oestrogen has been found in the Boston Collaborative Drug Surveillance Program. This makes the *in vitro* data on coagulation factors difficult to assess. However, the latter data refer to oestrogens only, piperazine oestrone sulphate (Harmogen) and oestradiol valerate (Progynova). High-dose sequential preparations have been studied, but at the lower doses only mestranol/norethisterone in a sequence designed to simulate the pre-menopausal steroid pattern (Menophase) have been evaluated. Although the latter showed an initial significant rise in Factor X and significant decrease in Factors IX, VIII, anti-X and anti-thrombin III during six months' therapy, other low-dose sequential preparations have not been studied *in vitro*. Nevertheless, in view of the US epidemiological data there seems no compelling reason to regard thrombosis as a worrisome feature.

B. DRUG TREATMENT

ORAL

Oestrogens and combined oestrogen/progestogen

The usual mode of administration is oral and there is a considerable number of preparations available. Ethinyloestradiol and mestranol are interconverted in the liver and metabolically there is nothing to choose between them. The Glasgow osteoporosis studies have been done with a mean dose of 25 micrograms mestranol but ethinyloestradiol 25 micrograms (Lynoral – 10 microgram tabs) has been shown to maintain calcium balance in patients with crush fractures. Further, 15 micrograms ethinyloestradiol daily can cause highly significant reductions in menopausal symptom scores.

Assay of plasma concentrations of oestrone and oestrone sulphate, the principal post-menopausal circulating oestrogens, has shown that comparable levels can be achieved by a piperazine oestrone sulphate (Harmogen 1–2 × 1.5mg tabs), ethinyloestradiol (10–25 micrograms), oestradiol valerate (Progynova 2mg) and conjugated equine oestrogen (Premarin 1.25mg). Similarly, comparable plasma oestradiol concentrations are achieved by conjugated equine oestrogens, oestrone piperazine sulphate and oestradiol valerate and these interconversions are effected by gut-wall and hepatic metabolism.

The concentrations of oestrone and oestradiol in the peripheral circulation each reach a peak at about four hours and decline slowly by 24 hours, although they are still somewhat elevated. Interestingly, daily administration for 21 days does not seem to result in elevated basal plasma concentration nor can this be demonstrated over a year or more. Concentrations in response to continuous oral therapy, however, are not known and it is perhaps a reason for endometrial proliferation in the face of long-term unopposed oestrogen. The other reason for potential stimulation is the very high peak concentration reached by oral administration – a level five to ten times those found at mid-cycle in pre-menopausal women.

That the doses used are excessive may be shown by the fact that hepatic synthesis of sex hormone binding globulin is grossly stimulated in post-menopausal women treated with standard preparations and reaches higher concentrations than are found in pre-menopausal women. Similarly, even a small dose of conjugated equine oestrogen (0.3mg Premarin) causes excessive hepatic synthesis of the protein renin substrate. Yet this dose is required to show a significant reduction in the calcium/creatinine ratio indicative of the calcium-retaining effect. Increasing doses, however, cause little additional change in the degree of keratinisation of the vaginal mucosa or further reduction in plasma FSH and LH concentrations.

Oestriol has been claimed as having minimal uterotrophic effects and therefore to be non-carcinogenic. Doses of up to 6mg are also converted to circulating serum oestrone and oestradiol but these concentrations are much lower than those achieved by the other oestrogens already described and there is no massive peak shortly after administration. Administration of 2mg eight-hourly, however, does result in endometrial stimulation. It seems then that the benign effect of oestriol is a function of both the concentration of potent oestrogen achieved in the circulation and the infrequent administration (once daily) flattening the plasma profile. In the light of these data it is interesting that oestriol is presented as 0.25mg tabs (Ovestin) with a recommended one to two tablets daily schedule. It seems that many times this dose would be safe and would be needed for efficacy.

Two other single oral preparations available are quinestradol (Pentovis 0.25mg) which appears not to have been studied recently and chlorotrianisene (Tace, 12mg) which is stored in fat depots and is released slowly. This means that it is contra-indicated in women who still have a uterus. An attempt to achieve peripheral plasma concentrations of the same hormones that occur endogenously in the human is made by a formulation containing oestriol 0.27mg, oestradiol 0.6mg and oestrone 1.4mg (Hormonin), but this seems not to be an advance as the concentration of oestrone alone is similar to that in oestrone piperazine sulphate (Harmogen 1.5mg) which reaches the high concentrations described above.

Developments in this area will be watched with interest as preparations of defined small particle size ('micronised') are orally absorbed as free steroids and if given in small doses every eight hours can maintain plasma levels constantly throughout 24 hours at low levels.

INDUCTION OF PUBERTY

For the very young patient deprived of oestrogen before puberty, the need may arise for the induction of puberty. Evidence has recently accumulated that suggests that the body-weight at which puberty begins is 47kg although menarche and indeed resumption of menstruation after amenorrhoea is related to body-weight other than adipose tissue i.e. bone and muscle.

The optimum time to start treatment may be difficult to decide if the young girl is quite small as a result of malnourishment due to her underlying disease (e.g. ulcerative colitis and delayed puberty). As the process of puberty takes perhaps two to three years and involves a resetting of the sensitivity of the hypothalamic control centre for gonadotrophins, a suitable plan for artificial progress through puberty is also slow. A pubertal growth spurt is simulated to some extent and this can be used to advantage in those of genetically short stature such as Turner's syndrome, although it can also be a problem in a tall girl with gonadal agenesis.

A convenient regimen is to give ethinyloestradiol 10 micrograms daily orally for three weeks out of four for three months. On review there is usually a much happier girl as early signs of breast development are evident. This is often the prime reason for presenting, as peer group differences in breast development become exaggerated as the girls grow older. These differences should be recorded and can be staged according to the description of normal pubertal breast development by Tanner (Grades I to V). The ethinyloestradiol should be increased to 20 micrograms daily on the same regimen and withdrawal vaginal bleeding may even start by the six-month stage. After six months' total treatment so far (three months of each) the third three-month phase of 30 micrograms ethinyloestradiol should begin. At the nine-month stage progestogen should be added and this can conveniently be given as a single tablet oral contraceptive formulation using the new low-dose ethinyloestradiol preparations (Eugynon 30, Ovran 30, ethinyloestradiol 30 micrograms/ levonorgestrel 250 micrograms; Microgynon, Ovranette, ethinyloestradiol 30 micrograms/ levonorgestrel 150 micrograms; Brevinor, Ovysmen, ethinyloestradiol 35 micrograms/norethisterone 0.5mg; Norimin, ethinyloestradiol 35 micrograms/ norethisterone 1mg). The progestogen component is of considerable importance in continuing breast growth even after the onset of regular withdrawal bleeding.

Subsequent withdrawal of the medication causes loss of breast size in addition to other menopausal symptoms. Plasma FSH and LH concentrations are usually very low in the pre-pubertal state even without gonads but subsequent withdrawal of the medication causes a rise within a few weeks.

This medication should probably be continued until the age of 35, subject to the usual caution arising from risk factors such as smoking, obesity, diabetes, hypertension. As contraception is not relevant to these women, the steroid dosage could then be dropped to ethinyloestradiol 20 micrograms/norethisterone acetate 1mg (Loestrin) until the time seems appropriate to change to a sequential preparation. Experience of such prolonged medication in these young women has, of course, not been obtained. Nevertheless, osteoporosis in untreated women with Turner's syndrome at long-term follow-up is well documented.

Similar regimens are recommended for management of transsexual males who undergo castration, amputation of the external genitalia and have an artificial vagina constructed. The regimen will cause breast development that is acceptable without breast prostheses. Combined oestrogen/progestogen combinations are also appropriate for young women under the age of 35 who have had both ovaries removed surgically, been irradiated post-puberty or developed primary ovarian failure, i.e. after previously experiencing regular menses. The low-dose combined oestrogen/progestogen preparations already described (Eugynon 30, Ovran 30, Microgynon, Ovranette, Brevinor, Ovysmen, Norimin) are ideal. If a uterus is still present as in primary ovarian failure, or if only a small amount of oestrogen has ever been secreted (but sufficient to cause some breast development as in some patients with gonadal dysgenesis) regular vaginal bleeding can be instituted. By the age of 35, the cut-off point designated by the Royal College of General Practitioners' study as bestowing greater risk of death from cardiovascular disease, these patients will still need some systemic hormonal support. They have no need to turn to non-hormonal methods of contraception as do other women, so Loestrin or sequential preparations are appropriate.

(b) Progestogen-only
Progestogens alone may be used to suppress menopausal symptoms and may be helpful where oestrogens are contra-indicated, for example in a patient with a history of a deep venous thrombosis or following surgical treatment of endometriosis. Norethisterone 5mg daily (Primolut N, Utovlan) is efficacious for hot flushes, but in the absence of oestrogen the vaginal dryness or dyspareunia are not relieved. A new progestogen, norgestrel, may be given at a lower dose. Levonorgestrel alone (Microval, Norgeston, 30 micrograms) has the same efficacy as a mixture of the d-and l-isomers (Neogest, 75 micrograms) and is quite effective for hot flushes, but again not in remedying the vaginal changes.

(c) Sequential oestrogen/progestogens
Unlike oral contraceptive formulations, the progestogen is not given during the first half of the regimen. Oestrogen doses used in the treatment of menopausal symptoms are not required to suppress ovulation, so lower doses of oestrogen are used; similarly progestogen, which increases the effectiveness of ovulation suppression when given in the first half of a course, is not required and its absence reduces the cost. To reduce neoplastic change in the endometrium on long-term administration 10 days' progestogen each month is optimally required. Oestradiol valerate 21 days (1 or 2mg) and levonorgestrel 0.25mg 10 days (Cyclo-progynova) meet this requirement. The lower oestradiol dosage is usually all that is required for relief of symptoms. To conjugated equine oestrogens (the major components of which are oestrone sulphate and equilin, a potent oestrogen not found in the human) 0.625mg or 1.25mg for 21 days have been added seven days norgestrel 0.5mg (Prempak). This is equally effective in relieving symptoms.

The other formulations differ from this simple sequential scheme by attempting to match the tableted components with endogenous oestrogen/progesterone patterns. These are shown in Table 2.

Table 2 Composition of two sequential preparations

Menophase		Trisequens		
mestranol	12.5 micrograms –5	oestradiol	2mg	} –12
mestranol	25 micrograms –8	oestriol	1mg	
mestranol	25 micrograms } –3	oestradiol	2mg	} –10
norethisterone	1mg	oestriol	1mg	
mestranol	30 micrograms } –6	norethisterone acetate	1mg	
norethisterone	1.5mg	oestradiol	1mg	} –6
mestranol	20 micrograms } –4	oestriol	0.5mg	
norethisterone	0.75mg			

Different combinations of steroids are differently coloured so that the correct sequence is taken by the patient. There has been no evidence produced to show that these preparations are superior to other formulations. That they are sequential would be advantageous and compatible with normal endometrial histology. Symptomatic relief has not been shown to be better but the total steroid dose is less and this is presumably better on theoretical grounds. The Trisequens (Table 2) makes use of the micronised oestrogens and so is able to use the same oestrogens as found in the human. *In vitro* studies suggest that no coagulation abnormality after Trisequens is associated with these oestrogens, but as stated above the *in vivo* evidence obtained epidemiologically does not suggest that clotting is a significant problem with menopausal hormone therapy. The effect of fluctuating doses on overall calcium balance is unknown nor is it known what is the effect of the micronised form of the oestrogens.

(d) Oestrogen/androgen combinations

Some years ago these combinations were widely used as it was thought that the androgen was anabolic for bone and it also increased libido. Since the newer techniques of assessing bone density have become available these combinations have not been reassessed. There is also often an increase in hair growth amounting to hirsutism peri-menopausally as the ovarian stroma produces an increased amount of androstenedione and testosterone, although much of this is converted into oestrogen in other tissues such as muscle, liver and adipose tissue. Finally, methyltestosterone can cause cholestatic jaundice. For these reasons ethinyloestradiol 4.4 micrograms/methyl testosterone 3.6mg (Mixogen) is little used.

(e) Other agents affecting bone

After the menopause calcium absorption is reduced. In the first few years after the menopause oestrogen alone is probably all that is required to retard bone loss, but as malabsorption due to vitamin D deficiency and dietary calcium deficiency exacerbate post-menopausal bone loss, supplementary calcium may have a greater effect than oestrogen alone. Calcium lactate gluconate (Sandocal providing 400mg of calcium) 800mg daily provides adequate supplementation.

Vitamin D metabolism is influenced by oestrogen therapy and it can be shown that serum 1,25 dihydroxy D_3 and immunoreactive parathormone are increased and correlate with each other and in turn with increased calcium absorption. Metabolically vitamin D_3 (cholecalciferol) is converted in the liver into 25 hydroxy D_3 and then under the influence of parathormone and low inorganic phosphate is 1-hydroxylated in the kidney to 1,25 dihydroxy D_3 a compound which acts on the gut and on bone. Similarly, the kidney may first hydroxylate 25 hydroxy D_3 in the 24 position before continuing to 1,24,25 trihydroxy D_3 which also acts on the gut.

Synthetic 25 hydroxy D_3 increases 1,25 and 24,25 dihydroxy D_3 levels in serum and also increases intestinal calcium absorption. It is therefore of considerable interest that 1α-hydroxy vitamin D_3 (1α-hydroxy cholecaliferol) is commercially available as alfacalcidol (One-alpha, 0.25 microgram). At a dose of 1–2 micrograms daily it has been shown to maintain calcium balance in women with spinal crush factors when used with ethinyloestradiol 25 micrograms or norethisterone 5mg daily, whereas it is unable to do so alone. It is not yet clear whether the effect will be greater with combined therapy than with sex steroid therapy alone, especially in older patients or whether the steroid dose can be reduced for the same effect. This will require long-term study. However, if it allows a reduction in sex steroid dosage to reduce the other unwanted side-effects of oestrogen such as increased hepatic protein synthesis or endometrial proliferation and the need for cyclic bleeding it will be particularly worthwhile.

New anabolic steroids with only weak sex steroid action also show promise on the same basis but these are not yet generally available.

(f) Other agents affecting early symptoms

Although clonidine (Catapres) is used at doses of 0.4–2.0mg daily as an anti-hypertensive agent having a central action (probably of α-adrenergenic-receptor stimulation inhibitory to sympathetic activity) it is used in lower doses to treat menopausal flushing. At doses of 50–100 micrograms (Dixarit, 25 micrograms) twice daily it has been shown to be effective against placebo. Its mode of action is unclear except that it has no hypotensive action at that dose.

Another non-hormonal mixture that has been shown in placebo-controlled studies to be effective in reducing the impact of menopausal symptoms is that containing total alkaloids of belladonna 0.1mg, ergotamine tartrate 0.3mg and phenobarbitone 20mg (Bellergal) administered as two tablets three times daily. A retard preparation containing twice the dose may be given as one tablet twice daily remembering that it is contra-indicated in glaucoma (atropine) and in the presence of cardiovascular disease (ergotamine, sympathomimetic vasocontrictor).

VAGINAL CREAMS

Vaginal dryness may be treated by local oestrogen cream but systemic absorption is efficient and pre-menopausal plasma levels are readily achieved. Conjugated equine oestrogen cream containing 0.625mg/g (Premarin vaginal cream) may be administered in doses of 1–2g daily, intravaginally, using a calibrated applicator. When 2g daily are administered the plasma levels do not achieve such high levels during the first week and this is thought to be due to poorer absorption through the atrophic mucosa. The vaginal mucosa keratinises during that week and, as it does so, its absorptive capacity increases so that normal pre-menopausal plasma and urinary excretion of oestrogens occurs. The plasma oestrone and oestradiol concentrations are higher than that reached by a corresponding oral dose, as less metabolism of the administered steroid occurs following vaginal administration.

Dienoestrol cream 0.16% (Hormofemin cream) presumably is equally well absorbed but no data appear to be available.

This recent information on absorption should stop the previous practice of using vaginal oestrogen cream in those patients thought to be at risk from systemic oestrogens. Local action only without systemic absorption was adduced as the rationale.

Stilboestrol pessaries (0.5mg with lactic acid5%– Tampovagan) are still available. They have not been studied recently but appear to offer no obvious advantage.

If vaginal dryness is a major complaint then vaginal administration of oestrogen may give a more rapid local improvement in symptoms but, of course, oral administration of oestrogen at the same time should be stopped. Doses of 0.5g daily are probably adequate or at least the dose could be divided into morning and evening components. Use when the patient is walking about may be messy, however, unless a tampon is also used. The duration of treatment should be tailored in a similar way to the oral medication, three weeks on and one week off, if the proliferative effects on the endometrium are to be avoided. Prolonged use of the cream still presents a problem as no sequential progestogen is used, so unless one were to use supplementary oral norethisterone 5mg daily (Primolut N) as a sequential regimen it is probably better to change to an oral sequential formulation.

Vaginal medication may be helpful when a ring pessary is inserted long term for prolapse, but it also seems rational to give intermittent courses subsequently if the patient can manage (remembering that the reason for inserting the pessary is that she is unfit for operation). This coupled with regular changing of the pessary would minimise the risk of vaginal ulceration.

Pre-operatively before prolapse repair an atrophic mucosa can be improved considerably to provide a better healing capacity, yet this is little practised nowadays. It was common practice before the higher circulating oestrogens were linked to postoperative deep venous thrombosis and pulmonary embolism; these older patients, often relatively immobile after operation with a urinary catheter in situ, are likely to be at increased risk of this complication.

Stress incontinence has sometimes been treated in post-menopausal women with vaginal oestrogens as post-menopausal urethral and vaginal laxity increase. Cytological evidence of oestrogen lack can be obtained from exfoliated bladder cells passed in urine. However, a more rational approach to the stress incontinence is to exclude a urinary tract infection by culture and perform a urodynamic assessment to understand any component of urgency due to detrusor instability. The role of surgery should then be clear. An oral sequential preparation may be preferable for more general treatment of post-menopausal symptoms, but a much older woman may find the return of regular withdrawal bleeding unwelcome.

INTRAMUSCULAR INJECTIONS

Oestradiol benzoate 25mg is available as an intramuscular injection but as its duration of action cannot be precisely controlled and yet is not sufficient to last for three to four weeks, it is not used in menopause therapy.

If oestrogens are to be avoided then a progestogen may be used on the same basis as the oral progestogens, i.e. if there is no relief from complaints of vaginal dryness or dyspareunia, recourse must be had to simple lubricants such as KY jelly. Intramuscular medroxy-progesterone acetate (Depo-Provera 50mg/ml) will relieve other menopausal symptoms for eight weeks and 150mg for up to 20 weeks. The only side-effects are withdrawal bleeding which may be unpredictable and is related to storage of the steroid in adipose tissue.

IMPLANTS

Because of the prolonged action of implants the patient who still has her uterus should not be treated by this method. Attempts have been made to give intermittent progestogen in an effort to induce regular withdrawal bleeding but a significant number of endometrial abnormalities still emerge. Even in patients without a uterus one should perhaps consider that cyclic administration of combined or sequential preparations may be theoretically better for the breast tissue, and there is, as yet, no evidence that long-term exposure to oral contraceptive formulations increases the risk of breast cancer.

Implants inserted under local analgesia into the buttock or subfascially into the lateral parts of the abdominal wall over one iliac fossa are widely used. Microcrystalline oestradiol may be inserted through a special trocar and cannula as 25mg pellets, 25mg being effective for three months although 100mg may be inserted. This probably lasts six to nine months; there appears to be some fibrosis around the pellet but there is fairly constant release of steroid during this time. This method is sometimes used at hysterectomy when the ovaries are removed and the implant is inserted into the adipose tissue at the edge of the abdominal incision. Younger women who have no uterus, such as one with testicular feminisation after the testes have been removed for their carcinogenic risk, would also be suitable for oestradiol implants, particularly if the motivation to sustain oral therapy was not good. These women have good breast development which is not sustained if their testicular oestrogen is not replaced.

OTHER METHODS

A number of other methods of administering steroids are being developed, but are not yet readily available. Percutaneous absorption of oestradiol can be readily achieved by topical application of 3mg of oestradiol in 5g of gel. After a few days, pre-menopausal concentrations of oestrone and oestradiol are achieved.

Oestrone-releasing vaginal rings have been used effectively, the advantage being that the ring can be removed at any time.

A variation of the implant is the silastic implant which needs to be removed whereas the microcrystalline oestradiol alone is slowly but completely absorbed. Nevertheless, the silastic capsule implant provides a sustained rate of release for up to two years. Removal of the empty capsule at two years can be done under local analgesia.

CONCLUSION

Routine long-term hormone therapy at the menopause at present is probably best given orally as a sequential preparation for three weeks out of four. After initial history taking, physical examination, screening and counselling, long-term surveillance is required. This is primarily at present for regular endometrial aspiration if the patient has a uterus. The regular induced withdrawal bleeding should reduce substantially the need for occasional curettage in response to irregular vaginal bleeding.

The degree of long-term compliance in these women is not yet clear but, to sustain therapy for up to 15 years with its regular vaginal bleeding, a philosophical objective based on the belief that treatment prevents osteoporosis needs to be presented repeatedly. More experience of long-term therapy needs to be obtained before we know whether a British population has an adequate long-term compliance rate, whether any complications of therapy become significant and whether the projected long-term improvement in well-being, morbidity and mortality is a reality. At present this is only a hope, but adequate methods are now available to achieve the objective and a better understanding of the pathophysiology has made a major contribution to this. Perhaps new preparations or combinations of approach will enable selective therapy of symptoms and prevention of osteoporosis to be achieved with a further reduction in side-effects and greater compliance. But the most important determinants of long-term therapy are the doctor's interest in and understanding of the subject area and the way in which he communicates this to his patient.

Chapter 23   Common drug interactions

D. I. R. JONES MD, MRCGP

INTRODUCTION

Although this chapter deals principally with unexpected and unwanted drug interactions, it should not
be forgotten that the careful use of drugs in combination is an important part of the prescribing art.
Hypotensive regimens are based rationally and sci-
entifically on potentiation of one drug by others. In
contrast, the use of multiple drug therapy in epilepsy is
hallowed more by custom than good sense (Shorvon et
al, 1978).

PROPER USE OF DRUG COMBINATIONS

There are several good reasons for using drugs in combination:

1. When the patient has more than one disease.
2. When different aspects of the same disease require
   different treatment.
3. When a greater effect can be obtained by using
   drugs in combination than when they are used
   alone.
4. When the incidence of unwanted effects can be
   reduced by the use of smaller doses of individual
   drugs.
5. To overcome the unwanted effects of other drugs.
6. To prolong drug action.

Interaction between drugs may result in:
1. Antagonism
2. Potentiation
3. An unusual or unexpected effect which cannot be
   predicted from the known actions of the individual
   drugs.

Clinically important drug interactions occur most
frequently with drugs having a steep dose-response
curve and a small therapeutic ratio. These include
anti-arrhythmics, anti-cancer drugs, anticoagulants,
anticonvulsants, cardiac glycosides, oral hypoglycaemic agents and sympathomimetics.

INCIDENCE OF DRUG INTERACTIONS

'Every time a physician adds to the number of drugs a
patient is taking he may devise a novel combination
that has a special risk' (Dollery, 1965).

In a hospital study over 40 per cent of patients were
receiving over six drugs and the incidence of unwanted
effects was seven times greater than in those who were
taking fewer than six preparations (Wade, 1970). In
another hospital study (May et al, 1977) the incidence
of unwanted reactions ranged from four per cent in
patients taking fewer than five drugs daily to 54 per
cent in those taking 16 to 20 drugs per day.

Doctors are frequently unaware of the pharmacological nature of the preparations which they prescribe
(Biron, 1973), awareness of the possibility of drug
interaction may be poor (Howie et al, 1977) and ability
to recognise unwanted reactions may also be suspect
(Petrie et al, 1974).

Because of species variability, animal studies are not
good predictors of drug interaction in man (Brodie,
1962). The accuracy and reliability of many drug-
interaction reports is questionable; they are all too
frequently based on anecdotal evidence or single case
reports (Sjoqvist and Alexanderson, 1972). There is a
great deal of variability, and interaction may occur in
some individuals and not in others (Vessell et al, 1975).
An interaction involving one drug may be wrongly
assumed to involve related drugs. While the anticoagulant effect of warfarin is always potentiated by
phenylbutazone, there is considerable variability in the
extent to which this occurs (Bull and Mackinnon,
1975; Aggeler et al, 1967). Genetic factors and
individual differences in metabolism are sometimes
important and some interactions involving
monoamine-oxidase inhibitors occur in only a minority
of patients. Interactions may be considerably modified
by disease and the elderly are particularly vulnerable.

RECOGNISING DRUG INTERACTIONS

Many lengthy lists of drug interactions have been compiled (e.g. Swidler, 1971). Useful reference sources
include Stockley, 1974; Wade and Beeley, 1976 and

Beeley, 1979. Clinical aids such as the Medidisc (Whiting et al, 1973) may be helpful, though some comprehensive tables are bewildering in their complexity.

The appearance of a drug interaction in a list may not necessarily mean that the interaction has been reported or confirmed. It may only have been suspected on theoretical grounds. This must constantly be borne in mind in using such data. It is clearly impossible to remember all possible drug interactions. The deficiencies of the various data-bases have been pointed out and the most efficient way of avoiding drug interaction is to acquire a thorough knowledge of the mechanisms underlying them and the circumstances in which they are likely to occur.

PRINCIPAL MECHANISMS INVOLVED IN DRUG INTERACTIONS

Drug interactions are of three basic types:

1. *Pharmaceutical interactions* occur when drugs are inappropriately mixed. In clinical practice this usually means in syringes and infusions.
2. *Pharmacodynamic interactions* occur when drugs act on the same physiological systems or site of action.
3. *Pharmacokinetic interactions* are those in which one drug interferes with the absorption, transport, distribution or elimination of another.

The most important mechanisms responsible for drug interactions are listed in Table 1.

Table 1 Principal mechanisms responsible for drug interactions

A. INTERACTIONS OCCURRING OUTSIDE THE BODY (PHARMACEUTICAL INTERACTIONS)

B. INTERACTIONS OCCURRING INSIDE THE BODY:

1. **Interference with transport of the drug to the site of action:**
   (a) Altered absorption
   (b) Altered distribution – protein binding
   (c) Altered tissue binding
   (d) Interference with intracellular transport
   (e) Gastro-intestinal toxic effects – malabsorption syndrome.

2. **Altered effect at the site of action:**
   (a) Competition for receptor-binding sites
   (b) Interaction between drugs which act at the same site or on the same physiological systems.

3. **Interference with removal of the drug from the site of action:**
   (a) Altered renal excretion
   (b) Altered biliary excretion
   (c) Altered metabolism:
      (i) Enzyme induction
      (ii) Enzyme inhibition
      (iii) Changes in hepatic blood flow
      (iv) Monoamine-oxidase inhibiters.

4. **Alterations in fluid and electrolyte balance**

5. **Mutual toxicity**

6. **Miscellaneous**

INTERACTIONS OCCURRING OUTSIDE THE BODY (PHARMACEUTICAL INTERACTIONS)

It is never wise to mix more than one drug together in a syringe or to add drugs to infusions of blood or parenteral food solutions. At best, the drug is likely to be unstable and inactivation or precipitation may occur with loss of therapeutic effect, e.g. both benzyl penicillin and heparin are both quickly inactivated in dextrose or dextrose/saline.

INTERACTIONS OCCURRING INSIDE THE BODY

1. Interference with transport of the drug to the site of action

(A) ALTERED ABSORPTION

(i) *Gastric Acidity:* Gastric pH affects the dissolution rate of drugs, acid drugs being more soluble in alkaline solutions and vice versa. For this reason aspirin dissolves more readily in the presence of sodium bicarbonate.

(ii) *Gastro-intestinal Motility:* The principal site of drug absorption is from the upper small intestine and not from the stomach. Drugs which delay gastric emptying (e.g. propantheline) reduce the rate of absorption of moderately soluble drugs like paracetamol, while accelerated absorption follows the administration of metoclopramide (Maxolon), which increases gastric motility and emptying (Nimmo et al, 1973). Conversely, rapid gastric emptying reduces absorption of poorly-soluble drugs like digoxin, by limiting the time available for the drug to dissolve (Manninen et al, 1973).

(iii) *Drug Binding:* Drugs may interact in the gut to form insoluble complexes which cannot be absorbed. The anion exchange resin cholestyramine reduces the absorption of many drugs including thyroxine and warfarin in this way. The concurrent administration of tetracycline and preparations of iron, magnesium and calcium results in the formation of non-absorbable complexes (Neuvonen et al, 1970). Tetracycline may, therefore, be largely inactivated if it is swallowed together with a glass of milk.

(iv) *Competition for Active Absorption Mechanisms:* Drugs which bear a close structural resemblance to certain food constituents, e.g. amino acids, purines, pyrimidines and sugars may be absorbed by active transport mechanisms in the small intestine. A high-protein diet, by competing for the absorption pathway, may decrease the therapeutic effect of L-dopa while a low-protein diet may increase it (Mena and Cotzias, 1975).

(B) ALTERED DISTRIBUTION – PROTEIN BINDING

The majority of acidic drugs are transported partially bound to plasma proteins. The free drug exists in equilibrium with that which is protein bound and only the former is able to diffuse out of the vascular compartment and exert a pharmacological effect. The concentration of the drug also determines the rate of elimination.

Many drugs will displace one another from protein-binding sites (Koch-Weser and Sellers, 1976). This may only be important if the displaced drug is highly protein bound, if binding sites are easily saturated at therapeutic blood levels, if the volume of distribution is small and if the usual rate of elimination is slow.

Clinically significant interactions usually occur only when accurate control of the plasma concentration of one drug is important, e.g. anticoagulants and hypoglycaemic agents.

(C) ALTERED TISSUE BINDING

Drugs frequently become bound to tissues and while it is possible that competition for non-receptor binding sites may occur, this has not been demonstrated to be a significant cause of drug interaction. The increased toxicity of primaquine and pamaquine in patients who have already received mepacrine may be due to this phenomenon, and the increased plasma digoxin levels in patients treated with quinidine may also be explained in this way (Ejvinsson, 1978).

(D) INTRACELLULAR TRANSPORT

An active transport mechanism is involved in the uptake of the postganglionic adrenergic hypotensive agents guanethidine, bethanidine and debrisoquine. This is inhibited by tricyclic antidepressants and some sympathomimetic agents (Oates et al, 1971). Control of hypertension may be lost in patients stabilised on these drugs, if treated with normal doses of tricyclic antidepressants. Many over-the-counter common cold remedies containing ephedrine and phenylpropanolamine may have the same effect.

Tricyclic antidepressants also block the uptake of noradrenaline at adrenergic nerve terminals and potentiate the pressor effect of systemic noradrenaline. This has resulted in severe hypertensive reactions in dentistry when local anaesthetics containing noradrenaline have been given (Boakes et al, 1972).

(E) GASTRO-INTESTINAL TOXIC EFFECTS

A malabsorption syndrome can be caused by chronic administration of colchicine, mefenamic acid, para-aminosalicylic acid (PAS), phenformin or neomycin. Thus neomycin may reduce the absorption of phenoxymethylpenicillin, and colchicine may cause a megaloblastic anaemia through interference with vitamin B_{12} absorption.

2. Altered effect at the site of action

(A) COMPETITION AT RECEPTOR LEVEL

Competition for receptor binding sites is a common cause of drug interaction. *d*-Tubocurarine, for instance, combines reversibly with receptors and, in doing so, blocks acetylcholine the normal transmitter. Neostigmine, by inhibiting cholinesterase and increasing the concentration of acetylcholine at the receptors, can reverse this effect. The antagonism of narcotic analgesics by naloxone and of propranolol by isoprenaline are mediated by a similar mechanism.

Oral anticoagulants act by competitive inhibition of vitamin K in the synthesis of clotting factors by the liver and an excessively long prothrombin time can be restored to normal by vitamin K.

Tricyclic antidepressants, antihistamines and the anticholinergic drugs used in parkinsonism all inhibit the autonomic effects of acetylcholine and produce atropinic side-effects, including blurred vision, constipation and a dry mouth. When two preparations are given together, as when anticholinergic preparations are used to prevent the extrapyramidal effects of phenothiazines, a marked increase in the atropinic effects may be noted. An acute confusional reaction may also result when patients on tricyclic antidepressants are given anticholinergic drugs.

(B) DRUGS ACTING ON THE SAME PHYSIOLOGICAL SYSTEM

Drugs which share the same site of action or which act on the same physiological system frequently interact. Both antagonism and potentiation occur.

Many sedatives, including alcohol, hypnotics, antidepressants and tranquillisers interact in this way and produce central nervous system depression.

Many sedatives, tranquillisers and antidepressants also produce vasodilation and so postural hypotension may be caused in patients under treatment for hypertension.

The autonomic reflex control of cardiac function is abolished by atropine and propranolol, and anaesthetic agents (e.g. ether) may cause a marked reduction in cardiac output.

3. Interference with removal from the site of action

(A) ALTERED RENAL EXCRETION

The kidney excretes water-soluble drugs by two mechanisms, glomerular filtration or active secretion in the proximal tubule.

(i) *Effect of Urinary pH:* The secretion of weak acids and bases depends upon the pH. Excretion by glomerular filtration is dependent on the glomerular filtration rate and the degree of protein binding. Alkalinisation of the urine may prolong the effect of quinidine, a basic drug, while forced alkaline diuresis is useful in the treatment of acute salicylate poisoning. Normal doses of antacids may also reduce the serum level of salicylates because of increased renal clearance caused by the rise in urinary pH.

(ii) *Competition for Active Renal Tubular Secretion:* Probenecid delays the excretion of penicillin by competing for the same transport mechanism in the proximal tubule and use of this may be made to achieve high tissue levels. Probenecid interferes with the excretion of dapsone, PAS and indomethacin, and toxicity may result when they are given together. Similarly, phenylbutazone competes with chlorpropamide and may cause hypoglycaemia (Thomsen et al, 1970).

(B) INTERFERENCE WITH BILIARY EXCRETION

Many drugs are excreted in the bile or are converted to water-soluble conjugates which can then be eliminated by the kidney. Competition is known to occur between probenecid and rifampicin, the former reducing the excretion of the latter.

Some conjugated drugs are hydrolysed by intestinal bacteria and the active drug formed is re-absorbed into the entero-hepatic circulation. Neomycin, by suppressing the intestinal flora, may interrupt this cycle (Brewster et al, 1977).

(C) ALTERED METABOLISM

(i) *Stimulation of Metabolism–Enzyme Induction:* Many lipid-soluble drugs stimulate hepatic microsomal enzyme production. Those which have been demonstrated to cause significant interactions in man include barbiturates, carbamazepine, alcohol, glutethimide, phenytoin and primidone. The inducing drug stimulates both its own metabolism and that of many other unrelated drugs which are metabolised in the liver.

Enzyme induction may lead to either increased or decreased drug effect depending upon whether active or inactive metabolites are produced.

The most important examples of enzyme inductions are the stimulation of warfarin and steroid metabolism by barbiturates. Complex interactions also occur between anticonvulsants (Richens, 1977).

(ii) *Inhibition of Metabolism:* Although relatively few drugs are known to inhibit hepatic microsomal enzymes, several important interactions are caused in this way. Inhibition results in prolonged action and an increased rate of toxicity. Phenylbutazone inhibits the metabolism of tolbutamide, and isoniazid and sulthiame of phenytoin, dicoumarol, tolbutamide and chlorpropamide. Acute alcoholic intoxication also inhibits warfarin metabolism in contrast to the stimulation which may occur in the chronic alcoholic.

A few interactions are the result of inhibition of other enzymes. For example, allopurinol inhibits xanthine oxidase and potentiates azathioprine and 6-mercaptopurine, and anticholinesterases inhibit pseudocholinesterase and potentiate suxamethomium.

(iii) *Changes in Hepatic Blood Flow:* The elimination of drugs which are metabolised in the liver may be affected by drugs which alter hepatic blood flow. Propranolol reduces cardiac output and hepatic blood flow and thereby affects both its own plasma clearance and that of other drugs, e.g. lignocaine.

On the other hand glucagon, phenobarbitone and isoprenaline may increase hepatic blood flow and the rate of elimination of propranolol and lignocaine. In the case of phenobarbitone this may sometimes be a more important effect than enzyme induction.

The significance of these possible interactions is not clear, but there are important implications for patients receiving intensive care with intravenous anti-arrhythmics.

(iv) *Interactions Involving Monoamine-Oxidase Inhibitors:* Monoamine-oxidase inhibitors cause several serious interactions (Sjoqvist, 1965). Dietary tyramine, present in such diverse foods as cheese, Marmite, pickled herrings or Chianti, is normally metabolised by monoamine-oxidase in the intestinal wall. More tyramine is therefore absorbed when this enzyme is inhibited. In addition, inhibition within the neurone results in the accumulation of noradrenaline in adrenergic nerve terminals. This may be released by indirectly-acting sympathomimetic amines, including amphetamine, ephedrine, phenylpropanolamine and tyramine, resulting in a hypertensive crisis characterised by severe headache and sometimes left ventricular failure and cerebral haemorrhage (Blackwell et al, 1967).

Other drugs, including tricyclic antidepressants, anaesthetics and pethidine, may produce hyperpyrexia, hypotension, tachycardia and coma, when given to patients receiving monoamine-oxidase inhibitors (Goldberg and Thornton, 1978).

4. Alterations in fluid and electrolyte balance
The effects of drugs which act upon the kidney, myocardium and neuromuscular transmission, may be profoundly altered by changes in electrolyte balance.

The best known example is the potentiation of digitalis derivatives by diuretic-induced hypokalaemia (Binnion, 1978).

Hypokalaemia may also antagonise the anti-arrhythmic properties of lignocaine, phenytoin and procainamide, and sudden release of potassium from muscle following suxamethonium injection may cause ventricular arrhythmias (Dreifus et al, 1974). Hypokalaemia causes hyperpolarisation of the motor end-plate and antagonises the action of acetylcholine, while non-depolarising muscle relaxants may produce prolonged paralysis in the presence of hypokalaemia in patients taking thiazide diuretics or carbenoxolone. The combination of potassium-retaining diuretics and potassium chloride has caused fatal hyperkalaemia in patients with renal failure (Greenblatt and Koch-Weser, 1973).

Lithium intoxication can be caused by diuretics since lithium excretion is dependent on sodium balance (Himmelhoch et al, 1977).

5. Mutual toxicity
It should come as no surprise that drugs having similar unwanted effects are more toxic when given together. Some common examples include the enhanced oto-toxicity of ethacrynic acid and streptomycin and the nephrotoxicity of aminoglycoside antibiotics.

6. Miscellaneous
Finally, a few interactions cannot be readily categorised. Examples include the antagonism of L-dopa by pyridoxine and the potentiation of tricyclic antidepressants by thyroxine.

CLINICALLY IMPORTANT INTERACTIONS

The drugs most frequently prescribed by the general practitioner are antibiotics, tranquillisers, analgesics and hypnotics. He is closely involved in the long-term management of hypertension, diabetes and epilepsy. While he must be aware of the catastrophic interactions which may occur in patients receiving oral anticoagulants and monoamine-oxidase inhibitors, it is the less dramatic but nevertheless important interactions which he must, most frequently, seek to avoid.

Drug interactions involving antibiotics
Antibiotics are frequently given together. There are only two good reasons for doing so, (1) to prevent the development of resistance, as in antituberculous therapy, and (2) when the antibacterial preparations are synergistic (e.g. trimethoprim and sulphonamides).

[handwritten notes in margins:]

Carbenoxolone Sod is in Biogastrone
Biople\
Biolal
Duogastrone / Pyrogastrone

. SEPTRIN — not so according to Marilyn Ramsden

Antagonism results when bactericidal (e.g. penicillin) and bacteriostatic (e.g. tetracycline) drugs are given together and such combinations are best avoided. In general practice it is rarely necessary to prescribe more than one antibiotic simultaneously and although there are many interactions involving the lesser-known antibiotics, these are only likely to be of interest to the specialist.

Drug interactions involving hypotensive agents

Modern hypotensive drug therapy is based upon the potentiation of one drug by another. A large number of drugs are capable of interfering with control (Nies, 1975).

Drugs which cause fluid retention may interfere with hypotensive therapy. These include oestrogens, carbenoxolone, phenylbutazone and indomethacin. Tricyclic antidepressants block the anti-hypertensive effect of bethanidine, debrisoquine and guanethedine by inhibiting the noradrenaline pump.

There is some evidence that tricyclic antidepressants also antagonise the action of methyldopa and desipramine antagonises the hypotensive action of clonidine. Amphetamine-like drugs antagonise adrenergic neurone blockers.

β-receptor stimulants (e.g. isoprenaline) also interfere with anti-hypertensive therapy, but their effect is rarely significant.

Drug interactions with oral hypoglycaemic drugs

Several drugs, notably phenylbutazone, increase the effect of sulphonylureas, but in most cases where hypoglycaemic coma has resulted other contributing factors such as advanced age, poor nutrition or renal or hepatic impairment have been important.

Intolerance of alcohol with facial flushing similar to that caused by disulfiram (Antabuse) has been reported with chlorpropamide.

Drug interactions involving oral contraceptives

Several drugs induce the hepatic enzymes responsible for metabolising oral contraceptives and cause reduced effectiveness. They include barbiturates, phenytoin and rifampicin (Skolnick et al, 1976). Break-through bleeding may be a warning sign (Hempel and Klinger, 1976; Robertson and Johnson, 1976). Oral contraceptives have also been demonstrated to inhibit the metabolism of other drugs (Homeida et al, 1978).

Ampicillin, neomycin and phenoxymethylpenicillin all reduce the urinary excretion of oestriol in pregnant women, although only ampicillin has been documented as a probable cause of contraceptive failure (Dossetor, 1975).

Oral contraceptives elevate blood pressure and should not be prescribed in patients with a raised blood pressure.

Drug interactions involving anaesthetic agents

Until recently it was believed that treatment with hypotensive drugs increased the risk of cardiovascular collapse during anaesthesia, but it has now been shown that the converse is true and that while hypertensive patients have a greater anaesthetic risk than normotensive patients, this risk is reduced by adequate drug treatment of the hypertension. Patients who have been receiving cortisone within two months of surgery should be given supplements to cover operation, and treatment with monoamine-oxidase inhibitors should be withdrawn at least a week before surgery.

Tricyclic antidepressants increase the risk of cardiac arrhythmias during anaesthesia and several antibiotics including streptomycin and the tetracyclines enhance the action of neuromuscular blocking agents.

Noradrenaline used for haemostasis in local dental anaesthetics, may increase blood pressure in patients on hypotensive therapy.

Drug interactions involving anti-epileptic drugs

Whenever possible epilepsy should be treated with a single drug. Almost all anticonvulsants are enzyme inducers and since unwanted effects are also potentiated, inadequate control and excessive toxicity may result.

While induction of metabolism is the most common drug interaction, benzodiazepines and isoniazid have been shown to antagonise the metabolism of phenytoin, and this may result in toxicity. Aspirin also displaces phenytoin from protein-binding sites and leads to an increase in the proportion of pharmacologically active drug in the blood, again leading to increased toxicity.

Drug interactions involving anticoagulants

Oral anticoagulants are frequently used for long periods and many other drugs may be given concurrently. In practice, few serious interactions occur (principally phenylbutazone derivatives, clofibrate and barbiturates). Barbiturates induce coumarine metabolism and reduce anticoagulant effect. Sudden withdrawal of the inducing drug may lead to disastrous haemorrhage. Displacement interactions are also important and therapeutic doses of phenylbutazone can double the plasma concentration of warfarin.

CONCLUSIONS

Although there is an impossibly large number of potential drug interactions, the number of situations likely to be met with in everyday practice are relatively few. Most can be avoided by a sound knowledge of the mechanisms involved, sensible prescribing from a selective personal pharmacopeia, the avoidance of unnecessary polypharmacy, and the application of common sense.

Finally, we may take comfort in the knowledge that, if all else fails, the patient may well remind us by asking: 'Will it go with what I'm on already, doctor?'

REFERENCES

Aggeler, P. M., O'Reilly, R. A., Leong, L. and Kowitz, P. E. (1967). Potentiation of anticoagulant effect of warfarin by phenylbutazone. *New England Journal of Medicine*, **276**, 496.

Beeley, L. (1979). *Safer Prescribing: a Guide to Some Problems in the Use of Drugs*, 2nd edition. Blackwell Scientific Publications Limited, Oxford.

Binnion, P. F. (1978). Drug interactions with digitalis glycosides. *Drugs*, **15**, 369.

Biron, P. (1973). A hopefully biased pilot survey of physicians' knowledge of the content of drug combinations. *Canadian Medical Association Journal*, **109**, 36.

Blackwell, B., Marley, E., Price, J. and Taylor, D. (1967). Hypertensive interactions between monoamine oxidase inhibitors and foodstuffs. *British Journal of Psychiatry*, **113**, 349.

Boakes, A. J., Laurence, D. R., Lovel, K. W., O'Neill, R. and Verill, P. J. (1972). Adverse reaction to local anaesthetics/vasoconstrictor preparations. *British Dental Journal*, **133**, 137.

Brewster, D., Jones, R. S. and Symons, A. M. (1977). Effects of neomycin on the biliary excretion and entero-hepatic circulation of mestranol and 17-β-oestradiol. *Biochemical Pharmacology*, **26**, 943.

Brodie, B. B. (1962). Difficulties in extrapolating data on metabolism of drugs from animals to man. *Clinical Pharmacology and Therapeutics*, **3**, 374.

Bull, J. and Mackinnon, J. (1975). Phenylbutazone and anticoagulant control. *Practitioner*, **215**, 767.

Dollery, C. T. (1965). Physiological and pharmacological interactions of antihypertensive drugs. *Proceedings of the Royal Society of Medicine*, **58**, 983.

Dossetor, E. J. (1975). Drug interactions with oral contraceptives. *British Medical Journal*, **4**, 467.

Dreifus, L. S., de Azevedo, I. M. and Watanabe, Y. (1974). Electrolyte and anti-arrhythmic drug interaction. *American Heart Journal*, **88**, 95.

Ejvinsson, G. (1978). Effect of quinidine on plasma concentrations of digoxin. *British Medical Journal*, **1**, 279.

Goldberg, R. F. and Thornton, W. E. (1978). Combined tricyclic-MAOI therapy for refractory depression: a review with guidelines for appropriate usage. *Journal of Clinical Pharmacology*, **18**, 143.

Greenblatt, D. J. and Koch-Weser, J. (1973). Adverse reactions to spironolactone: a report from the Boston Collaborative Drug Surveillance Program. *Journal of the American Medical Association*, **225**, 40.

Hempel, E. and Klinger, W. (1976). Drug-stimulated biotransformation of hormonal steroid contraceptives: clinical implications. *Practical Therapeutics, Drugs*, **12**, 442.

Himmelhoch, J. M., Foust, R. I., Mallinger, A. G., Hamin, I. and Neil, J. F. (1977). Adjustment of lithium dose during lithium-chlorothiazide therapy. *Clinical Pharmacology and Therapeutics*, **33**, 225.

Homeida, M., Halliwell, M. and Branch, R. A. (1978). Effects of an oral contraceptive on hepatic size and antipyrine metabolism in premenopausal women. *Clinical Pharmacology and Therapeutics*, **24**, 228.

Howie, J. G. R., Jeffers, T. A., Millar, H. R. and Petrie, J. C. (1977). Prevention of adverse drug interactions. *British Journal of Clinical Pharmacology*, **4**, 611.

Koch-Weser, J. and Sellers, E. M. (1976). Binding of drugs to serum albumin. *New England Journal of Medicine*, **294**, 311, 526.

Manninen, V., Apajalahti, A., Simonen, H. and Reissel, P. (1973). Effect of propantheline and metoclopramide on absorption of digoxin. *Lancet*, **1**, 1118.

May, F. E., Stewart, R. B. and Cluff, L. E. (1977). Drug interactions and multiple drug administration. *Clinical Pharmacology and Therapeutics*, **22**, 322.

Mena, I. and Cotzias, G. C. (1975). Protein intake and treatment of Parkinson's disease with levodopa. *New England Journal of Medicine*, **292**, 181.

Neuvonen, P. J., Gothoni, G., Hackman, R. and Bjorksten, K. (1970). Interference of iron with the absorption of tetracyclines in man. *British Medical Journal*, **4**, 532.

Nies, A. S. (1975). Adverse reactions and interactions limiting the use of antihypertensive drugs. *American Journal of Medicine*, **58**, 495.

Nimmo, J., Heading, R. C., Tothill, P. and Prescott, L. F. (1973). Pharmacological modification of gastric emptying: effects of propantheline and metoclopramide on paracetamol absorption. *British Medical Journal*, **1**, 587.

Oates, J. A., Mitchell, J. R., Feagin, O. T., Kaufmann, J. S. and Shand, D. G. (1971). Distribution of quanidium antihypertensives: mechanism of their selective action. *Annals of New York Academy of Sciences*, **179**, 302.

Petrie, J. C., Howie, J. G. R. and Dumo, D. (1974). Awareness and experience of general practitioners of selected drug interactions. *British Medical Journal*, **2**, 262.

Richens, A. (1977). Interactions with anti-epileptic drugs. *Drugs*, **13**, 266.

Robertson, Y. R. and Johnson, E. S. (1976). Interactions between oral contraceptives and other drugs; a review. *Current Medical Research and Opinion*, **3**, 647.

Shorvon, S. D., Chadwick, D., Galbraith, A. W. and Reynolds, E. H. (1978). One drug for epilepsy. *British Medical Journal*, **1**, 474.

Sjoqvist, F. (1965). Interaction between monoamine-oxidase inhibitors and other drugs. *Proceedings of the Royal Society of Medicine*, **58** (2), 967.

Sjoqvist, F. and Alexanderson, B. (1972). *Drug interactions; A critical look at their documentation and clinical importance.* In Baker and Neuhaus (Eds) *Proceedings of the European Society for the Study of Drug Toxicity, Vol. 13, Toxicological Problems of Drug Combinations*, p 167. Excerpta Medica, Amsterdam.

Skolnick, J. L., Stoler, B. S., Katz, D. B. and Anderson, W. H. (1976). Rifampin, oral contraceptives and pregnancy. *Journal of the American Medical Association*, **236**, 1382.

Stockley, I. (1974). *Drug Interactions and Their Mechanisms.* Re-printed by the Pharmaceutical Journal.

Swidler, G. (1971). *Handbook of Drug Interactions.* John Wiley and Sons, Inc, New York.

Thomsen, P. E. B., Ostenfeld, H. O. L. and Kristensen, M. (1970). Chlorpropamide-phenylbutazone as the cause of hypoglycaemia. A case of an unfortunate drug combination. *Ugeskrift for Laeger*, **137**, 1722.

Vessell, E. S., Passanati, G. T. and Glenwright, P. (1975). Anomalous results of studies of drug interaction in man. *Pharmacology*, **13**, 481.

Wade, O. L. (1970). A pattern of drug-induced disease in the community. An unsolved enigma. *British Medical Bulletin*, **26**, 240.

Wade, O. L. and Beeley, L. (1976). *Adverse Reactions to Drugs*, 2nd edition. William Heinemann Medical Books Limited, London.

Whiting, B., Goldberg, A. and Waldie, P. (1973). The drug disc. Warning system for drug interactions. *Lancet*, **1**, 1037–8.

Index

Proprietary names

Wherever possible approved names of drugs have been used within the text. The following Trade Names (Proprietary names) will, however, be found within the text.